SCHOOL HEALTH PRACTICE

SCHOOL HEALTH PRACTICE

WILLIAM H. CRESWELL, Jr., A.B., M.S., Ed.D.

Professor and former Head,
Department of Health and Safety Studies,
University of Illinois, Champaign, Illinois

IAN M. NEWMAN, M.S., Ph.D

Professor of Health Education,
University of Nebraska, Lincoln, Nebraska

NINTH EDITION

With 122 illustrations

TIMES MIRROR/MOSBY COLLEGE PUBLISHING

St. Louis • Toronto • Boston • Los Altos   1989

Publisher: Nancy Roberson
Editor: Pat Coryell
Editorial Assistant: Shannon Ruyle
Project Manager: Kathleen L. Teal
Manuscript Editor: Carl Masthay
Book Designer: Susan E. Lane
Production: Ginny Douglas, Teresa Breckwoldt

NINTH EDITION

Library of Congress Cataloging in Publication Data

Creswell, William H., 1920-
   School health practice.

   Includes bibliographies and index.
   1. School hygiene—United States.   I. Newman, Ian M.
II. Title.   [DNLM: 1. School Health Services.
WA 350 C923s]
LB3409.U5C69 1989   371.7′1   88-31547
ISBN 0-8016-2560-2

TSI/D/D   9 8 7 6 5 4

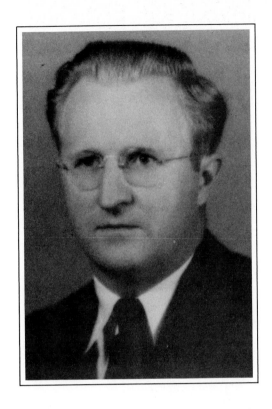

IN MEMORIAM

Carl Leonard Anderson, B.S., M.S., Dr. P.H.
Corvallis, Oregon

Preface

Since the eighth edition of *School Health Practice,* the United States Department of Health and Human Services has published a "midcourse review," a progress report on achieving the nation's 1990 health objectives. The report is both encouraging and optimistic that many of the objectives relating to the 15 priority areas will be achieved by 1990.

The report also stresses the fact that continued vigilence must be maintained if progress is to be sustained in the areas of immunization and injury control. We are reminded that each new generation of school children must be "reeducated" on the importance of practicing health behaviors that will assure continued progress toward optimum levels of health and education development. Problems persist, and they are not only a threat to youth but also to the health of the nation. The misuse and abuse of drugs, teenage pregnancies, and sexually transmitted diseases are some of the most prevalent threats. The unanticipated problem of AIDS may indeed become the major health threat of this age.

Conditions that were unheard of a few years ago and could now be defined as epidemic, such as sexually transmitted disease, have received increased attention since the last edition of this text. It is difficult for teachers to remain abreast of these new developments when they do have much of the crucial technical information at their disposal. But because they are spreading rapidly in some segments of the community, the above conditions characterize an especially difficult and critical problem for schools.

New data on teaching effectiveness are emerging from the research being conducted on substance and drug use and abuse. Although there is the need to inform each new generation about the health hazards of these substances, information alone is not effective. Psychosocial approaches emphasizing social, communications, and peer-resistance skills are proving to be effective. Teaching students social skills together with coping and problem-solving skills will prove effective not only in drug education but also in serving to strengthen student academic performance in schools.

AUDIENCE

Like its predecessors, the ninth edition is based on the assumption that an effectively functioning school health program calls for a clear vision of the total school health program.

Because the program described is school based, the primary audience for which the book is written includes elementary and secondary school teachers, specialists in school health education, school health services, and school administration.

NEW TO THIS EDITION

In this edition of *School Health Practice,* greater emphasis has been placed on contemporary issues that have a direct bearing upon the school health program—policies and practices required in meeting the health needs of today's school-age population. Specific changes are as follows:

- The original Chapter 6 has been revised and brought forward as Chapter 2 in a revised sequence of chapters for this edition.

- A new Chapter 15 has been added, "Policies and Practices in Health Teaching." In this chapter, policies governing controversial issues relating to drugs, alcohol, tobacco, and sex education are discussed to help clarify the issues and to give school administrators and teachers guidance in the formulation of the school's goals and educational objectives. In this chapter, schools are also urged to accept the challenge of a smoke-free environment.

- New material in this edition includes more emphasis on health problems such as substance use, anorexia nervosa, bulimia, and sexual behavior, which are often disproportionately affected by social pressure.

- The matter of child abuse is now recognized as a major health issue and one in which the school can play an important role. In the ninth edition of *School Health Practice,* teachers are urged to recognize the existence of the problem and the need to develop policies and practices that address this issue.

- Renewed emphasis is placed on the concept of a comprehensive school health program. To this end, the establishment of school-based clinics, a rapidly developing trend, is discussed as an example, showing how school health services can be effectively integrated with the school health education program.

- Chapter 9, "Safety, Emergency Care, and First Aid," has been rewritten and updated by Dr. Alan Braslow, a special consultant to the American National Red Cross. Dr. Braslow's revision of the chapter reflects modern concepts of injury control that are consistent with community emergency medical services.

ACKNOWLEDGMENTS

As has been typical of previous editions, many persons have made important contributions to this edition of *School Health Practice*. To each of these persons who have made sacrifices and accommodations in order to allow us to pursue the tasks required to meet deadlines, we express our gratitude.

Also, there are those persons who have made special contributions to this revision and who we wish to publicly recognize. Dr. Alan Braslow, a specialist in health education and emergency health care services, carried out the major revision of Chapter 9. Those who have provided special editorial, technical, and photographic services include Amy Knox Brown, Jean Creswell, Katherine Farrell, David Riecks, and Bill Weigand. Thanks go to Harriet Hinderer, Mary McLauflin, and Michelle Wiese for their typing of the manuscript. To Peter Mulhall, who contributed to the revision in a variety of ways through research, technical reviews, and special knowledge of the subjects, we are especially grateful.

We give special thanks to the following professionals who lent their expertise in reviewing this text:

Tom Hurt
James Madison University

Leslie Oganowski
University of Wisconsin–La Crosse

Janice Young
Iowa State University

We wish to thank Mrs. Carl (Alyce Stapleton) Anderson for providing us with the biographical information that has enabled us to dedicate this edition to the memory of Dr. C.L. Anderson and his many contributions to the field of health education. We also wish to thank Shannon Ruyle and Carl Masthay for their advice, patience, and gentle urgings that have kept the project moving.

Finally, we wish to acknowledge the contributions of our wives, who, despite the disruption to family life, have remained steadfast and committed in their support of our efforts.

William H. Creswell, Jr.

Ian M. Newman

BIOGRAPHIES OF EARLY LEADERS IN SCHOOL HEALTH

Contents

APPENDIXES

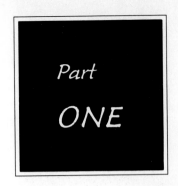

THE SCHOOL-AGED CHILD

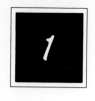

1   School Health and Health Education
The Challenge and the Source of Inspiration

OVERVIEW   *From the beginning of time human beings have sought to protect their health by controlling disease, improving the environment, caring for the sick, and protecting food and water supplies. Passing accumulated knowledge from one generation to another through formal and informal education has led to significant advances in humankind's abilities to protect and maintain health.*

This chapter demonstrates that health is a concern, integrated into social mores, and illustrates how health knowledge has accumulated over the centuries. Health knowledge, because of the great scientific advances over the last 100 years, has increased dramatically, but society's ability to share and implement this knowledge has lagged. To benefit from this new knowledge, we must share it through education. Adolescents today may not share the practical benefits of this new knowledge to the same degree as other age groups, since their death rates have not declined to the extent others have. Education's challenge is clear: (1) find new ways to help students protect their health and to help them use education to advance their health, (2) identify ways that poor health detracts from educational efforts and help school personnel overcome these forces, (3) identify how students' health influences the benefits gained from this investment in education, and (4) help school personnel accept options available to improve the school environment, school health services, and health education.

OBJECTIVES   **After reading this chapter, the student should be able to:**

1. Identify the principal health problems faced by children and adolescents
2. Describe the development of public health through the ages, identifying the specific contributions of various eras and individuals
3. Explain why the modern philosophy of health and disease as natural and therefore understandable processes has affected the rate of knowledge in the health field
4. Identify the most important elements directed specifically at developing or improving school health programs of the last 50 years
5. Present an argument that shows how health directly affects the outcome of educational efforts

THE CHALLENGE

Despite significant gains made in the quality of health in the United States, further progress is possible. Young people, as a group, will benefit more from improved health than other age groups, and no group has a greater potential for health improvement than do the young. The later years of childhood and the early years of adolescence are noted as the healthiest in a person's life. Knowledge gained and habit patterns established in this period will influence a person's health for the rest of his or her life.

All is not well with the health of children and adolescents. Consider the following: Americans 15 to 24 years of age have a death rate higher than that of 20 years ago, which means that proportionally more people in this age group die each year than were dying 20 years ago. In 1960 the death rate for adolescents and young adults was 106 deaths per 100,000 people. By 1970 the death rate was 128 per 100,000, and according to the U.S. Surgeon General, in the report *Healthy People* (1979), the rate was down somewhat to 113 deaths per 100,000 by 1977, but it was still higher than two decades earlier. The death rate of 113 per 100,000 equaled 48,000 deaths among young people 15 to 24 years of age. How does the U.S. rate compare to that of other countries? Our rate of adolescent and young adult deaths is higher than England's, Japan's, and Sweden's. Furthermore, these deaths are among people who have just completed their education and whose lost contributions to society are immeasurable.

The challenge to school personnel is twofold: first, to help overcome the unnecessarily high mortality and, second, to provide the best possible foundation on which young people can build their health knowledge and practices and so increase the quality of their lives.

So important is the health of the people to the well-being of the nation that the U.S. Department of Health and Human Services (formerly the U.S. Department of Health, Education, and Welfare) has established specific health-related national objectives to be reached by the year 1990 (*Healthy People*, 1979).

Healthy children

attitudes are formed here seen in later yrs.

> Goal: to improve child health, foster optimal childhood development, and by 1990 reduce deaths among children aged 1 to 14 by at least 20%, to fewer than 34 per 100,000 (*Healthy People*, 1979)

In 1900 the death rate for children 1 to 14 years of age was 870 per 100,000 with most deaths occurring from infectious diseases caused by poor nutrition, sanitation, and housing. These diseases posed a special threat because of the absence of vaccines and antibiotics. By 1925 mortality had fallen to 330 per 100,000, and today it is 43 per 100,000. Yet, according to the U.S. Surgeon General, black American children have a 30% higher death rate than whites, and the death rate for children 1 to 14 years of age is significantly higher than that found in several other countries.

promote accident prevention in the classroom

The leading cause of death for this age group is accidents, which result in approximately 10,000 deaths per year. Motor vehicles account for 24% of these accidents, drownings 8%, and fires 6%. Although accidents kill some persons outright, they also injure, maim, and reduce the life potential for others.

Vaccines have eliminated many contagious diseases, and yet unnecessary cases of preventable diseases still occur. As recently as 1977, 57,000 cases of measles were reported.

Although measles is a completely preventable disease, society pays the cost for neglected immunization with permanent brain damage and retardation in 1 child in every 1000 infected, and approximately 1 in every 10,000 dies of measles complications.

Rubella (German measles) occurred an estimated 40,000 times in 1977. The gravest threat from rubella is fetal damage. Other disease, such as mumps, diphtheria, and tetanus, still occur, though the recent national childhood immunization effort has greatly decreased the incidence of these diseases.

Dental care continues to be a problem. At age 11 the average American child has three teeth permanently damaged by decay. By age 17 the average student has nine permanent teeth either decayed, missing, or filled.

Poor nutrition, as indicated by obesity, and the early evidence of coronary artery disease among otherwise healthy children is another area of concern.

Child abuse, mental retardation, and learning disabilities are significant problems for young people. Approximately 20% of school-aged children have some type of learning disability. The effectiveness of the school and its investment in learning are greatly depreciated by learning disabilities, which may go undetected and untreated unless the school has an adequate health service program.

Because children are likely to spend more active learning time with teachers and school personnel in their formative years than they do with their parents, the potential for the schools to contribute to the health of young people is enormous. This book clearly outlines the many ways school personnel and school resources can improve the health and health knowledge of all school-aged individuals to increase the quality of students' lives.

Healthy adolescents and young adults

Goal: to improve the health and health habits of adolescents and young adults and by 1990 to reduce deaths among people aged 15 to 24 by at least 20% to fewer than 93 per 100,000 (*Healthy People,* 1979)

By the time young people reach 15 years of age the behavioral characteristics of adolescence are reflected in their mortality. Death rates for adolescents and young adults ages 15 to 24 are more than twice as high as those for children, and for young men the rate is triple that of young women. As young people gain freedom from family and school, their life-styles and behaviors determine their degree of health. As children move into adolescence, their health results from their own volitional behavior, whereas in childhood their health was the result of the behavior of others, principally their parents. Greater freedom from parental supervision is clearly reflected in health, disease, and mortality patterns.

In 1985 36% of all deaths in the 15- to 24-year age range were the result of motor vehicle accidents. When young people this age are involved in automobile accidents, they are almost twice as likely to die as persons 25 years and older are. Excessive speed is the principal cause of 50% of all fatal automobile accidents in young people 15 to 19 years of age. Eighty percent of young people never use seat belts; 30% of all motorcycle accidents occur in young people under 20 years of age. Alcohol is involved in an unknown number of automobile accidents. However, it is known that 50% of all alcohol-related highway fatalities are among young people.

Teen-aged pregnancy brings special risks to the young mother and to her baby. One fourth of American teen-aged girls have been pregnant at least once by 19 years of age. Approximately 10% of all teen-aged girls become pregnant each year.

Sexually transmitted diseases infect millions of teenagers. Although such diseases are sometimes difficult to detect and often unreported, it is estimated that 8 to 12 million cases of sexually transmitted diseases are contracted each year. Young people ages 15 to 24 account for approximately 75% of all cases, which affect not only young people themselves, but also induce conditions that are passed on to the next generation.

Suicides and homicides also contribute to teen-aged mortality. Of all suicides, approximately 20% occur among those under 20 years of age. Murder accounts for 10% of all adolescent and young adult deaths. The American adolescent homicide rate is much greater than that of most other industrialized nations.

Education is costly but promises great returns for society's investment. For schools and school personnel to ignore the health concerns of their students while focusing only on the educational concerns is to waste not only enormously valuable educational resources, but also valuable young lives.

Although humanity's attempt to promote health is age old, only recently has the school been incorporated into the general program of health promotion. Even more recently has the school health program demonstrated a positive, measurable effect on the health of citizens. However, the present-day school health program still falls short of realizing its opportunities.

Throughout history, in the attempt to understand disease and health, people have studied the phenomena of the universe, attempted to control the forces of nature, developed specialized languages, invented devices, instituted new practices, written laws and regulations, established institutions, and spent fortunes on research.

Progress in health has always been associated with advancement in various pursuits of learning and with improvement in providing for material needs. When health has been neglected, civilization has declined and humanity has retrogressed. The times of greatest health progress have always been associated with other advances in a civilization.

THE QUEST FOR HEALTH

Certain periods in the history of the health movement serve as landmarks of progress in health promotion. Increased understanding of health and changing concepts of health promotion are reflected in the pertinent contributions of various periods. The school became one of the principal agencies for health promotion, and health education developed its own history. To understand the role of the school in the health field, it is important to understand the background of school health.

For centuries people have faced the basic problems of public health: controlling communicable disease, improving the physical environment, providing care and medical assistance to the sick, and maintaining safe and adequate supplies of food and water. What each generation learned was passed on to the next, and knowledge accumulated and was further refined.

Greek contributions

The Greek concept of the human body was dominated by the idea of balance: balance of the individual and the environment, balance of mind and body, balance of nutrition and excretion, and balance of exercise and rest. Greek learning was concerned with cleansing and exercising not only the mind but also the body. Hygiene and physical fitness at the height of Greek culture were implemented to a degree unparalleled in later history.

The Greeks considered a disease a natural, not a supernatural, process; therefore disease was understandable and potentially manageable and had little to do with a person's spiritual condition. Epidemiology, the study of disease, was developed by the Greeks. The first clear accounts of clinical characteristics of communicable diseases, such as mumps, pneumonia, malarial fevers, and diphtheria, are present in their literature.

The idea of the balance between man and nature was best expressed by Hippocrates in his *On Airs, Waters and Places* (1939). Noting that human well-being depended on climate, soil, water, mode of life, and nutrition, Hippocrates drew the distinction betweeen endemic and epidemic diseases. The Hippocratic writings remained the underpinnings of public health practice until the nineteenth century when microbiology and bacteriology developed. The development of scientific medicine notwithstanding, the Greek physician and the modern public health physician have much in common in their humane approach to their patients and to illness (Figs. 1-1 and 1-2).

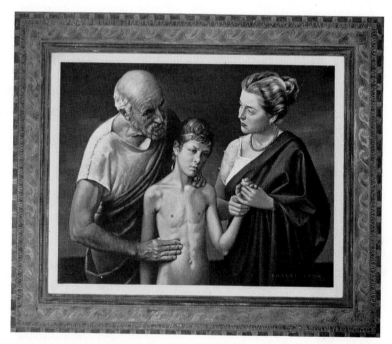

FIG. 1-1. Hippocrates. His aphorism "Where there is love for mankind, there is love for the art of healing" is reflected in the face of this revered physician, scientist, and teacher.
(Copyright, Parke, Davis & Company, and reproduced by special permission of Parke, Davis & Company, who commissioned the original oil paintings for the series "A History of Medicine," a project written and directed by George A. Bender and painted by Robert A. Thom.)

iatreion

Greek medicine and public health focused on disease prevention, but the Greeks also paid close attention to curative medicine. The Greek physician often practiced his craft while wandering from town to town. If he found enough work in a town, he would settle there and open a shop, called an *iatreion*. The town councils of large communities often employed physicians and supposedly guaranteed medical care for all residents—an early form of socialized medical care. The town councils paid the physicians a base salary but allowed them to charge residents additional fees.

The Greeks are responsible for the following concepts:

1. The first application of scientific thinking to matters of health
2. The recognition of the relationship between environment and health
3. The development of personal hygiene based on the concept of a balanced life
4. The provision of basic health services by the state

Despite the great idealism and concern for the health of the average citizen exhibited by Greek culture, the benefits derived from Greek medicine and hygiene remained the domain of the wealthy, the privileged, and the powerful and were not shared universally with the masses. Idealism and democratic intent aside, matters related to health were a privilege, not a right, in Greek society.

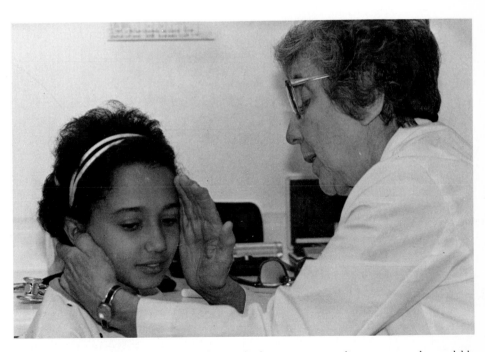

FIG. 1-2.   The modern physician, like the Greek physician, accepts disease as an understandable and therefore potentially treatable condition. Health is the result of appropriate life-style, an adequate environment, and prudent care. The title "doctor," from the Latin *doctōr,* means 'teacher'—a concept well understood by medical practitioners throughout time.
(Copyright 1983 by David Riecks.)

Roman contributions

Rome conquered the Mediterranean world and, with the destruction of Corinth in 146 BC, took over the legacy of Greece. The Romans accepted almost completely the Greek ideas of health and medicine but did little to advance them in the ensuing years. The Romans' outstanding contributions to public health were in the areas of engineering and administration. Aqueducts that provided an organized system of water supply, sewage disposal systems, refinements in the delivery of health services, and improved patterns of health administration make up the extensive legacy left for the modern world.

With the migration of Greek physicians to Rome, the practice of medicine in Rome shifted from a spiritual to a secular base, from the priests to the physicians. By AD 200 Rome had established a public medical service patterned after that of Greece. Public physicians were appointed by town councils. Salaried physicians were expected to provide free care for all who could not afford to pay. Private practicing physicians were also available to people of means. These aspects of Roman medical service followed the Greek precedents. Rome, however, set an important new precedent by establishing an elaborate system of public hospitals. In fact, Rome established two parallel systems of hospitals, one for the general public and one for the military.

Rome's efficient system of public administration directly benefited public health. In addition to the administrative water boards responsible for the maintenance of the aqueducts, there were special officers who supervised public baths, whose duties included testing of the heating apparatus and cleaning and policing of these facilities. Other officers supervised the cleaning and maintenance of streets, and yet others controlled the storage and distribution of food supplies.

With the fall of Rome many aspects of its public health organization and practice were lost. The health teachings of the Greek physicians were essentially discarded except in the Christian monasteries, where some persisted. Also, these teachings were kept alive by the Arabs of the eastern edges of the Roman Empire, who absorbed and translated vast amounts of Greek and Roman writings, adding their own contributions to the development of public health over the next few centuries. Later these learnings would be "rediscovered" and reintroduced to Europe as part of the Renaissance.

The Middle Ages (476 to 1453)

During the period from the fall of Rome to the Renaissance, the Middle Ages, health was not the concern it was during the Greek and Roman times. Laws and administrative practices relative to health continued to evolve during medieval times but failed to keep pace with ever-increasing health problems.

The evolution of medieval towns with congestion on the inner sides of city walls and squatters' slums on the outside directly contributed to the decline in community hygiene standards. The walled cities were ideal environments for the spread of contagious diseases. Many who moved to the towns brought with them not only their country ways but also their livestock. Barns were as common in Paris as were houses, and it was not until 1641 that the citizens of Berlin, for example, introduced a law to forbid the building of pigpens adjacent to streets.

Against the background of early urbanization developed the first of the three great eras of pestilence or plague that swept the world in the Middle Ages. The first of these was leprosy, the second, black death, and the third, syphilis.

Leprosy marked the onset of the Middle Ages, and black death marked the waning of the Middle Ages. During this period, Europe and the Mediterranean countries were also ravaged by a variety of communicable diseases; smallpox, diphtheria, measles, influenza, tuberculosis, scabies, anthrax, and trachoma were but a few. None of these diseases, however, caused as much suffering and death as leprosy and black death.

Leprosy.   During medieval times, no disease aroused more fear than leprosy, based on the facts that (1) it spread rapidly, (2) caused physical disfigurement, and (3) was regarded as a sign of spiritual impurity.

Long before the principles of contagion were validated, the practice of isolation was introduced in an attempt to control the spread of the disease. In fact, the ceremonial instructions of the Book of Leviticus (13:1-59 and 14:1-57), as well as other early writings, contain explicit references to quarantine and other means of combating leprosy. The biblical references indicate that the principle of isolation and quarantine was at first as much a religious concept as a medical concept.

The treatment of leprosy was the first clear example of what is now called a *prophylaxis*, that is, the control of a disease by systematic treatment: isolating or quarantining the carrier of a disease and thereby preventing the contagion from spreading. Despite these efforts, however, leprosy was not eradicated. Even today, leprosy persists in many parts of the world.

Black plague.   From the wild rodents of the steppes of Asia, a plague swept westward and reached the Black Sea around 1346. The plague was referred to as the "black death" because of the hemorrhaging of its victims. From the Black Sea the plague was carried on shipboard to the ports of Europe. By 1348 the first of many successive waves of black plague blanketed Europe. Individuals afflicted with leprosy were especially susceptible to the plague, and the majority of lepers died, which precipitated a decline in the prevalence and severity of leprosy.

Panic, flight, prayer, and penance were initial reactions to this plague. More rational thinking soon followed. Stringent standards of quarantine were established, much like those set down for the leprosy control. The gates of cities were closed to outsiders, houses of the sick were marked, and food and water supplies were carried in only by authorized people who themselves were then quarantined to ensure no contagion. Venice, for example, in 1348 held ships and their crews at an isolated island in the harbor for 40 days before entry to the dock to unload, a practice that was then widely adopted. The term *quarantine* means 'pertaining to 40.'

Some 20 to 35 million people, one third to one half of the European population, died from the plague. The effects were devastating. In England, for example, the labor supply became so short and the economy so restricted that Parliament in 1350 had to freeze prices and forbid laborers to migrate to other towns.

Syphilis.   The last of the great plagues of the Middle Ages was syphilis. Although there is some debate as to where syphilis originated, there is no disagreement with the fact that syphilis reached epidemic proportions in Europe in the late 1400s. By 1497 the spread of syphilis was well documented and was reported to have spread as far as remote areas of Scotland. At that time syphilis was an acute and often fatal disease. This acute version seems to have attenuated into the less virulent chronic condition present today. The decreasing virulence of the disease no doubt reduced its threat and the chance of widespread prophylaxis. Unlike leprosy and the plague, syphilis is still present in epidemic proportions.

The Renaissance

In the period extending roughly from the fourteenth century through the sixteenth century, a rebirth of interest in the learning, literature, and artistic achievements of classical Greece and Rome, called the *Renaissance,* began in Italy and then spread throughout western Europe.

Among the forces that led to the Renaissance were the invention of the printing press, which allowed for the widespread distribution of ideas, and the introduction of gunpowder, which led city planners to cease building walls around cities, opening them to free passage of people. This rebirth of learning extended into areas related to public health and medicine. Many people contributed new ideas that now went beyond those of the Greeks and Romans, and the increasing movement of people and ideas meant that again knowledge was being shared widely. Scholars at centers of learning in Paris, Oxford, and Cambridge began to reorder knowledge into the classical disciplines of law, medicine, theology, and philosophy. Humanists, with their emphasis on the natural, began to accept sickness and disease as phenomena to be investigated and understood.

Mercantilism

With the humanism of the Renaissance, the seventeenth, and eighteenth centuries also came the rise of commerce and industry and the development of the new economic theory of mercantilism. Increased economic activity and trade resulted in increased wealth and led to the clear identification of the nation state. As a nation's wealth became important, so the value of the nation's workers increased. This fact, along with the spirit of humanism, led to a concerted interest in solving the health problems of the day, especially as they affected the workers. After all, a sick and ailing work force meant less production and therefore less wealth. The positive results for the work force, however, were lost temporarily in the Industrial Revolution as it developed later in the 1800s.

Beginning of the modern era

In seventeenth century London, bills of mortality were published weekly. These were basically an account of the causes of death, an early example of biostatistics. John Graunt (1620-1674) made the first systematic study of these bills of mortality and in 1662 published *Natural and Political Observation upon the Bills of Mortality,* a text that indicated some of the real meaning of mortality in his society. He observed that more boys than girls were born but that the ratio of the sexes was soon equalized because the rate of death during childhood was higher for boys than for girls. Graunt also noted that death rates were higher in urban areas than in rural areas and that death rates varied by season.

William Petty (1623-1687) went beyond Graunt in the analysis of numeric data on population, education, disease, revenue, and economic structure. Petty established the statistical basis for health planning, which involved the identification of existing needs, medical work force, medical care, and ancillary medical services designed to satisfy those needs. Petty's efforts to relate statistics to the real needs of the day became known as "political arithmetic" (Petty, 1699).

Humanism, mercantilism, and the pioneering work of Graunt and Petty led to a gradual increase in community involvement in matters related to their own health. The quality of medical practice however, available to the average citizen changed little.

The eighteenth century marked an early triumph of preventive medicine. The practice of inoculation had been known in India and China for hundreds of years. This practice was first introduced into Europe around 1713 and made famous by Lady Mary Wortley Montague, wife of the English Ambassador to Turkey, who had her 3-year-old son inoculated against smallpox in Constantinople in 1718.

The lag between the development of a medical or preventive technique and its eventual success in the eradication of a worldwide health problem is a lesson of history worth noting. Edward Jenner (1749-1823), a British physician, made inoculation with smallpox obsolete by discovering that the application of cowpox virus to scratched human skin produced an immunity to smallpox. According to WHO, smallpox was eliminated in 1979.

The era of modern bacteriology ushered in by the work of Louis Pasteur and Robert Koch marked the first major redirection of medicine since the time of the Greeks. The discovery that a specific organism causes a specific disease transferred attention from the general environment to specific elements in the environment. The recognition that the spread of disease could be prevented by blocking routes over which the disease traveled resulted in emphasis on the sanitation of water, milk, and other foods, the elimination of insects, and the disposal of sewage. Sanitary engineers, sanitary inspectors, bacteriologists, and laboratory technicians became essential to the health program. This era reestablished many of the important principles first identified by the early Greek physicians. These developments, from earliest times until today, are summarized in Fig. 1-3.

Control of the ill person, who was the source of the disease, became an established practice. Isolation and quarantine measures were enforced. Progress in the prevention and control of infectious diseases included immunization, antiseptic procedures, and chemical treatment. Immunization was a natural outcome of the interest in bacteriology. In 1883 Pasteur developed the inoculation against rabies. Von Behring's development of diphtheria antitoxin was first used in 1894. Wright developed typhoid inoculations in 1904. Lord Lister's development of carbolic acid (phenol) and Ehrlich's discovery of the value of arsenic compounds in the treatment of syphilis lowered the death rate from communicable diseases.

The dramatic progress of this era made it seem as though with time all disease could be conquered. By environmental management, improved care, and the widespread use of the dramatically successful inoculations, anything seemed possible. Public health focused its

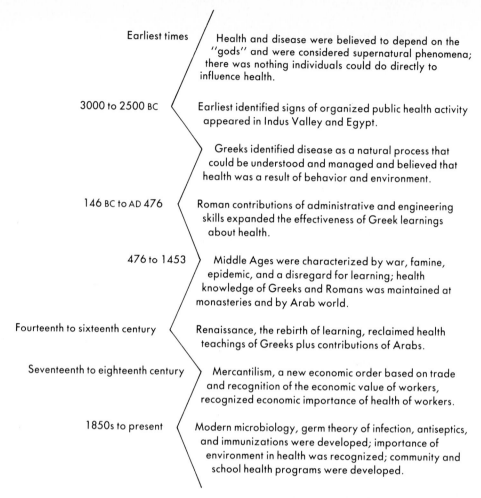

Earliest times	Health and disease were believed to depend on the "gods" and were considered supernatural phenomena; there was nothing individuals could do directly to influence health.
3000 to 2500 BC	Earliest identified signs of organized public health activity appeared in Indus Valley and Egypt.
	Greeks identified disease as a natural process that could be understood and managed and believed that health was a result of behavior and environment.
146 BC to AD 476	Roman contributions of administrative and engineering skills expanded the effectiveness of Greek learnings about health.
476 to 1453	Middle Ages were characterized by war, famine, epidemic, and a disregard for learning; health knowledge of Greeks and Romans was maintained at monasteries and by Arab world.
Fourteenth to sixteenth century	Renaissance, the rebirth of learning, reclaimed health teachings of Greeks plus contributions of Arabs.
Seventeenth to eighteenth century	Mercantilism, a new economic order based on trade and recognition of the economic value of workers, recognized economic importance of health of workers.
1850s to present	Modern microbiology, germ theory of infection, antiseptics, and immunizations were developed; importance of environment in health was recognized; community and school health programs were developed.

FIG. 1-3. Major periods in public health history. Moving from an era of complete acceptance of disease as supernatural, humankind has come to view disease as a natural and therefore understandable phenomenon. The Greeks believed that if disease could be understood it could be limited. Many of the Greek notions of balance, moderation, and recognition of the importance of environment were lost during the Dark Ages only to reemerge during the Renaissance as important principles in modern public health thinking.

efforts on doing things to and for people. Only gradually did it become clear that the people themselves must be involved in their own health. Basic education about hygiene and nutrition developed. To become more responsible, people needed greater knowledge and greater encouragement to exercise that knowledge.

As communicable diseases were controlled and the environment improved, there emerged new patterns of disease that emphasized the need for new knowledge and new levels of personal responsibility for improved health. Today the principal causes of death result in varying degrees from the way persons act, from what they do to and for themselves.

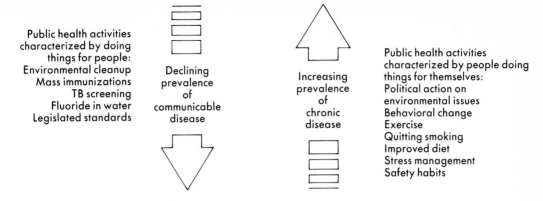

Public health activities characterized by doing things for people:
Environmental cleanup
Mass immunizations
TB screening
Fluoride in water
Legislated standards

Declining prevalence of communicable disease

Increasing prevalence of chronic disease

Public health activities characterized by people doing things for themselves:
Political action on environmental issues
Behavioral change
Exercise
Quitting smoking
Improved diet
Stress management
Safety habits

FIG. 1-4. The changing nature of public health problems results from and involves changes in strategies used to improve health. Control of chronic diseases was achieved largely by doing things *to* the environment and *to* people. To reduce and delay modern causes of death (i.e., degenerative diseases and accidents) public health workers will have to work *with* people to bring about changes in individual health practices and in political action to improve community health.

To reduce today's diseases the public needs not only knowledge, but also help to behave in a responsible way, thus reducing their individual risk of disease and death. Changing and improving behavior is the objective of education (Fig. 1-4).

THE SCHOOL HEALTH MOVEMENT

Children's health has long been a concern of the public, and history is replete with individual and group efforts to improve their lot. It is logical that early contributions to the school health movement came from Europe.

European heritage of school health

As early as 1790 Bavaria provided free school lunches for the underprivileged. The eminent European scientist Johann Peter Frank (1745-1821) published a series of papers dealing with the general subject of school health. In 1832 Edwin Chadwick, an assistant commissioner, studied the operation of the poor laws of England. A year later he became secretary of the Factory Commission. From his studies of the conditions of child employment came reforms recognizing the health needs of children.

Physicians were placed on public school staffs in Sweden in 1868, Germany in 1869, Russia in 1871, and Austria in 1873. In Brussels, Belgium, the first organized, regular medical inspection system was instituted in 1874. Every 3 months all schools were inspected by a physician. Later dentists and vision specialists were added to the inspection staff.

It is significant that all these early school health activities in Europe were directed toward doing something *for* the child. The concept of preparing the child to do something for himself or herself had not yet evolved because the essentials for health education did not exist. An extensive knowledge of health, plus universal education, is essential for health education.

1700s	Evolving philosophies reflecting new appreciations for the value of people and their welfare.
1868-1873	Physicians placed on school staffs in Sweden, Germany, Russia, and Austria.
1850	Shattuck's report of the Sanitary Commission of Massachusetts outlined a plan for health instruction in school.
1885-1899	Increasing support for physical education including the employment of speciality teachers and passage of laws requiring physical education in schools.
1910-1911	First White House Conference on Child Health and Families of Joint Committee of the American Medical Association and National Education Association.
1918	Commission on the Reorganization of Secondary Schools named health as one of the seven cardinal objectives of education.
1948-1955	A series of national conferences on competencies for health education sponsored by U.S. Office of Education.
1964	First Surgeon General's Report on Smoking and Health leads to direct allocation of money for research and educational intervention with high school aged students.
1967	School Health Education Study provides first nationwide accounting of the status of school health.
1973	Report of the President's Committee on Health Education outlined future governmental and private sector developments leading to the creation of the USPHS Bureau of Health Education (1984) and the National Center for Health Education (1975).
1970s	School Health Curriculum Project sets new standards for scope of health education and preparation of teachers.
1978-1982	National Forward Plan for Health in fiscal years 1978-1982 identifies health education as prominent part of federal health policy.
1980s	Centers for Disease Control includes a Center for Health Promotion and Education. Increased emphasis on evaluating school health programs. Federal government support becomes more evident. Some of the National Institutes for Health begin to fund school-based research initiatives.

FIG. 1-5. In the modern period it became increasingly clear that human behaviors were major contributors to disease and death. There was an increased interest of the federal government and of schools to teach people to value and protect their health.

Beginning of the modern school health era

The modern school health program is based on the fundamental concept that schools can prepare people to protect, preserve, and promote their own health. The modern program retains the school's responsibility for supervising the child's health and promoting school sanitation, inherited from Europe, but also has added the all-important objective of preparing each young person to make decisions necessary for his or her own health (Fig. 1-5).

Before 1850 the schools in the United States were dominated by the church. The type of imposed pedagogy that prevailed before 1850 did not lend itself to health education. However, in 1850 tax-supported public schools became a reality in most of the United States, particularly in the north.

A second fortunate development was the publication of the *Report of the Sanitary Commission of Massachusetts* (Shattuck, 1850). The awakening concern for health led this commission to study and make recommendations on matters affecting public health. The report, which dealt with a large number of health topics, included a plan for school health instruction. A Boston bookseller and politician, Lemuel Shattuck, wrote the report, which included the following classic concept of education about health:

> Every child should be taught, early in life, that to preserve his own life and his own health and the lives and health of others, is one of his most important and constantly abiding duties. Some measure is needed which shall compel children to make a sanitary examination of themselves and their associates, and thus elicit a practical application of the lessons of sanitary science in the everyday duties of life. The recommendation now under consideration is designed to furnish this measure. It is to be carried into operation in the use of a blank schedule, which is to be printed on a letter sheet, in the form prescribed in the appendix, and furnished to the teacher of each school. He is to appoint a sanitary committee of the scholars, at the commencement of school, and on the first day of each month, to fill it out under his superintendence. . . . Such a measure is simple, would take but a few minutes each day, and cannot operate otherwise than usefully upon the children, in forming habits of exact observation, and in making a personal application of the laws of health and life to themselves. This is education of an eminently practical character, and of the highest importance.

Because the report was the most important health pronouncement in an era of increasing health interest, it attracted much attention. It recognized the school as an agency for health promotion. For the next 20 years this seed of recognition was nourished by influential European leaders in education such as Rousseau, Pestalozzi, and Froebel. This influence, which stressed education as growth from within, not imposed from without, stimulated an interest in understanding children, their needs, and the best means to meet these needs.

Beginning in 1880, pioneering work in problems relating to children's health was inaugurated. These developed a diversity of concepts concerning which body of information constituted school health and the school's responsibilities for students' health. Educators studied the physical and psychologic characteristics of child development as the basis for the school program. by the early 1900s child study was an established basis for all school planning and activities.

Physical education experienced a robust expansion during this period. To promote physical conditioning and efficiency, calisthenics made up a considerable part of the program. Kansas City, Missouri, schools had a director of physical education as early as 1885, and during the next 10 years physical education was widely adopted by schools in the Middle West. By 1892, Ohio law *required* that physical education be taught in the schools of all first- and second-class cities. In 1899 North Dakota law *required* the teaching of physical education in all public schools. Schools in other sections of the nation were slower to accept physical education.

Physical education and health were considered identical; apparently not until 1910 did this point of view change. In that year the seventeenth meeting of the American Physical Education Association used "School Hygiene and Physical Education" as its theme. Not until 1937 did the American Physical Education Association become the American Association for Health and Physical Education and thus recognize the distinction between health and physical education.

The end of the first decade of the 1990s marked two important developments in the school health movement. The first White House Conference on Child Health and Protection was held in 1910, and in 1911 the Joint Committee of the National Education Association and the American Medical Association was appointed. This committee, representing the official position of the two parent bodies on health programs affecting schools, became an authoritative source of recommended policies and practice for health programs.

Health examinations in schools began in 1894 when Dr. Samuel Durgin, Health Commissioner of Boston, introduced the first regular program for medical inspection in the United States. Similar programs began in Chicago in 1895, New York in 1897, and Philadelphia in 1898. Connecticut law required teachers to test students' vision. Reading, Pennsylvania, employed a school dentist in 1903, and in 1904 Vermont initiated compulsory eye, ear, nose, and throat examinations in the public schools. By 1910 more than 300 cities required medical inspections in their schools.

In 1918 the Commission on the Reorganization of Secondary Education named health as the first of the seven cardinal objectives of education.

In 1922 in Malden, Massachusetts, under the direction of Dr. C.E. Turner and with the support of the Massachusetts Institute of Technology, a 2-year school health demonstration program was conducted. Incorporating the best activities in school health, Dr. Turner developed a relatively complete program. At the termination of the demonstration, a critical analysis of the results showed that not only had the students' health behavior improved, but also their health, growth, and development had been affected favorably.

From 1922 to 1925, the American Red Cross sponsored a similar demonstration with similar results in Mansfield and Richland Counties in Ohio. In Fargo, North Dakota, the Commonwealth Fund conducted a school health demonstration from 1923 to 1927. With the Milbank Memorial Fund assisting financially, Cattaraugus County, New York, conducted a school health demonstration program. Each of these studies contributed to the school health movement by pointing out strengths and weaknesses, suggesting methods and techniques, explaining appropriate procedures, and showing results obtained from a school health program.

In 1930 the Second White House Conference on Child Health and Protection grappled with the task of synthesizing various aspects of child health and its concomitant problems. The conference report served as a guide for two decades. The Midcentury White House Conference on Children and Youth in 1950 submitted a further report. With time, school health programs evolved from multiphasic programs identifying elements such as health examination, health guidance, prevention and correlation of physical defects, control of communicable diseases, mental health, health instruction, and the maintenance of school sanitation to the modern threefold program focusing on health education, health services, and healthful environment.

One single publication figures predominantly in shaping schools' policies regarding school health. *Suggested School Health Policies* was first issued in 1940 by the American Public Health Association with a second edition published in 1946 by the National Conference for Cooperation in Health Education. This national conference included representatives from all the leading educational, health, and medical organizations concerned with school health. *Suggested School Health Policies* was published by the Health and Education Committee on School and College Health of the American Medical Association.

Beginning in 1948 a series of national conferences sponsored by professional groups and the Office of Education was held to define functions and competencies needed by the school health educator. These conferences were held in Jackson's Mill, Weston, West Virginia, in 1948; in Père Marquette State Park, Illinois, in 1950; and in Washington, D.C., in 1949, 1953, and 1955. The interest in professional preparation was also evident during the 1960s when the American Association for Health, Physical Education, and Recreation sponsored national conferences to develope standards for accrediting colleges and universities offering training in health education (Means, 1975). In 1974 the American Association for Health, Physical Education, and Recreation issued a report on competencies for school health and safety education; in 1976 a committee of the American School Health Association issued a report on professional preparation; and in 1977 the Society for Public Health Education (SOPHE) published guidelines for professional health education practice. Schaller (1978), summarizing several of these reports, identified common areas of professional preparation in health education: (1) the physical and biologic sciences, (2) the behavioral sciences, (3) a core of health content courses, and (4) the skills of professional practice. The preamble of the SOPHE guidelines report contains an appropriate statement of purposes and methodologies of the health educator:

> Health education is concerned with the health-related behavior of people. Therefore, it must take into account the forces that affect those behaviors and the role of human behavior in the prevention of disease. As a profession, it uses educational processes to stimulate desirable change or to reinforce health practices of individuals, families, groups, organizations, communities, and larger social systems. Its intent is the development of health knowledge, the exploration of behavior change options, and the consequence of these changes.

Government support

In 1971 President Nixon appointed the National Committee on Health Education. Earlier that year, in his health message to Congress, the President had stated that there was no national instrument, no central force to stimulate and coordinate a comprehensive health program (*Report of the President's Committee on Health Education,* 1973). Accordingly, the committee was charged with doing the following:

1. Describe the state of the art in health education
2. Define the nation's need for health education
3. Establish goals, priorities, and objectives for health education
4. Determine the most appropriate structure, organization, and function for a national health education foundation

The President's report led directly to the establishment of the Bureau of Health Education in 1974 as a part of the U.S. Public Health Service. The bureau provided a focal point for health education within the federal government and encouraged industry to build health education into existing programs. Another purpose for the bureau was to fund the training of health education specialists.

A further outgrowth of the President's report was the establishment in 1975 of the National Center for Health Education. As stated in its 1978 brochure, the primary mission of the center is:

> . . . improving and increasing the education of the American public about health matters, encouraging people about health matters, encouraging people to place greater value on their health, emphasizing health rather than sickness . . . and [creating] better understanding of how to shape those forces which influence our health.

In 1983 the National Center for Health Education relocated its central office to New York City.

Besides the creation of the Bureau of Health Education, the *Report of the President's Committee on Health Education* triggered other federal activities. For example, Congress has written new charters for the National Cancer Institute and the National Heart, Lung, and Blood Institute. In addition to their traditional biomedical research missions, it is now mandated that more attention be given to prevention, education, and control measures.

Federal legislation authorizing the establishment of health maintenance organizations (HMOs) required health education as one of their basic functions. The 1974 Health Planning and Development Act, the National Consumer Health Information Act, and the Health Promotion Act each highlighted health education needs.

In 1978 the Bureau of Health Manpower of the U.S. Public Health Service sponsored a workshop on the preparation and practice of professional health educators. The workshop's purpose was to identify the roles and functions of health educators in their various occupational settings. Conclusions from the conference held that the commonalities of professional preparation and practice in health education would be the basis for developing national standards to establish health educators' credentials.

This work, the Role Delineation Project, was continued by the National Center for Health Education and resulted in a precise listing of skills and competencies basic to entry-level health education practice (*Focal Points,* 1980).

For the first time, health education became a prominent part of a federal policy statement when the National Forward Plan for Health, FY 1978-1982, issued in 1976 by the Chief Health Officers of the U.S. Department of Health, Education and Welfare, offered several recommendations directly related to school health education. The Public Health Service was charged to give priority attention to the following:

1. Foster research and pilot programs aimed at improving health education principles and techniques
2. Conduct specific health education activities in accident prevention
3. Conduct research to determine the best methods of teaching children about the harmful effects of smoking, alcohol, drug abuse, and careless driving
4. Emphasize the development of lifelong attitudes toward health and the improvement of health in later years as a major goal of child health. Health activities cited in this report were immunizations, nutrition, dental health, and mental health.

The decade of the 1970s was characterized by a visible involvement of the federal government in school health–related activities. In addition, each state education department nurtured the development of school health activities. Because health and education are the responsibilities of different state agencies, state health departments also suported school health programs. County governments were also frequently involved in school health programs as were local school boards. During the 1970s, a period of economic growth, concern for adolescent health problems such as drug abuse and an increasing awareness of health risks caused school health programs to expand significantly. The early 1980s, however, with a less robust economy and a federal government philosophy characterized by decreasing involvement, meant that many initiatives supporting school health programs were curtailed. The Department of Education, for example, was marked for reduction and possible elimination, and accordingly the Office of School Health was phased out. The visible presence of other school health programs also declined.

Federal support for school health focused on two principal agencies, both parts of the Department of Health and Human Services. These two agencies were the Center for Disease Control in Atlanta, Georgia, and the Office of Disease Prevention and Health Promotion, a part of the office of the Assistant Secretary of Health, Department of Health and Human Services, in Washington, D.C.

In 1980 the Center for Disease Control reorganized into the Centers for Disease Control. These six centers are the Center for Prevention Services, the Center for Environmental Health, the National Institute for Occupational Safety and Health, the Center for Health Promotion and Education, the Center for Professional Development and Training, and the Center for Infectious Diseases.

The Center for Health Promotion and Education includes the Division on Nutrition, the Division of Reproductive Health, and the Division of Health Education, which is now the major health education coordinating and supporting mechanism for school programs.

The second major focus of the federal government having a direct bearing on school health programs is the Office of Disease Prevention and Health Promotion. The mandate of this office is one of coordination and policy development in health promotion matters. This office provides leadership, coordination, and support for the aims of the Department of Health and Human Services outlined in *Healthy People*.

It would be incorrect, however, to assume that these two offices and their programs represent the nation's commitment to school health. A 1983 report at a meeting of several U.S. government departments showed that practically all cabinet-level departments had some interest and involvement in school health–related programs. Most of the programs were located in either the Department of Education, which in this particular document listed 26 separate programs, or the Department of Health and Human Services, which identified 61 separate programs. Because of rapidly changing conditions, no single reporting of projects or budgets reflects an accurate accounting of priorities or programs.

School health education: evaluation activities

The curriculum reform of the 1960s, prompted by Russia's launching of Sputnik in 1957, created a new interest in the school curriculum. In addition to national curriculum projects in science and mathematics, the nationwide *School Health Education Study: a Conceptual Design for Curriculum Development* (SHES) (1967) was carried out. The first phase of this study began in 1961 with a national survey of health instruction in U.S. elementary and secondary schools that revealed a need for young people to acquire new levels of health knowledge. Also revealed was a considerable level of health misinformation in need of correction. The second phase involved the development of a comprehensive curriculum covering the full range of health topics with appropriate instructional materials for various grade levels (see Chapter 12).

Adding to this interest in health education was the publication of the first *Surgeon General's Report on Smoking and Health* (1964) and the resulting public concern over youth smoking.

At about the same time in California, an experimental program was begun to teach intermediate-grade children about the heart and circulatory system. Known first as the "Berkeley Project" and later as the "School Health Curriculum Project" (SHCP), this curriculum helped young people recognize the body as their greatest natural resource. The School Health Curriculum Project was unique in the way the curriculum was organized and in the way teachers were prepared.

The curriculum included a common organizational pattern that involved seven stages: (1) an introduction to arouse curiosity and motivate students to learn more, (2) an overview of all the body systems, (3) activities to increase personal appreciation of the body systems and their unique function, (4) exercises to teach structure and function of the body system, (5) a discussion of diseases and problems of the body system, (6) instruction and care of the body system and the prevention of disease, (7) and finally, group activities to provide a culmination: synthesis for the total unit.

Starting with a focus on the heart and circulatory system, stimulated by the increasing recognition of the dangers of cigarette smoking, this curriculum expanded to include materials for grades 4 through 7. Grade 4 lessons focused on digestion and nutrition, grade 5 lessons on lungs and respiration, grade 6 lessons on heart and circulation, and grade 7 lessons on the nervous system.

The special attention devoted to preparing instructors to teach this curriculum represented a unique initiative. Schools wishing to participate in the *School Health Curriculum Project* were required to send a team of four or five members to special training centers. Teams were composed of at least two classroom teachers, who would better teach the curriculum, one administrator, preferably a principal, and two other persons such as school nurses, curriculum specialists or counselors. This team participated in 60 hours of training that involved them in all of the curriculum activities, just as they would expect students to participate. Upon return to their districts, these teams were expected to train additional personnel to teach this program.

Considerable federal government support for this project led to its wide adoption and to several attempts to evaluate its effectiveness. The apparent success of this project led to the development of an additional project called the "Primary Grades Health Curriculum Project," which addressed the needs of students in grades kindergarten through 3. Involving a shorter but equally intense teacher-training program following the same team concept, the Primary Grades Health Curriculum Project devoted 20 to 30 minutes a day over an 8- to 10-week period and introduced kindergarten students to the notions of happiness and health. Grade 1 students learned to value themselves as "super me," grade 2 students learned about "sights and sounds," and grade 3 students learned about "the body: its framework and movement."

Based on many evaluation reports of varying quality of the School Health Education Project, the Centers for Disease Control and the Office of Disease Prevention and Health Promotion contracted with ABT Associates, a private consulting company, to conduct a 3-year study of four different health education programs. The intent of this study was to establish well-founded measures of health education efforts. More than 30,000 students in grades 4 and 7 in a thousand classrooms in 20 states were involved.

This project measured the outcomes of four different health education curricula that met a variety of important educational criteria. The programs evaluated were Project Prevention, Know Your Body (both examples of multifocused curricula), Three R's and HBP, and Chicago Heart Health Curriculum Project (both examples of limited-focus curricula). Each of these curricula met the standards of specificity, measurable objectives, and teacher preparation.

Although there were many specific measures, the results clearly indicated that students in health classes significantly increased their knowledge, developed much healthier attitudes, and reported health skills and practices in support of their greater knowledge and positive attitudes.

In addition to these general outcomes, more specific results suggested that to get the largest benefit from the educational programs at least 50 classroom hours were needed and that with a commitment equal to or greater than 50 hours significant changes in knowledge, attitudes, and practices could be achieved and would maintain stable levels over a period of time.

These data gave clear-cut data-based guidelines for school officials planning health instruction programs.

Emerging issues

Three emerging issues will have great impact in school health education curricula developments in the 1980s. The present secretary of education has highlighted the need for schools to address drug abuse and has supported the development of a wide range of school and community programs. It will be some time before the long-term benefits of these programs are evident. However, these initiatives resulted from a reasonably well-developed surveillance system that presented a clear picture of adolescent substance abuse, and they should prove effective in the long run.

AIDS (acquired immunodeficiency syndrome) and the high level of public concern and fear of this disease will also have a clear impact on the future of school health programs. The need to teach about sexually transmitted diseases (STDs) has been brought to a level of public priority by AIDS that was never achieved by the concern about syphilis and gonorrhea, which are much more widespread. AIDS has fueled the debate about how far schools can go in discussing sexually transmitted diseases and sharing knowledge on how to prevent the spread of these diseases.

Debate over the school's role in controlling AIDS has also highlighted the possible roles schools can play in providing counseling and school-based clinic services. Discussion on school-based clinics frequently polarizes communities into groups that support and do not support an increased role for the schools in providing health information and health services.

This debate is also fueled by the high incidence of teen pregnancies. The need to teach about the management of sexual behavior, the prevention of pregnancy, and the care of persons in the earliest stages of pregnancy is a medical necessity not yet viewed as an educational necessity. With an estimated 3000 teen-age pregnancies occurring daily, the condition is epidemic. The challenge at the community level is to assist those already pregnant while encouraging others to prevent pregnancy.

Some argue that schools provide the best chance to help young people avoid disease and prevent pregnancy. Education is an avenue to achieve this end. The school-based clinic is another.

SUMMARY

Health has concerned pepole from earliest times. Even before the great empires of Greece and Rome it was clear that people had explicit rules to protect health and knew that behavior affected their health. If individual actions affected health, it was clearly understood that others could learn to reduce illness, that the environment could be changed to reduce health risks, and that medical services could reduce the duration of disease.

Although much of the health-related knowledge of the Greeks and Romans was disregarded during the Middle Ages, many of their principles are now important again. Supplementing the rediscovery of old knowledge has been an enormous quantity of new scientific health-related findings within the last 100 years. Despite these advances in knowledge, one fact continues to be clear: what individuals do to and for themselves in terms of personal behavior has the greatest influence on health. Education, especially education in schools, therefore becomes critical. What individuals do to and for the environment also affects health, as does the quality and quantity of health services and the way they are used. The basic elements of the school health program (i.e., education, environment, and services) are, in fact, microcosms of all that is critical to the health of our community, our country, and our world.

Although the earliest emphasis for school health education in America is evident in Shattuck's report to the Sanitary Commission of Massachusetts, it was the developing philosophies of education leaders in Europe in the late 1800s that provided early substantial support for school health education.

After World War II, participants in a series of conferences explored and defined the nature and contribution of school health education. In the 1960s it became increasingly clear that behavior was a major contributor to disease and death, and the federal government became more directly interested and involved in and supportive of school health programs. Major curriculum initiatives—the School Health Curriculum Study and the School Health Curriculum Project—and recent efforts to evaluate and compare the effectiveness of well-designed health curricula have provided both data and experience upon which to build. Although notions of balance and moderation first expounded by the Greeks are still relevant, current knowledge about what effectively improves behaviors indicates that future school health programs may be more focused, more accountable, and more responsive to changing health needs.

The next decade holds promise to be one of the most exciting for school health programs. Recognizing how much schools can contribute to the achievement of the nation's health goals and how controversial the schools' role in providing critical information and services in areas such as sexually transmitted diseases, AIDS, and teenage pregnancy can become means that those entering this important field will face challenges never before experienced. School health personnel stand to make some significant contributions to the improvement of the nation's health.

STUDY QUESTIONS

1. Why are the nations with the highest level of health also the nations with the greatest political, economic, and social advances, and, conversely, what are the political, economic, and social advances for the nations with the highest level of health?

2. What was the significance of Shattuck's 1850 *Report of the Sanitary Commission of Massachusetts* with respect to the development of school health in the United States?

3. Why did the early interest in child study hasten the promotion of the school health movement?

4. Which developments in the past decade do you consider to be of major importance to health education?

5. What are the purposes on which a school health program should be based?

6. Differentiate between natural and supernatural and relate the two concepts to the development of public health history.

7. What are the major health risks facing today's children and adolescents?

8. The Roman contributions to public health differ from those of the Greeks in which important dimensions?

9. The Middle Ages were characterized by a rejection of learning and a lack of knowledge. Who was responsible for the protection of health and medical knowledge?

10. What is the basis for the practice of quarantine? Explain why quarantine was practiced long before the principles of infection were understood.

11. Why was the development of mercantilism so important to the development of public health practice?

12. Why did it take so long for the principles of immunization first introduced by Jenner in the late 1700s to be used to eliminate smallpox?

13. What role has AIDS played in (1) promoting school health education and (2) creating opposition to school health education?

14. What characteristics were unique about the School Health Curriculum Project?

15. What contributions will be made by recent attempts to carefully evaluate school health education programs?

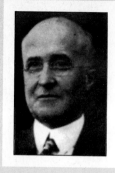

Thomas Denison Wood

BORN   August 2, 1865, Sycamore, Illinois
DIED   March 19, 1951, Taunton, Massachusetts
EDUCATION   B.A., Oberlin College, 1888; M.D., Columbia University, 1891

Thomas D. Wood became the first professor of health education (1927) in the United States and initiated the first graduate program in the field as well as the first school health program. He was trained as a physician and as a physical educator, and he combined these disciplines in his emphasis on health as a fundamental condition to meet the aims of education. After graduating from Oberlin (Ohio) College in 1888, he studied physical education with Dudley Sartent at the Normal School of Physical Training in Boston and worked at the Boston Young Men's Christian Association. He studied medicine at Columbia University, graduating with a doctorate of medicine in 1891.

On graduation, Wood went to the newly established Stanford (California) University as a professor of hygiene and physical training, director of physical education, and college physician. He established a program that was the first in the United States to award credit for physical education. In 1901 he returned to Columbia University to organize a department of physical education and to improve the student health services program. He remained there until his retirement in 1931, becoming known as the Father of the Natural Idea of Play. He developed purposes, content, and methods for school and college physical education programs centering on games, sports, dancing, outdoor activities, and general skills instead of the regimented exercises formerly advocated.

Dr. Wood organized the Joint Committee on Health Problems in Education of the American Medical Association and the National Education Association and chaired it for more than 25 years (1911-1938). Wood was the first person to discuss health instruction in *Health and Education,* the ninth yearbook of the Society for the Study of Education (1910). His books include *Healthful Schools, The Child in School, Course of Study in Health Education, Health Through Prevention and Control of Disease, Physical Education, Health Behavior,* and many others. He was active in professional organizations, was instrumental in the development of the American Child Health Association, the health section of the International Federation of Home and School (1928-1936), and was chairman of the Committee on the School Child of the White House Conference on Child Health and Protection (1930). He was a fellow of the American Academy of Medicine, the American Academy of Physical Education, and three times received the Gulick Award for distinguished professional service.

REFERENCES

Allensworth, D.D., and Kolbe, L.J.: The Comprehensive School Health Program: exploring an expanded concept, J. Sch. Health 57:409, 1987.

Bruess, C.E., editor: Professional preparation of the health educator: report of the ASHA Committee on Professional Preparation and College Health Education Conference at Towson State University, Jan. 29-30, 1976, J. Sch. Health 46(7):418, 1976.

Burton, L.E., and Hollingsworth Smith, H.: Public health and community medicine, Baltimore, 1970, The Williams & Wilkins Co.

Chadwick, E.: Report on an inquiry into the sanitary condition of the laboring population of Great Britain (poor law commissioners), London, 1842, W. Clowes for Her Majesty's Stationery Office.

Connell, D.B., and Turner, R.R.: The impact of instructional experience and the effects of cumulative instruction, J. Sch. Health 55:324, 1985.

Connell, D.B., Turner, R.R., and Mason, E.F.: Summary of findings of the School Health Education Evaluation: health promotion effectiveness, implementation and costs, J. Sch. Health 55:316, 1985.

Focal points, Atlanta, July 1980, Bureau of Health Education, U.S. Department of Health and Human Services, Public Health Service.

Healthy people: the surgeon general's report on health promotion and disease prevention, DHEW (PHS) Pub. No. 79-55071, Washington, D.C., 1979, U.S. Department of Health, Education and Welfare, Public Health Service, U.S. Government Printing Office.

Hippocrates: On airs, waters, and places. In The genuine works of Hippocrates, Baltimore, 1939, The Williams & Wilkins Co. (Translated by Francis Adams.)

Kirby, D.: Comprehensive school-based health clinics: a growing movement to improve adolescent health and reduce teenage pregnancy, J. Sch. Health 56:289, 1986.

Means, R.K.: A history of health education in the United States, Philadelphia, 1962, Lea & Febiger.

Means, R.K.: Historical perspectives on school health, Thorofare, N.J., 1975, Charles B. Slack, Inc.

Newman, I.M.: Comments from the field, J. Sch. Health 55:343, 1985.

Petty, W.: Political arithmetic or a discourse concerning the extent and value of lands, people, buildings, etc., ed. 3, London, 1699, Robert Clavel.

Porter, P.J.: School health is a place, not a discipline, J. Sch. Health 57:417, 1987.

Report of the President's Committee on Health Education, Washington, D.C., 1973, U.S. Government Printing Office.

Schaller, W.E.: Professional preparation and curriculum planning, J. Sch. Health 48(4):236, 1978.

School health education study: a conceptual design for curriculum development, St. Paul, 1961, 3M Education Press.

School health education study: a summary report, Washington, D.C., 1967, National Education Association Publications.

Shattuck, L.: The report of the sanitary commission of Massachusetts, Cambridge, Mass., 1948, Harvard University Press. (Originally published in 1850.)

Smoking and health—report of the Advisory Committee to the Surgeon General of the Public Health Service, Washington, D.C., 1979, U.S. Government Printing Office.

Society for Public Health Education Ad Hoc Task Force on Professional Preparation and Practice: Guidelines for the preparation and practice of professional health educators, S.O.P.H.E. Health Education Monographs 5(1):75, 1977.

U.S. Department of Health and Human Services: Health USA, Hyattsville, Md., 1988, Public Health Service, Centers for Disease Control, National Center for Health Statistics.

U.S. Department of Health and Human Services: The 1990 health objectives for the nation: a mid-course review, Washington, D.C., 1986, U.S. Government Printing Office.

U.S. Department of Health, Education and Welfare: The health consequences of smoking: a report to the Surgeon General, Washington, D.C., 1964, U.S. Government Printing Office.

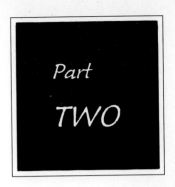

Part

TWO

ORGANIZATION OF THE SCHOOL HEALTH PROGRAM

2 Basic Plan of the Health Program

OVERVIEW   *Strongly organized and effectively coordinated programs are essential to the goal of furthering school health education. The two facets of a school health plan, services and education, must be integrated to serve adequately the changing needs of a modern society. Based on these precepts, this chapter outlines the organization of health services and the organization of health instruction within the schools. The importance of integrating health services and health education is stressed while recognizing that the programs offered by the school have important ties to health agencies in the community.*

The chapter is divided into five sections: (1) the organization of health services, (2) the authorization of school health programs, (3) the basic divisions of the school health program, and (4) the integration of health services and health education, with school-based clinics providing an example of how school health services are integrated with health education.

The first three sections deal with the organization of health programs. Organizational studies of public health for all levels of government are presented, including international, federal, state, and local health agencies. This larger perspective of health services provides a context for the school health program and reveals some of the origins of its health activities. The organizational part of the chapter concludes with a discussion of the three basic divisions of the school health program.

The final two sections of the chapter deal with the importance of integrating not only school and community projects but also health service and health education programs if educators are to meet the health needs of the school-aged child.

OBJECTIVES   After reading this chapter, the student should be able to:

1. Describe the organization of health services at an international, federal, state, and local level
2. Identify the five major services of the World Health Organization (WHO)
3. Describe the major functions and organization of the U.S. Public Health Service
4. Explain the state's role in public health
5. Chart the process of authorizing school health programs
6. Distinguish between permissive and mandatory state legislation
7. Explain the roles of state education departments and local boards of education in the authorization process
8. Outline the benefits of programs that combine health services and education
9. Explain the purpose of school-based clinics
10. Cite Newman's six principles for integrating programs

A basic plan or blueprint is essential to any important undertaking, particularly one such as the school health program, which is expected to deal with the diversity of factors and situations related to human well-being. Although the plan for school health must have a basic pattern or framework, it should be sufficiently flexible to adapt to any situation or need. To be functional it must be practical. It should be adjusted to the needs of the students and must be in harmony with the background of both the school and the community.

There is no such thing as a single school health program. Many plans have their merits. However, it is important to recognize that school health programs in the United States are legal responsibilities of both public education and public health. School health laws in the state of Illinois reveal the shared legal relationship of the two community governmental agencies of education and health. The school code pertaining to physical examination states in part that "physical examinations as prescribed by the Department of Public Health including vision screening tests, shall be required." The Critical Health Problems and Comprehensive Health Education Act for Illinois Schools states that the office of the Superintendent of Public Instruction (Illinois Office of Education) "shall establish the minimum amount of instruction time to be devoted to comprehensive health education at all elementary and secondary grade levels."

Because of this mutual concern, several different administrative patterns of school health programs are often employed. The school health service aspect of the program may be placed under the jurisdiction of the local health department. Some schools operate under a joint administration of school health shared by the board of education and the health department. The most common pattern places the school health services under an associate superintendent for special services or associate superintendent for pupil personnel services.

How the program is administered is not of great importance so long as agreement on program objectives and a very real and cooperative working relationship exists between the school personnel and the health professionals. Serious difficulties have arisen in schools that have not had the benefit of leadership from professionally trained school health nurses and school health educators. Without such leadership, misunderstandings may arise over program priorities, based on a failure to understand the difference between the educators' objective to teach and the health professionals' goal to treat or to correct. Although the objectives of school personnel and health professionals are different, they are not mutually exclusive but instead serve to complement and strengthen each other. The student's full effectiveness in the teaching and learning situation cannot be achieved if he or she is not at optimal health, and optimal health cannot be achieved or maintained without benefit of education.

THE CONTEXT OF HEALTH PROGRAMS

The school health program must be understood in the total context of health programs and services. To be effective, the goals and functions of school health must be integrally related to all levels of health service, including the international, federal, state, and local levels.

Government health services have been concerned primarily with those functions that require organized community action, rather than services that can be easily provided on an individual basis. Government health agencies have undergone and continue to undergo considerable change. Earlier activities were concerned primarily with the prevention and control of communicable diseases on the local, national, or international level. This emphasis is changing to meet new health problems and the evolving needs of people.

Modern public health organizations have a variety of responsibilities that go far beyond efforts to control communicable diseases. Such diverse activities as mental health, crippled children's services, health hazards of the environment, medical care of the indigent, home health services, and the ever-increasing problems of chronic disease are now included. With the growing number of older citizens in U.S. society comes a need to devote more services to those with chronic illness.

International health services

The World Health Organization (WHO) is the major international health agency; its headquarters is in Geneva, Switzerland. Several regional WHO offices are located around the globe. The Western Regional Office, known as the Pan-American Health Organization (PAHO), is located in Washington, D.C., and has responsibilities for the western hemisphere. The major health service functions of WHO are as follows:

1. Supplying technical assistance to countries throughout the world to improve their own health services. For example, WHO may send a team of public health specialists to help a country control a malaria problem.
2. Coordinating a world wide health program by encouraging nations to assist each other in raising their health standards.
3. Providing a variety of special services to member nations, such as epidemiologic reporting, collection and dissemination of statistical data on prevention of diseases, standardization of public health and drug usage data, and dissemination of health information procedures.
4. Operating an extensive program of education and training in public health. For example, WHO may assign a public health specialist to a country to serve as a university instructor in order to help strengthen that country's program of professional education in the public health field. WHO has assisted the University of Ibadan in Nigeria in establishing a school of public health where public health education specialists are trained for service in Africa.
5. Carrying out a variety of research programs to acquire new knowledge of communicable diseases, nutritional methods, and public health administration.

Federal health services

In recent years, government health organizations and public health agencies have undergone many changes because of the federal government's growing involvement in such programs as Medicare and the delivery of health services.

As shown in Fig. 2-1, the U.S. Public Health Service has six major operating agencies, which carry out the principal activities of public health. Each of these agencies is under the administrative authority of the Assistant Secretary of Health, who in turn is responsible to the Secretary for Health and Human Services (HHS). The U.S. Public Health Service is administratively divided into 10 regional offices. Each of the regions has an administrator and staff that are representatives of the Assistant Secretary for Health. According to Grant (1981),

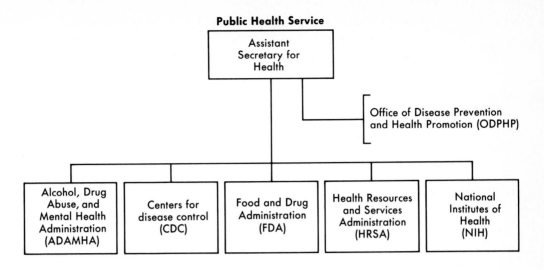

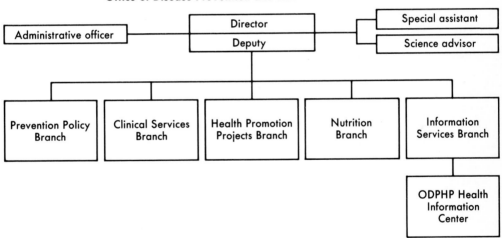

FIG. 2-1. U.S. Public Health Service.

"Public Health Services is the federal agency charged by law to promote and to assure the highest level of health attainable for every person in the United States and develop cooperation in health programs with other nations."

The major functions of the U.S. Public Health Service are as follows:
1. To stimulate and assist states and communities with the development of local health resources and to further the development of education for the health professions
2. To help improve the delivery of health services for all Americans
3. To conduct and support research in medical and related health sciences and to disseminate this scientific information

4. To protect the health of the nation against unsafe drugs and other potential community hazards

5. To provide leadership in the prevention and control of communicable diseases

State health services

Each state is responsible for the protection of the health of its citizens. The state, in fact, is the sovereign power. According to the U.S. Constitution, the federal government possesses only those powers in the field of health that have been delegated to it by the state. Local governments also derive their power and authority from the state. Public health laws vary considerably from state to state. Typically states will have a board of health or some similar authority such as a department of public health that has specific public health responsibilities. These responsibilities may be advisory in nature, but they also may be policy making. The health authority may have the power to enact regulations that are to be implemented throughout the state.

State organizations, like federal agencies, have undergone many changes in the organization of health services. The nature of problems confronting public health agencies is also changing. Some states have created large, umbrella type of organizations, analogous to the U.S. Department of Health and Human Services structure at the national level. Such an organization may encompass all agencies having to do with human services, such as the department of welfare, department of mental health, and department of public health.

Because the state health department is the agency vested by law with responsibility for protecting and promoting the health of its citizens, much of the burden for providing services falls on the states. However, the federal government often provides special grants either for conducting or for assisting the state in providing the needed health services. Although state programs may vary considerably, state health departments usually are responsible for the recording of vital statistics and providing programs of environmental health and maternal and child health, public health laboratory services, communicable disease control, public health nursing, and health education.

With the emergence of new health problems in society, new structures and programs in state health departments have developed. Some of the more recent programs include special programs for mental health and retardation, chronic disease control, accident prevention, and medical care for the indigent, as well as special functions, such as the licensing of nursing homes for the aged.

Local health services

As at the other levels of public health, recent developments have had a profound effect on the local health department. Populations have shifted, with the more affluent citizens moving out of the cities and rural dwellers moving into the cities. Many people are moving to the southern and southwestern regions of the country. The resultant changes in racial, ethnic, and age distribution in the population present new problems for public health. Many city health departments now have to provide a disproportionate share of services for the elderly, the very young, and the poor. At the same time, local tax resources are being reduced because the more productive members of the cities' population have moved away.

AUTHORIZATION OF SCHOOL HEALTH PROGRAMS

Inherent in the American system of schools is the principle that the local board of education is responsible for the schools of its district. This principle acknowledges that the closer a government agency is to the people, the more likely it is to be in tune with the situation in which it functions. Accordingly, extensive authority and responsibility have been delegated to the local school board. However, as illustrated in the Illinois situation, state laws make certain requirements of the school districts. In addition, state departments of education, through regulation, have set standards that local school districts must meet. Such legislative and regulative requirements have applied to school health programs.

State legislation

States pass two forms of legislation that affect the school health program: permissive laws and mandatory laws. In practical terms, permissive legislation simply recommends or encourages the local board of education to institute certain procedures that are beneficial to the health and well-being of schoolchildren. Permissive laws are couched in such language as "school districts should provide" or "are encouraged to provide." The conditions or procedures outlined in the law are recommended but not required. Therefore the school board has the option to accept or not accept the recommendation set forth in the law.

However, in the case of mandatory legislation, laws are authoritatively ordered. The state requires the local districts to carry out the provisions of the law. This requirement is obligatory, meaning that no exceptions to the law are permitted. Ideally, such legislation is drafted in broad outlines so that the state department of education can interpret the legislation and write guidelines to schools for implementing the requirements. Such guidelines are usually developed by persons who have had extensive school experience and who are recognized for sound administrative judgment and knowledge of successful school practices. The terminology of mandatory legislation contains such phrases as "The school district shall provide" or "must include." Statutes may further indicate the areas of health instruction and charge the state superintendent of instruction with responsibility for providing materials and advisory services for the schools throughout the state. The state department of education in cooperation with the state department of health may also be required to prescribe a program of health examinations of students in the elementary and secondary schools. The state superintendent of public instruction is charged with the implementation and enforcement of these statutes. Enforcement is exercised through school standardization requirements.

Among other requirements, in order to qualify as standard, the school district must meet the state standards for health services, health instruction, and school sanitation. Failure to meet these requirements may place the district in a probationary status for a specified period of time. Failure to meet requirements within this time period may disqualify the district from participation in certain state school aid funds.

Advocates of legislation to ensure health protection and promotion for *every* schoolchild in the state assert that many school boards have very little understanding of school health work. The thinking of board members and administrators is conditioned by the old classical education they received. The practical value of health in the school may not be fully appreciated. State recognition of the importance of health in the school will assure *every* schoolchild of at least a minimum of health promotion and health education.

State education department initiative

Some states seek to achieve the same goal through prescription by the state board of education. The state board sets up standards for school health services, health instruction, and a healthful school environment. Again, those districts failing to meet requirements may be declared substandard and ineligible for certain state financial aid.

In practice, these provisions are not carried out ruthlessly and dictatorially. Great leniency is granted by giving ample time for the development of health programs. Only in those districts in which the school board or administration actually resists the development of an adequate school health program will the ultimate in enforcement be exercised. The important thing is the health of the students, not the state aid or the prerogative of school boards and administrators.

Responsibilities of the local board of education

Sovereignty, or ultimate authority, rests with the people. Except for such authority as the states have granted to the federal government through the federal constitution, the people have vested their authority in the 50 states to be exercised within their own borders. Local government units have only such authority as has been granted to them by the state legislature through specific legislation and accepted practice. Unless otherwise specified or prohibited, local school boards have broad authority to make such provisions for their schools as they deem necessary to discharge their responsibilities to the school-aged children of their district. From common practice, certain authority and responsibility of the school for health promotion have become generally accepted.

1. School health promotion is vested in the board of education. Although in practice the superintendent and his or her professional staff propose the program, such proposal is merely a recommendation to the board. Only as the board approves the plan can the program have official status. The board can make the program as extensive as it sees fit. It can appropriate such funds as it deems necessary for the health program.

2. All phases of the school health program must comply with state laws and their implementing regulations. In practice, the state provisions serve as minimal standards. A board of education properly may set standards or requirements higher than the state provisions, but not lower. If a state statute provides that all students participating in interscholastic athletics must have a health examination before the season in which they are to compete, the local board on its own initiative may also require such an examination of all who participate in intramural sports.

3. A board of education has the authority to require every child to have a health examination before entering school and at such other times as it deems reasonable. Some boards have made provisions for exceptions on religious grounds. Other boards have made no exceptions, contending that a health examination does not constitute medication. The Washington State Supreme Court has upheld this point of view.

4. A school board can require immunization against a particular disease as a condition for admission to school. Here religious rights definitely do enter in, and provisions for exceptions should be made. In the event of an epidemic or threatened epidemic, the board may exclude those children from school whose parents refuse permission for immunization on religious grounds.

5. The school can pass rules governing school attendance. It can extend this authority to include provisions for exclusion and readmission in control of communicable diseases. Although legal isolation and quarantine are functions of the health department, the school can assert control of communicable diseases insofar as this control is part of the school program.

6. A board may require daily inspections for indications of communicable disease.

7. A child may be excused from sex education if the parents of that child object to the instruction on the basis of religious belief.

8. School boards may specify the areas of health instruction, going beyond any requirements of the state but including the state requirements in the program.

BASIC DIVISIONS OF THE HEALTH PROGRAM

In a world that gets progressively more complicated, it is refreshing to find a group, especially an education group, that is striving to simplify its program. Two decades ago the school health program in general use consisted of seven phases or divisions. Repeated reassessment and realignment have sifted down to the following three basic divisions: (1) school health services, (2) health instruction, and (3) healthful school living (Fig. 2-2).

In a well-integrated school health program no pronounced demarcation of the divisions exists. They are interdependent and support and supplement each other. In actual operation the divisions do not exist; they are essentially creations for organizational and administrative convenience. There is *one* school health program with three different aspects.

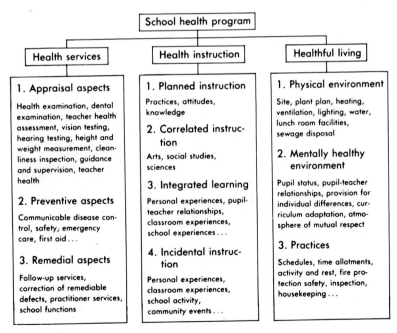

FIG. 2-2. Organization of the school health program. For purposes of planning and administration, three distinct phases of the program are recognized, but in actual function the three phases constitute a cohesive integrated contribution to the total school program.

Whether a particular activity belongs under one aspect or division is primarily academic. How effectively it functions is the significant consideration.

SCHOOL HEALTH SERVICES

School health services constitute those school activities directly concerned with the present health status of the schoolchild. It is only natural that the school should concern itself with the health condition of children because the health of the students and the type of education program in which they participate are interdependent. The children can do their best work only if their health will permit them to participate to the extent that the school program requires. A child with low vitality will have little interest in any school program. A school program in turn must be adapted to the physiologic and emotional health levels as well as the intellectual level of the child. More than this, the program should be designed to develop the highest possible level of physical and emotional health in the child.

School health services can reinforce the efforts of the parents and the family physician in promoting the health and well-being of children. The school setting provides an unusually good vantage point from which to observe and assess the health of children. Teachers and nurses, because of their experience of observing many children, have a ready-made standard against which to compare and evaluate a child's health status and behavior. Those children who deviate from the expected normal range of health status or behavior are readily apparent to teachers and nurses. As Eisner and Callan (1974) have stated:

> The classroom teacher should become the focus of case finding and the child's behavior and functioning should become the primary indicators of his or her health. If this were done, school physicians could devote their time and attention to those children who have been identified as having problems.

School health services of this type can have a profound effect on children's health and their eventual development as healthy and mature adults. The healthy adult whose preadult years were marked by proper supervision of health, growth, and development enjoys a high level of well-being built on a solid foundation of two decades of planned health promotion. An accumulation of 12 years of organized school health services will have a beneficial effect on a person's health for the remaining years of life. The healthy, well-educated student in school becomes the effective and happy adult citizen of the community, freely giving of his or her services and influence to neighbors and the nation.

Scope

The school has a fundamental concern for all aspects of the child's health and well-being. No child should suffer the burdens of illness or defects resulting from conditions that are preventable or correctable. Although the parents have primary responsibility for the health care and supervision of their children, the school cannot ignore the needs of children who are neglected or abused. In fact, when parents fail in these responsibilities, the school must be the child's advocate as well as defender.

Traditionally, school health services have been considered a part of preventive medicine. Emphasis is given to health appraisal activities that identify those conditions or problems interfering with the child's educational progress, and the results of that appraisal are used to inform the parents about their children's health needs. Such programs have operated on the assumption that any treatment needed by the child should be provided by the family physician. Unfortunately, large numbers of children today come from families and homes that do not have or cannot afford the cost of private medical care. Nevertheless, the emphasis on prevention is still the proper role for school health programs in the total health care scheme.

School officials have had a tendency to view their child health responsibilities too narrowly. As a consequence, school health services have, in too many instances, become isolated and unrelated to the community health program. Even though the focus of such services is on preventive activities, it is essential that they be related to and coordinated with other agencies in the community so that comprehensive and continuous health care may be available for children and families.

New patterns of health care have been developing. Title XIX of the Social Security Act is intended to make comprehensive medical services available for those families who are unable to pay for them. This program is popularly known as Medicaid. For services to be effectively used, the interrelationship of school and community health programs must be fully understood so that the necessary cooperation as well as coordination can be achieved (Fig. 2-3).

Appraisal

Complete evaluation of each child's health includes health examinations by a physician, dental examinations, health assessments and observations by the teachers and nurses, screening of vision and hearing by the teachers, weighing and measuring, and inspections of cleanliness.

Health guidance and supervision

In a well-conducted school health program, provision is made for aiding students in directing their own health. This includes all processes necessary to acquaint students with their health status and the sources and channels for developing their health assets. It aims to help the students in their health self-direction. The school supervises the children in caring for their own health. An important part of the health education program includes individual and small group counseling of both students and parents. Such supervision must be planned, be well organized, and have recognized spheres of responsibility.

Recommendations of the Education Commission of the States

One of the most important and authoritative policy statements supporting school health education was issued by an educational task force representing the education commissions of the 50 states. The task force was appointed as a mechanism to study educational policy and to offer recommendations on behalf of the 50 state school offices. The health education task force was charged with conducting a review of current school health practices in order to identify the issues and problems hampering the implementation of effective school health education programs. After these deliberations, a series of recommendations that the task force deemed essential to establish these recommendations called for each state education agency to:

1. Take the lead in encouraging local school boards and administrators to include health education as an integral part of the elementary and secondary school curriculum.

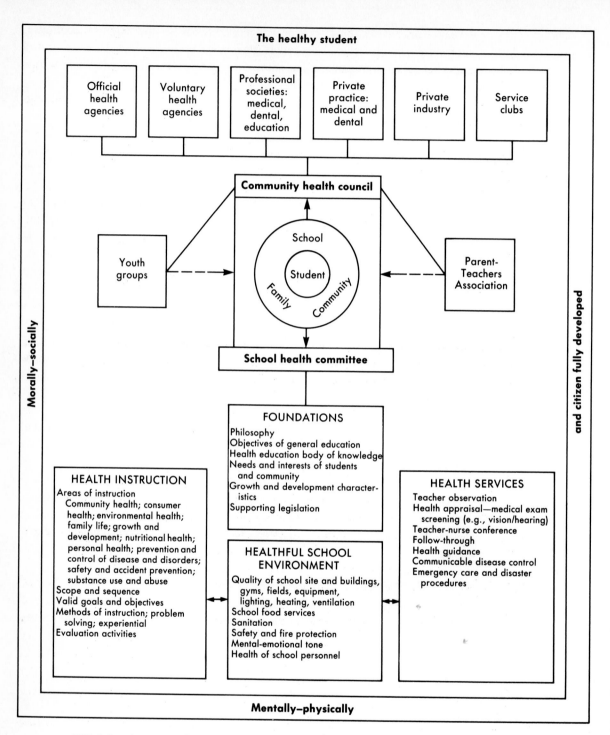

FIG. 2-3. A concept of a comprehensive school health program.
(From Killip, D., and others: J. Sch. Health **57**(10):437, 1987; adapted from Johns, E.B.: World Med. J., no. 5, 1973.)

2. Promote health education as a responsibility shared by the family, school, and community.
3. Support the development and improvement of school health education with whatever resources would be available.
4. Provide technical assistance to local districts in order to facilitate the planning necessary for the implementation of school health education programs and to "promote the development of comprehensive school health education programs."
5. Take the lead in establishing standards of preparation that would assure the availability of qualified teachers in health education.

To make clear the commission's intent the following definitive statements concerning health education and its reference to comprehensive programs were offered. In addition, Fig. 2-3 is presented as a conceptionalized model of the comprehensive school health program illustrating all elements of a total program and its integrated relationships to the school and to the community. It is in this theoretical construct that the comprehensive health education program can make its maximum contribution to the health and educational development of the school child.

Health education

Health education is a process with intellectual, psychologic, and social dimensions relating to activities that increase the abilities of people to make informed decisions affecting their personal, family, and community well-being.[1]

School health education

One component of a comprehensive school health program, school health education is a unified program of learning experiences:

- Planned by both school and community;
- Demonstrating scope, sequence, progression and continuity;
- Planned for grades kindergarten through 12;
- Taught by teachers trained and prepared in health education;
- Designed to develop critical thinking and individual responsibility for one's health;
- Structured to incorporate current and emerging health problems;
- Focused on the dynamic relationship between physical, mental, emotional and social well-being;
- Strengthened by integrating available community resources into classroom teaching.[2]

---

[1]"Report of the 1972-1973 Joint Committee on Health Education Terminology," by representatives of the American Academy of Pediatrics; American Association of Health, Physical Education, and Recreation; American College Health Association; American School Health Association; Public Health Education Section, American Public Health Association; School Health Section, American Public Health Association; Society for Public Health Education. *Health Education Monographs*, no. 33, pp. 65-66, 1973.

[2]Adapted from Northern California Chapter of the American Academy of Pediatrics paper cited in *Physician's Guide to the School Health Curriculum Process*, 1980, American Medical Association.

Prevention

Control of communicable diseases, safety promotion, first aid, and emergency care not only are opportunities for school service but also are responsibilities for doing everything reasonable to prevent unnecessary illness or injury.

Remedial measures

Although the school is not expected to treat or to correct defects, it does have a responsibility to assist the child and family in securing the necessary health care. Whether such services are provided by the private physician or through some community agency will depend on the circumstances of individual students and their families. Effective follow-up depends on school personnel. Health education can play a fundamental role in developing an understanding as to why health care is needed and where the needed service may be located.

HEALTH INSTRUCTION

Formal planned classroom health teaching is designed to prepare students to make the proper decisions throughout their lives on matters affecting their health. The very nature of health allows for a great variety of approaches in instruction.Diverse methods, techniques, and combinations have been effective in health instruction. In the final analysis any program of health instruction must be appraised in terms of the extent to which it modifies persons in their understanding and practice of health principles. Instruction that promotes the development of favorable attitudes and understanding and that results in a pattern of living enabling the individual to attain the highest possible level of health meets the true goal of all health teaching.

Elementary school

During the early years of school life health instruction is directed primarily to the establishment of recognized health practices and the inculcation of desirable health attitudes. Health knowledge may be used as a vehicle for promoting health practices and health attitudes. Elementary schoolchildren will acquire valuable health knowledge that may be associated with pleasant experiences, but health knowledge should always be considered a means to an end — better health. As such, health knowledge should be regarded as secondary to health attitudes and practices in promoting an effective elementary school health instruction program.

Middle school or junior high school

The idealism and group tendencies of junior high school students make an ideal setting for the promotion of community health interests and ideals. Interwoven with the concept of respect for the welfare of one's neighbors are the interrelationships that exist between personal and community health. Practices and attitudes are fortified with further knowledge.

Senior high school

Health attitudes and practices developed in the previous years are fortified by knowledge gained in the high school from a sound scientific basis. Since for many students this will be their last opportunity for formal health instruction, high school health teaching should prepare young people to accept their responsibilities of adulthood to care for and promote their own health and well-being as well as that of their future families and communities. Ideally, the health education experience should serve to sustain the individual's interest through self-directed study of health problems. Developing students' ability to select appropriate sources of health information, health services, and health products is of particular importance in high school health instruction.

HEALTHFUL SCHOOL LIVING

From the beginning of public school education in the United States, communities have shown a special pride in their new up-to-date school buildings. The school building denoted a monument to the culture of the community and the people's concern for their children. With this concept was the implication that the school environment consisted of the physical plant and that a costly building constituted an ideal environment for learning. However, physical structures per se are static concepts.

The present-day dynamic concept of the environmental factors in the school is well expressed in the designation *healthful school living*. It denotes a social situation in which children develop their potentialities in effective and enjoyable living. Children's educational, emotional, and physical development will have the stimulation and motivation essential to their fullest attainment. It is expressed in the atmosphere of the classroom, the corridors, the gymnasium, the playground, and every other place about the school. It incorporates factors that affect the physical, mental, and social health of the child. In so doing, it includes the physical plant, its equipment, the personnel, and the practices within the school.

If an atmosphere of wholesome living is to be created, all plans and activities must be focused on the child's need for wholesome development. The physical, esthetic, cultural, moral, emotional, social, and all other aspects of the experiences and needs of the child must be met by the school. It properly should create in every child a pride in being a part of the school.

The physical plant with its site, proper living conditions, ideal sanitary equipment, and general attractiveness represents a first essential in healthful school living. How the teaching staff uses and incorporates these assets into the life of the student will determine whether the school is truly a place of healthful living. To have a lunchroom with adequate space and sanitary equipment is not enough. The practices in the lunchroom and the general atmosphere are equally important. Children need guidance in learning to appreciate and live fully in even the most ideal physical environment. Out of this appreciation should evolve the social values so important to the present and future citizen.

When the physical plant is not of an acceptable standard, the intrepid teacher can instill in the children a desire to better the conditions under which they are learning. Even to appreciate what is and what is not commendable in the school is an achievement in personal growth. Out of these experiences can come improvements in school, home, and community.

After all, people are the most important elements in the school environment. The quality of these people can be noted in their values, attitudes, activities, and attainment. Healthful school living is an important aspect of the quality of life.

Responsibility for environmental health

Parents, school board members, architects, administrators, teachers, custodians, lunchroom personnel, and students are responsible for the environment of the school. United responsibility combined with collective effort produces the environmental conditions conducive to the atmosphere necessary for healthful school living.

Factors influencing environmental health

The attitude of the school community constitutes the all-important background for environmental health. First, those concepts that the parents hold as standards and put into effect by their own contribution and interest establish the pattern or mold for a healthful school environment. Through the board of education, this attitude will project itself into attractive, functional school buildings that are safe, efficient, sanitary, and commodious. It will lay the groundwork for an effective school program that will assure the children of an opportunity to develop their potentialities. This community support makes it possible for the school staff to create an atmosphere in which children can live effectively and enjoyably.

A second factor is a well-planned, well-constructed sanitary school plant. This implies a suitable site, functional architecture, adequate heating, ventilation, and lighting, safe water supply, approved disposal facilities, and essential accessory school equipment.

A third factor incorporates the practices of the school. From custodial housekeeping to lunchroom decorum, to group courtesy, to opportunities for self-status, many practices contribute vitally to healthful school living. Capable teachers can use fully the available facilities and opportunities to create a mentally and physically healthy environment.

Healthful school living can be reduced to a rather simple equation:

$$\frac{\text{Functional}}{\text{school plant}} + \frac{\text{Wholesome}}{\text{practices}} = \frac{\text{Healthful}}{\text{school living}}$$

Public health's relationship to school health

The titles of the six operating agencies of the U.S. Public Health Service (Fig. 2-1) illustrate the types of program activities that relate directly to the school health program. For example, the Alcohol, Drug Abuse, and Mental Health Administration provides scientific information as well as support and expert guidance to schools on alcohol and drug education and ways of handling problems stemming from the misuse of these substances. Also, the knowledge gained from the scientific study of disease prevention is ultimately translated into policies and program practices at the local health department level including the school health program.

The Health Services Administration has a great impact on schools through a variety of health care programs. The most visible programs are the Maternal and Child Health Act and Early Periodic Screening, Diagnosis and Treatment (EPSDT). Both of these programs provide health care services to children and youth of low-income families. These programs work in close coordination with the Education for all Handicapped Children Act, PL 94-142. This law recognizes the rights of all handicapped children and their need for special services. All these children, 3 to 21 years of age, are to receive "a free and appropriate education." Examples of the kinds of health services activities provided through these programs include comprehensive health assessments, immunizations, physical examinations, vision and hearing screening, laboratory tests such as those to detect the presence of lead in children's blood, diagnostic evaluation, and treatment and rehabilitation services for children who suffer from handicapping or chronic conditions. Other examples of services include physical, speech, and occupational therapy and the provision of dental care. New areas of service that are now receiving special attention are programs of adolescent health, child abuse, and mental health services including outpatient therapy.

Despite the problems faced by these programs, including a lack of resources and the difficulties of achieving effective coordination among various programs, a report (Better Health for Our Children, 1981) to Congress has cited significant accomplishment. A panel of experts has pointed to important progress in the effort to reduce disabilities of handicapped children. Medicaid and EPSDT programs have made health care available to more children. There has been a substantial increase in the availability of mental health services.

Because the need for health care is great and the ability to provide it where most needed is difficult at best, the weaknesses or shortcomings of these programs are often overemphasized. Nevertheless, these programs demonstrate effective participation in the provision of health services at all levels of government: federal, state, and local. Because schoolchildren and youth are the intended beneficiaries of many of these services, school officials should become informed about them to ensure that children receive needed services. The health of children is integrally linked to their success in school. Enhancing the health of children makes it possible for them to gain the fullest measure of benefit from their educational experience.

INTEGRATING HEALTH SERVICES AND HEALTH INSTRUCTION

Although it has been shown that both the education and the health of the public are legal responsibilities of the state, as specifically defined by the federal constitution, this does not guarantee adequate or equal development of both program areas. In fact, quite the opposite may be the case. Some communities may have a well-developed educational program with little in the way of school health services, whereas other school systems may have a strong health service program and an almost nonexistent health instruction program. In addition, some schools may have strong programs in both health services and health instruction, but these programs may operate independently and in isolation from each other.

Newman (1982) has spoken out forcefully against this separation of health services and education. He has reminded school officials that the justification for health services in schools rests on the assumption that such services contribute to the school's educational goal. Therefore, if health activities in the school are to be an educational experience, it is essential that health services and health education be integrated.

Such integration benefits the school in several distinct ways. Those in the health services can aid the educator by creating the best atmosphere for learning for both the student and the school as a whole. By identifying health problems or conditions that handicap the child's ability to learn, such as visual or auditory deficiencies, the health services staff promotes the health and learning potential of the child. By maintaining immunization levels that prevent or reduce school absenteeism, the health services program assists the goals of the educator.

The assistance of the health services staff may increase the effectiveness of teachers. The support and consultation of the health services staff can often help to identify the causes of student behaviors that disrupt the teaching-learning process. For instance, many student behavior problems stem from emotional difficulties that may require the assistance of a health professional to identify and treat.

Furthermore, the coordination of health services with health instruction makes a direct contribution to the students' health knowledge as well as health practices. When the health educator and the school nurse work with the school dietitian to improve student eating habits, the school lunch program becomes more than a food service; it becomes a laboratory for learning.

To help school officials achieve this objective, Newman has offered the following six guiding principles in the planning for integration of health services and health education.

1. *The means for integrating health services and health education should be clearly identified and stated as a set of program objectives.* There is also the need to inform the public or the community about these objectives. The reasons for health services in the school, the objectives, and program activities should be thoroughly understood. Moreover, if the program is to be effective, many different people should be involved.

2. *The program objectives should reflect the various interests of the community.* If these two programs are to be integrated, school administrators, teachers, students, parents, and health professionals should be involved.

By reducing absenteeism, by decreasing discipline problems, by improving teacher morale, and by improving the school's relationships with parents and the community at large, integrated health programs, when properly coordinated, can improve the school. To convince administrators of the importance of an integrated program, they need the opportunity to observe the benefits that result from the coordinated efforts of health and education personnel.

All too often teachers have only a superficial understanding of the health program and its impact on the school. How many teachers consider the state of the student's health as a possible contributing cause of classroom disruptive behavior or as a cause of learning problems? There is a failure, also, to appreciate the important relationship between the health of the teacher and that person's role as an educator. The problem of teacher burnout illustrates this point. Teachers who do not appreciate the importance of their own health can hardly be expected to be sensitive to the health of their students.

Parents and students both need to understand the role of school health in order to complement the efforts of the school in promoting the student's health. The role of parents and students is central to any follow-up efforts to ensure the students' optimal growth and development.

Medical and health professionals must understand the services and educational aspects of the school health program. A mutual support and trust between the school's and the health professionals' programs will strengthen the entire effort. To achieve this integration, all of the constituent groups must understand (1) the need for health education, (2) the importance of health services, and (3) how these programs can be mutually supportive.

3. *Knowing how young people use the school health services provides yet another basis for the integration of health services and health education.* Typically, more data are available at the

national level concerning the health problems of children than about the health problems of students in the schools. In this regard, Newman has reported on the recent study of school-children's use of school health services in which he was able to document the rate at which students use the nurse's office. One interesting observation reveals that there is a seasonal pattern to the use of health services, with headaches and gastrointestinal complaints most often occurring during the cold months and wounds, trauma, and skin problems occurring most frequently during the warm months. Conclusions drawn from these observations indicate, too, that many of the health service visits were unnecessary, at least from a medical perspective. Even at this early age, it appears that children have learned to play the "sick role" and use illness as a reason for visiting the nurse's office to avoid some other school activity. In this case the solution to an apparent health problem was found in the way classroom activities were being conducted. With the high cost of health care, misuse of health services is an important problem. Students, even at the elementary school level, can be taught the appropriate use of health care services.

Knowing that headaches and stomach problems occur more often in winter months and wounds and trauma are more likely to occur in the spring and fall provides an opportunity to structure the health education curriculum to address these trends so that students can anticipate and better manage these health problems. The important conclusion from this discussion is that school health service records, if carefully maintained and regularly analyzed, can serve as a useful basis for the development of a program of instruction.

4. *The integration of services in education will depend to a great degree on the quality of persons employed.* Unfortunately, not all schools will hire school nurse practitioners nor will they hire fully qualified health education teachers. In the best situation the school would have a staff of trained health teachers and trained school nurse practitioners. Anything less might compromise the quality of the program. However, despite limitations in the training of various personnel, nurses and teachers with appropriate administrative support can be encouraged and assisted to work together to develop good programs. If resources are lacking, obviously the scope of the program must also be reduced. It is still fundamentally important, however, to capitalize on the available staff resources and, in the most vital subjects, to maintain standards commensurate with those in better-staffed schools.

5. *The basis for integrating health personnel and education personnel is the clear delineation of responsibilities.* The integration of education and health personnel does not mean that each must learn the other's job. It should be evident that health professionals can best conduct health service programs and education professionals can best conduct the instructional program. The understanding and acceptance of this point are important to avoid confusing roles and unhappiness with responsibilities that may develop among staff members. Experience has shown that interdisciplinary programs do work when people are well trained and are confident in their roles and committed to the objectives of the program.

6. *To strike the best balance between services and education, clear data on program outcomes should be developed.* A search of the literature reveals a lack of scientific research on school health services and health education. In other words, there is a lack of scientific basis for school health services and little objective information available on the practice of school health services and the behavior of students who are using school-based services. Even less information is available on the problems and the benefits involved in the coordination of the

education and health service programs. If this information on the coordinated program and its outcomes is not made available to administrators, school boards, and the public, it will be all the more difficult to solicit their support for program development.

School-based clinics

School-based clinics are a rapidly developing trend that are designed to meet the special health care needs of the adolescent. Although teenagers have the usual health care needs of others, they also have special problems stemming from the physical and emotional changes they are undergoing. Over one fifth of the children under 17 years of age come from homes of the poor; however, less than one half of these poor or near-poor children were covered by Medicaid. Hence the economic factor is a serious obstacle to obtaining adequate health care for many adolescents. Contrary to popular belief that the adolescent age group is one of the healthiest in our society, in reality adolescents are one of the most medically underserved groups. The American Medical Association pointed out that until recently the age group 15 to 24 years was the only U.S. age group where the death rate actually increased over what it was 20 years ago.

As of 1987 there were 101 school-based clinics, representing a growth of over 200% since 1985. The principal objectives of school-based clinics as expressed in both state and federal legislative initiatives is to provide health care for the adolescent in or near the school site where such a site is most accessible to the student. There is a compelling interest to intervene in the adolescent health problems that are having especially adverse educational and social consequences causing an increase in the drop-out rate and a rise in adolescent dependency on public assistance.

The increase in the number of school-based clinics and the results of several national polls show strong support for the school-based clinics. Nationally, Congress has moved to amend the Public Health Service Aid by adding a new title, "School-based Adolescent Health Amendments." In addition to providing the usual health care services, this new amendment emphasizes health education and preventive services including prenatal care, mental health, family planning service, and screening and follow-up care for sexually transmitted diseases. The location of the clinics at or near the school makes them ideally suited for student counseling and follow-up observation over an extended period of time. Typically the program provides students with information and resources for avoiding unwanted pregnancy. The clinic staff often serve important educational functions by making presentations in health education classes and working closely with teachers to establish well-integrated sexuality education counseling and instructional programs. The clinic maintains student confidentiality while encouraging students to interact with parents and other adults. These clinics offer a truly comprehensive range of services relating to the physical and emotional well-being of adolescents.

SUMMARY

The school health program is presented as a formal entity and responsibility of two primary governmental agencies of the state — public health and public education.

The context of the school health program is examined in relationship to the larger picture of public health. School health is an aspect of the health and educational functions revealed in health organizations at all levels of government ranging from the local health department to the state national and international health organization.

Public health, as an arm of government concerned with school health, gained much of its momentum in the early days after passage of state and federal laws requiring compulsory attendance in the public or common schools. This influx of children into the public schools was soon followed with a series of communicable disease outbreaks, which called for a major public health effort to control epidemics such as smallpox. Large cities like New York, Boston, Philadelphia, and Chicago employed physicians and nurses to serve as medical visitors to examine children who were believed to be ill. Although the communicable disease threat has lessened, except for the problem of AIDS and sexually transmitted diseases, the control and prevention of the major chronic diseases are now receiving much attention. Because each of these agencies, health and education, has a legal responsibility for school health, the program often is administered under a variety of organizational patterns with some programs being jointly administered by education and health officials. Under such a divided authority pattern the school health services are administered by the local health department, and the school health instruction part of the program is administered by the school administration in charge of curriculum. In still other instances, the total program is under the direction of school district employees some of who may be physicians and nurses hired by the school district.

However, despite the fact that they may be fully qualified health specialists, they are technically and legally under the authority of the health department for all school health services relating to public health laws.

Regardless of the type of administrative organization, both of these official educational and health agencies have responsibilities that must be recognized. Carrying out these functions and the day-to-day activities calls for special administrative skills and knowledge of the interrelationships that exist. An inherent difficulty is the tendency to conduct the health instruction program as though it were separate and unrelated to the health services or, on the other hand, to conduct a health service activity like screening for visual defects without considering its implications for health education.

To avoid this pitfall special importance is given to an integrated approach for administrating health services and health instruction. Six guiding principles are offered to all school officials to achieve the goal of an integrated program.

A new development, the school-based clinic, is discussed as an example of a community's response to the special health needs of the adolescent. The success of such clinics is the planned coordination and integration of health services, follow-up student counseling, and health education of the adolescent.

John's conceptual model of the comprehensive school health program and its multifaceted interrelationship with the home, the school, and the community is a visualization of the goal to be achieved.

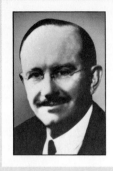

Clair Elsmere Turner

BORN   April 28, 1890, Harmony, Maine
DIED   November 27, 1974, Cambridge, Massachusetts
EDUCATION   A.B., Bates College, 1912; A.M., Harvard
University, 1913; Dr.P.H., Massachusetts
Institute of Technology, 1928; M.Ed., Boston
University, 1944; M.P.H., Harvard School of Public Health, 1948

Dr. Turner was a faculty member for 30 years at the Massachusetts Institute of Technology and later held a visiting professorship at the University of California. Because of his long tenure, his writing, and his extensive involvement in international work, he was one of the world's best-known personalities in health education. Among his international appointments was that of chief of health education for the World Health Organization and expert consultant to the United Nations Educational, Scientific, and Cultural Organization.

Dr. Turner gained early prominence for his research work as director of the Malden, Massachusetts, School Health Study, 1921 to 1931. This was one of the first major school educational studies to investigate the effects of a carefully developed school health education program. Findings from this study were used to examine the relationships of curriculum and textbook materials to the outcomes of student health knowledge, attitudes, and practices and the relationship of school health education to the growth patterns of children.

As a result of the reputation Dr. Turner gained from the Malden studies, he was invited to serve as a consultant and advisor to many school health education curriculum planning committees. He gave important leadership to school health education development in Cleveland, to the states of Illinois and Kansas, and to many national and international groups.

In addition to his work in school health, Dr. Turner played a key leadership role in professional societies. He was one of the first to serve as chair of the American Public Health Association's Committee on the Educational Qualifications of Community Health Educators. The work of this committee was important to the development of standards and the recognition of health education as a field of professional specialization. His leadership ability was acknowledged by his election as the first president of the Society for Public Health Education and through his election to the presidency of the American School Health Association.

STUDY QUESTIONS

1. What are the merits and demerits in the American system that places responsibility for public school education in a local board of education?
2. Compare the practice of having the state legislature set up standards for school health programs with that of having the state education department prescribe what the school health programs shall be.
3. Courts have held that, when a school requires that a child be immunized, the child's parents can object on religious grounds, but requiring a health examination is not an infringement on the child's religious rights. How do you explain the possible paradox?
4. Why should the school be concerned with the present health status of a child?
5. Which activities in the school health program are preventive measures?
6. Compare the relative merits of having a public health nurse serve the school and having a school nurse hired by the school district.
7. From an administrative and organizational perspective, explain why it is highly desirable for school officials to create a school health advisory council. Which groups or agencies should be represented on the council?
8. From a legal perspective, where does the ultimate authority rest for protecting and promoting the health of school-children?
9. Identify the three major areas of the school health program and explain the principal program activities in each of these areas.
10. Explain the apparent inconsistency of legislation that mandates certain health services and health instruction standards despite the fact that extensive authority and responsibility have been delegated to the local school board.
11. What are school-based clinics and what purposes do they serve?
12. Which programs at the federal level have a direct involvement in school health affairs?
13. What are some of the changes that are occurring in American society that are affecting public health today?
14. What is the basis for the statement that "children are learning to play the 'sick' role"?
15. Which steps can be taken to bring about a more effective integration of school health instruction with health services?

REFERENCES

American Academy of Pediatrics: School health: a guide for health professionals, Elk Grove Village, Ill., 1987, the Academy.

Better health for our children: a national strategy. The report of the Select Panel For the Promotion of Child Health to the United States Congress and the Secretary of Health and Human Services, DHHS (PHS) Pub. No. 79-55071. Washington, D.C., 1981.

Education Commission of the States: *Recommendation for school health education: a handbook for state policymakers,* Report no. 130, Denver, 1981, The Commission.

Eisner, V., and Callan, L.B.: Dimensions of school health, Springfield, Ill., 1974, Charles C Thomas, Publisher.

EPSDT: does it spell health care for poor children? A report by the Children's Defense Fund of the Washington Research Project, Inc., Washington, D.C., 1977, Children's Defense Fund.

Grant, M.: Handbook of community health, ed. 3, Philadelphia, 1981, Lea & Febiger.

Kirby, D., et al.: School-based health clinics: an emerging approach to improving adolescent health and addressing teenage pregnancy, Washington, D.C., 1985, Center for Population Options.

Lovick, S.R., The school-based clinic: update 1987, Washington, D.C., 1987, Center for Population Options.

Miller, D.F.: School health programs: their basis in law, New York, 1972, A.S. Barnes & Co., Inc.

Nader, P.R., et al.: Options for school health meeting community needs, Germantown, Md., 1978, Aspen Systems Corp.

Newman, I.M.: Integrating health services and health education: seeking a balance, J. Sch. Health **52**(8):498, 1982.

Preventive Medicine, U.S.A.: Theory, practices and application of prevention in personal health services: quality control and evaluation of preventive health services. Task force reports sponsored by The John E. Fogarty International Center for Advanced Study in the Health Sciences, National Institutes of Health, and the American College of Preventive Medicine, New York, 1976, Prodist, Division of Neale Watson Academic Publications, Inc.

School-based clinic policy initiatives around the country: 1986, Washington, D.C., 1986, Center for Population Options.

Wallace, H.M., et al.: Maternal and child health practices: problems, resources, and methods of delivery, ed. 2, New York, 1982, John Wiley & Sons, Inc.

3 Health and the Normal Child

OVERVIEW *Health no longer means only the absence of disease. Today's concept of health implies adaptability and incorporates the notion of reaching an optimal level of health that differs for each person. Teachers and school personnel need to understand that health implies normality but that all deviations from normal do not necessarily mean an absence of health or the presence of disease.*

Health results from the interaction of a person and the environment, which means that those interested in health must be sensitive to both personal and environmental concerns. History clearly shows that the greatest gains in health improvement result as much from changes in the environment as from changes in the quality of health care.

OBJECTIVES After reading this chapter, the student should be able to:

1. Describe and illustrate how a full understanding of the concept of normal will affect a teacher's approach to teaching and a school administrator's approach to facilitating the educational process
2. Describe health as a process of adaptation
3. Illustrate the differences between primary, secondary, and tertiary prevention and explain why these concepts are useful to school health personnel
4. Explain how the epidemiologic model of agent, host, and environment provides a useful framework for developing school health programs
5. Describe the basic characteristics of a healthy child in terms of physical and mental health

For teachers who dedicate their lives to student welfare and improvement, understanding the concept of health and translating its meaning into terms relevant to students is important for several reasons. First, increasing students' educational levels, more than any other social variable including increasing wealth, will increase the likelihood of better health and longevity. Second, teachers must be informed about their students' health and understand their students' growth and development in order to assist students with the rigors of growing up. Third, teachers present to their students a model in their own behavior and appearance; teachers must appreciate and maintain their own health at an optimal level. And fourth, because we lose our entire effort and investment in education if a person dies prematurely or greatly decrease the investment if a person is disabled or frequently ill, it is important to help students protect their own health. Health, indeed, has not only personal value but also economic value to the entire society.

Although it is not necessary that all teachers have a high level of health expertise, all teachers should know something about health, and some teachers in key positions must have considerable health knowledge. In addition, a comprehensive health planning group is recommended for each school district. Such a group could involve health teachers, nurses, parents, and students. These people should be expected to identify health problems and recommend solutions.

To be a competent health educator, the teacher does not need to be an expert. Experience indicates that certain basic knowledge is adequate for the position the teacher rightfully holds on the health team. Primarily, that knowledge includes an understanding of normal growth and development, normal health status, and common deviations from the normal. A study of deviations does not imply that the educator is to be a diagnostician, but rather a "suspectitian." The teacher may be in the best position to recognize first that a child does not appear to be normal in some respect.

Professional preparation should develop in the teacher an attitude toward health that focuses attention on the child and proceeds to identify existing health problems. Just as the lawyer must develop a certain frame of mind and approach to problems of law, the health educator must develop an approach to problems of health founded on an understanding and appreciation of the individual child's health.

THE CONCEPT OF NORMAL

Health is not a single static state. Neither is the concept of normal a single point on a scale. Teachers see a wide range of students and therefore will be expected to judge individuals' health from many perspectives.

"Normal" is that which we accept as the usual. It must be understood as encompassing a range of concepts rather than a single entity. "Normal" includes the average but extends considerably on both sides of average. No two persons are exactly alike; each is unique. A person may be clearly normal on a series of measures and abnormal by one measure, but the total outcome may still be healthy. A very short person, for example, may not be anything but healthy when viewed in total.

The range of normal can be illustrated by a statistically normal curve. In any group of persons, measures of health will tend to cluster around the average. The farther persons or measures of health move from the average, the more they will be outside the range of normal.

However, as Fig. 3-1 shows, the number of people who deviate greatly from normal declines as deviation increases. By definition, deviations are uncommon and therefore abnormal.

What constitutes the normal, or usual, is easy to determine in some instances but extremely difficult to ascertain in others. To say with assurance that the normal range of glucose in human blood is between 0.08 and 0.14 mg/100 ml is easy because in more than 96% of analyzed blood samples the glucose content falls in this range. Many physiologic norms are well established; yet the normal range for certain physical measurements is not so easily set down. For example, what is the normal range of height for American women? Should one arbitrarily say it is between 5 feet, 2 inches and 5 feet, 7 inches? What of the woman who is 6 feet, 1 inch in height? Should she be considered abnormal? According to Fig. 3-1 and its accompanying discussion, she should indeed. Deviations such as 6 feet, 1 inch are uncommon and therefore abnormal. Whether that woman is healthy is another matter.

If normal for physical factors is a precise quantity, consider how variable it can be when applied to social and psychologic phenomena. What is the normal range of emotional responses for junior high school boys frustrated by losing election to an office or to a group? Standards of normal social acceptance vary from community to community, from school to school, and from family to family. Yet determining what is normal usually does not pose too difficult a problem for the sensitive teacher.

In actual school practice most cases fall definitely in the normal range, whether physical, psychologic, or social. In the relatively few borderline instances the decision of an expert of the collective judgment of several competent teachers can usually serve the needs of the particular case. Even more important, many deviations from the normal are of little significance in terms of effective and enjoyable living. Every human being has imperfections, most of which go unnoticed or are accepted by this imperfect world of imperfect people. To be abnormal in some respects, perhaps, is normal.

THE CONCEPT OF HEALTH

"Health" is a word that is used frequently but it is difficult to define. The World Health Organization states that health is the "state of complete physical, mental, and social well-being and not merely the absence of disease." Health, in other words, represents a com-

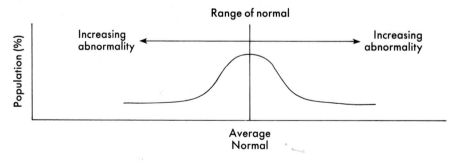

FIG. 3-1. The range of normal is a function of the tendency to cluster around the average. Average dictates normal, but deviation from the average (abnormality) does not necessarily imply anything in terms of health.

pleteness that goes beyond the simple absence of illness. The word *health* implies physical, mental, and social well–being, yet society tends to measure health in disease-oriented terms. If a physician cannot find anything wrong with the patient, the patient is likely to be declared "healthy." If a country has fewer deaths, a longer life span, and a lower incidence of disease, that country is considered to have a healthier population than one with a higher death rate, a higher incidence of disease, and a shorter life span. In other words, health is frequently measured against the quality and quantity of disease and not the quality or quantity of life.

The simplest way to think of health is as the absence of disease, but a person can experience many levels of health without exhibiting clinical signs of illness. Look at the structure of the word *disease:* dis-ease. Disease implies that for one reason or another a person is not "at ease." Disease, in this sense, may not necessarily represent a clinical illness such as what a physician would diagnose, but it may represent a departure from the ideal, or optimal, health. On any given day a person will experience varying degrees of "dis-ease" without actually being ill.

A person's optimal level of performance is limited only by genetic inheritance. Optimal health therefore does not mean that a person is simply stronger or taller or faster than others but that the person operates at a level close to his or her personal potential. All persons have a potential to achieve their optimum even after serious illness or injury greatly changes the dimensions of that goal. For example, an athlete may be seen as a "picture of health." An automobile accident may injure that same athlete so that she cannot walk. To the extent that the athlete adjusts to an injury, accepts a new level of optimal health, and works to improve herself within the new limitations, she could be described as healthy. The trauma of the accident greatly reduced certain potentials and caused enormous "dis-ease," but the potential to reestablish health exists. At some point, recovery will be complete, and physicians will no longer be able to find actual clinical illness—only a reduction in certain functions.

Remember also that health encompasses more than just physical dimensions. It is possible for an athlete, for example, to allow training to so affect her life and her behavior as to cause significant "dis-ease" and actual illness. In this case a person appearing physically healthy may actually be experiencing mental illness.

Health as ability to adapt

Health is a particularly delicate condition affected by tangible forces such as trauma, bacteria, and viruses and by less tangible forces such as stress and grief. Students are well aware that they can feel "dis-eased" before examinations and especially well (at ease) on receiving an "A" grade. Sudden fright can change the body temperature and the body metabolism in such a way as to represent disease. How well a person responds to changes, how well he or she adjusts, represents the state of health. Health, in other words, depends on an ability to adapt: to adapt to trauma, to pathogens of various types, to social stresses, to emotional crises, to varied foods, to different temperatures, and to all the forces in the world. To the extent that persons cannot adapt to these changes they are not "at ease"; they are "diseased." These varied levels of health and disease are shown in Fig. 3-2.

Fig. 3-2 illustrates a continuum of health that ranges from optimal to death. At the higher levels of health this continuum identifies mild discomforts, minor traumas, muscle

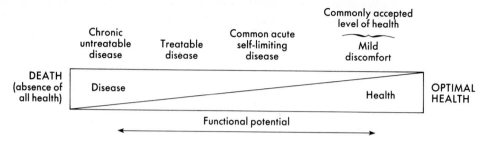

FIG. 3-2. A person's state of health is constantly varying in degree ranging from optimal health through varying degrees of disease to death — the total absence of health. At any given time, a person's health represents his or her ability to adapt to varying degrees of stress and pathoses.

soreness from overexertion, and common acute self-limiting diseases such as the common cold. In a general sense these conditions are accepted as normal; and persons do not think of themselves as diseased when they experience them. When a condition becomes serious enough to require medication, some type of remedial action, or diagnostic assistance from a physician, persons might recognize that they are not well but might not yet acknowledge that they are diseased. There is a clear indication, however, that functional potential has been reduced and that whatever is done to overcome these conditions will move a person back up the continuum of health toward the optimal level. Diseases that are chronic can seriously jeopardize function and are represented on the lower levels on this continuum. When these conditions continue and functional potential decreases, death results. It is important to note that a position on this continuum is not necessarily dictated by age. As persons get older, they tend to have more diseases and their ability to adapt declines, but increasing proportions of older people maintain high levels of health. Age alone does not imply disease. Age does affect the nature of one's optimal potential, but it is still possible to maintain optimal health.

The teacher's challenge is to help young people develop skills to facilitate their adaptation to a variety of stresses and to provide them with sufficient knowledge to deal with specific health-threatening situations. This should include knowledge to seek appropriate diagnosis and treatment to gain complete recovery from illness when it does strike. It also means helping young people avoid situations that will threaten health and make knowledgeable decisions that facilitate adaptation. One significant part of health education is to help young people accept their potentials and their limitations: their own range of normal. Recognizing strengths and weaknesses, playing to strengths, working to strengthen weaknesses, and developing a feeling of self-confidence are basic to both physical and mental health. In other words, the well-adjusted child with a good range of basic skills has the greatest potential for good health.

Most persons are born healthy and lose their health to disease through actions they or others take. There was a time when disease (i.e., infectious disease) could reach almost anyone. Today, however, with infectious diseases largely controlled in North America and most of Europe, diseases are largely self-inflicted or inflicted by the behaviors of others.

Heart disease, for example, is caused by five major risk factors: diet, exercise patterns, heredity, cigarette smoking, and stress. Only heredity is beyond a person's behavioral control. Cancer presents a similar picture, as do accidents, stroke, and suicide. Cancer also represents a good example of how the conscious or accidental behavior of others affects health. The release of a carcinogen into the environment, either intentionally or accidentally, contributes to cancer.

Because most persons are born healthy, the challenge is to protect that health and to prevent the onset of disease. Public health workers over the years have conceptualized several ways of thinking about prevention and how persons can increase their chances of preventing disease. Teachers generally deal with healthy populations and so an understanding of prevention is useful to envisage how education can contribute to the maintenance of health.

THE CONCEPT OF PREVENTION

Public health workers describe prevention as having three levels: *primary, secondary,* and *tertiary.* Primary prevention focuses on the environment and how the environment facilitates or prevents the spread of disease; secondary prevention focuses on individuals and how they react to the onset of disease; tertiary prevention relates to the complete process of rehabilitation so that the chances of reinfection or recurrence are minimized. Fig. 3-3 describes these levels.

Primary prevention

Primary prevention is best illustrated by considering diseases that were once common and are now relatively rare. For example, as recently as 100 years ago conditions such as malaria,

Primary prevention	Precedes the earliest signs of a disease and involves changes in the physical or social environment to reduce the likelihood that the disease can or will occur
Secondary prevention	Identifies diseases at their earliest stages and initiates appropriate treatment to limit the course and consequences of the disease
Tertiary prevention	Maintains appropriate treatment through its full course to complete rehabilitation and returns a person to optimal health, thereby minimizing the likelihood of recurrence

FIG. 3-3.   Three levels of prevention. Primary prevention attempts to prevent conditions from occurring. Secondary prevention and tertiary prevention attempt to prevent unnecessary development of health problems once they have been detected.

scarlet fever, tuberculosis, and diphtheria were commonplace in North America. These diseases are no longer prevalent, but simply identifying and treating people with these diseases could not account for their almost total elimination. Mortality from tuberculosis infections in England and Wales declined from almost 4000 cases per million population in 1838 to 2000 cases per million population in 1880. This decline was in advance of any modern treatment techniques and actually predated the identification of the tubercle bacillus in 1882. After the identification of the tubercle bacillus the incidence of the disease continued to decline. By 1944, when an effective chemotherapy was developed (*para*-aminosalicylic acid), the rate was down to about 500 cases per million population. Shortly thereafter, an even more effective treatment, isoniazid, was perfected.

Why did the incidence of tuberculosis decline so greatly before the introduction of effective treatment? The primary reason can be traced to major changes in the environment that occurred at the time. Noticeable improvements in housing, management of water and sewage, production and marketing of milk, quality and availability of food, and the work environment, took place in midcentury. From today's perspective it is hard to judge the years of the Industrial Revolution as a time of great improvement in living conditions, but in relative terms they were. In short, the decline in tuberculosis can be attributed mainly to improvements in the environment and not to increased capabilities for treating disease.

This same lesson is true for most of the other infectious diseases that are no longer present. Even something as common as dental caries is prevented only by changes in the environment. Careful attention to the care of teeth helps reduce dental caries, and frequent visits to a dentist leads to the early detection and treatment of caries and other dental problems. However, the introduction of fluoridated water contributed more to the decline of dental caries than any other measure. Primary prevention, in other words, means changes in the environment that reduce the likelihood of the condition's initial occurrence.

How does immunization contribute to the control of infectious diseases? Immunizations, particularly effective in reducing several infectious diseases, are an aspect of primary prevention. The immunizing agent changes the environment in which the disease occurs, namely, the body. The injected substance in the immunization process triggers a response that changes the body's environment so that the disease cannot occur. Even if the causative agent enters the body, the body's environment will not sustain it. Immunization is an excellent example of primary prevention, that is, a change in the environment.

The examples just cited are mostly of infectious diseases. Today, however, there are many diseases that are not infectious and can be attributed to life-style. Cancer, heart disease, strokes, accidents, suicide, homicide, and drug abuse are all problems of the modern age. These result to a large degree from decisions relating to behavior; the question arises of how primary prevention can apply. The answer is simple. Whereas tuberculosis and similar infectious diseases were related to the physical environment, the conditions of today, such as heart disease, are largely attributed to the social environment. Changing social attitudes toward behaviors such as eating, exercise, overindulgence in alcohol, and tobacco use will ultimately change the incidence of diseases to which these behaviors contribute.

Primary prevention relates to those actions that change the environment, physical and social, to reduce the likelihood that disease will occur or will be transmitted to another person.

Secondary prevention

Secondary prevention is the common practice of the majority of people. Secondary prevention indicates early detection and treatment. Most persons are more conscious of secondary prevention than primary prevention. When a person aches or feels ill or believes he or she has the early signs of disease, that person either initiates some type of treatment or seeks an expert opinion from a health professional to identify the disease and set a course of treatment. Early detection and treatment are effective ways to reduce the course and the cost of a disease. However, early detection, or secondary prevention, differs from primary prevention. Secondary prevention means the condition has occurred, has been detected, and will now likely be limited by effective treatment. The modern world has focused the majority of its health care efforts on early detection and treatment rather than on primary prevention.

Tertiary prevention

Assuming that early detection is carried out and treatment initiated, tertiary prevention implies the complete course of treatment through rehabilitation. A person who breaks off treatment before full recovery increases the chance of a relapse. Rehabilitation then is prevention, in this case the third level — tertiary prevention.

Prevention and the school health program

Health is a dynamic state, and these three levels of prevention (Fig. 3-3) offer three levels of opportunities to deal with the maintenance of health or the management of disease.

The school health program is most effective at the first two levels. The school's responsibility is to provide an environment conducive to health and to reduce the risks of disease, including accidents. The school's educational program is responsible for teaching knowledge and skills so that individuals can relate responsibly to their environment and, along with others, work to establish an environment that is conducive to health. This may involve knowledge about such things as air pollution; it may also involve knowledge to take political action to get air pollution levels changed. This may mean helping students gain the social skills to be able to say no in a social environment that encourages the use and abuse of substances or behaviors that increase the risk of disease. Schools should also help students develop sensitivity to provide a supportive environment to others who are potentially at risk or who are recovering from an illness.

Also, the school health program should provide opportunities, through screening, health appraisal, and teacher observation, for the early identification of persons who have initial signs of disability or disease so that specific diagnostic services can be sought and treatment initiated. Early intervention in certain health conditions means that treatment can be initiated so that the person can return to school. Left undetected, some conditions limit the potential to learn or severely handicap a person's ability to put that learning to productive use in later life.

THE HEALTHY CHILD

When health is regarded as the quality of well-being that enables people to live effectively and enjoyably, it must be considered a means to an end. To a person who is ill, health may be an end to be gained, but to the person who possesses health, it is a vehicle for effective and enjoyable living.

It is to the best interests of youngsters in a schoolroom that the teacher be conscious of the health status of every child, whether the child has normal health or is ill. The teacher must have a positive attitude and think in terms of the attributes or qualities of health each child possesses. This requires an evaluation of the natural endowment of each child. The constitutional makeup of one child may be such that he or she has great vitality and almost unlimited energy, endurance, and ability to recover, although neither the child nor the parents follow the accepted practices of good health. Another child may possess a constitution that is adequate for typical living but so near to inadequacy that every principle of health promotion must be practiced to maintain a normal level of health. Intergrades between these two types require thoughtful discrimination by teachers who strive to understand the health capacity, just as they seek to understand the intellectual capacity, of each child.

Normal health is appraised in terms neither of physical size nor of muscular strength. The small child who appears to be underweight may possess an optimal level of health. Often these children have boundless energy, are on the go constantly, and recover quickly from fatigue. It may be desirable to augment such a child's weight but only on a physician's advice.

In appraising schoolchildren's health, one must give consideration to the personality dynamics of individual youngsters. A student who is not aggressive, driving, and extremely active physically nevertheless may possess a high level of health, both physical and mental. The studious, industrious, methodical child may possess a level of health as optimal as that of the athletic child whose activity is obvious.

A child's capacity to measure up to life's demands should be the cardinal criterion used by a teacher who attempts to appraise the health of a child. Health is one overall condition of well-being encompassing the physical, mental, emotional, and social aspects of well-being. (See Fig. 3-4.)

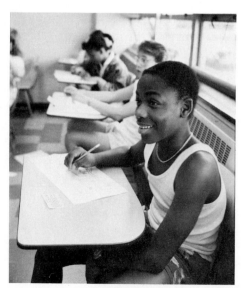

FIG. 3-4. Optimum physical growth and development is fundamental to the child's social, emotional, and intellectual development.

Indicators of physical health

A clinical examination by a physician, supplemented by laboratory tests, is necessary for a thorough inventory of a person's precise status of health, but for practical purposes a teacher can observe certain outward indices as a general gauge. These landmarks of health are of special significance in the school situation where the teacher observes the child daily. This day-to-day observation builds an inventory of each child's general pattern of health. Being familiar with the child's normal condition, the teacher can readily observe any deviation from normal. The teacher does not deal in the specifics of the diagnostician but in the child's overall condition.

Certain common indicators can be used to ascertain a child's health. Of necessity, these indices are interpreted in relative terms, as follows:

1. *Vigor.* Healthy children have bounce or a feeling of lightness. They have a zest for life and what sometimes appears as unlimited vigor.

2. *Awareness of the body.* Healthy children are interested in their bodies and enjoy learning about body parts and functions. For very young children, self is determined by the body almost exclusively. Children at play, however, seem to ignore the limits of their bodies and quite naturally are prone to accidents.

3. *Pleasure in activity.* Every normal child delights in physical action. Restraint, either physical or psychologic, both irritates and frustrates a child. Teachers soon recognize that the solution to most restlessness in the classroom is physical action. A child who prefers inactivity usually is a child who is not well physically or mentally.

4. *Sleeps well and recovers from the day's fatigue.* Not all children function maximally at 9 o'clock in the morning. Some have a constitutional makeup that is slow to accelerate; others have been socially conditioned by the home or other influence to a slow pace in the morning. An alert teacher will quickly identify these differences and take them into account.

5. *Relaxation.* Being at ease in the school situation is both necessary for and an indication of good health. An occasional short-lived display of tension is to be expected in most children, but a constantly tense child is not a healthy child.

6. *Appetite steady and not capricious.* A finicky appetite may be the product of improper or negligent rearing in the home but more often is associated with a low level of health. Which is cause and which is effect is for a physician to determine, but a poor appetite is a symptom that demands constructive attention by the school.

7. *No appreciable variation in weight.* During his or her school-aged years a child experiences a steady increase in weight. Variation in the rate of increase is to be expected, but a child whose weight fluctuates appreciably is in need of a thorough physical checkup. Included in this category are children who lose 3 to 4 pounds (1.36 to 1.81 kg) in a week for no discernible cause and may regain the weight just as mysteriously, only to go through the same down-and-up cycle again. Failure to maintain a stabilized body weight is a symptom of a lack of constitutional stability or of inappropriate behavior.

8. *Adaptation to disability.* As discussed earlier, a person can achieve optimal health even when disability exists. The central issue in health is adaptability. Healthy children learn to adapt and should be encouraged to live up to their potential, which may mean adapting to certain disabilities.

Most defects that are overlooked in schoolchildren are minor ones that are not noticeably disabling. Through the years, however, their cumulative effect can be considerable, though they do not become more aggravated. The presence of a so-called minor disabling defect lowers the child's health level, perhaps even to subnormal levels, and should not be overlooked.

Attributes of mental health

Because every child is unique, it would seem that an evaluation of mental health would have to be an individual matter applied to each child. Strictly speaking, this would be true for detailed or specialized purposes, but children, though different, are not tremendously different. Certain optimal attributes should be identifiable in every child. Although each child in his or her normal maturation exhibits variations in emotional responsiveness, the same fundamental attributes provide the framework of mentally healthy persons. By the same token these are the qualities the school should strive to develop in each child to ensure a high level of adjustment during both childhood and adulthood.

1. *Self-esteem*. All children should have a feeling of worthiness and believe that others regard them highly. Children should know that they have something to live up to rather than something to live down.
2. *Obtain self-gratification through avenues approved by society*. Children are self-centered and seek to gratify their egos. Society recognizes this desire for self-gratification but also lays down rules by which this gratification may be attained.
3. *Security*. No person attains absolute security, but normal children seek and need acceptance by their own group.
4. *Confidence*. All children have a feeling of inferiority, but through the acquisition of skill and experience much of this feeling can be replaced with confidence.
5. *Courage*. Children with the courage to face new situations and difficult tasks have a valuable asset for effective and enjoyable living. In contrast, fear of failure is a liability in both childhood and adulthood.
6. *Stability*. No person is perfectly stable, but mood and conduct should fluctuate within a relatively narrow range.
7. *Orderliness*. Some degree of order is essential for both efficient and gratifying living.
8. *Adaptability*. Life changes constantly, and good mental health requires flexibility to adjust to changes with a minimum of friction and disturbance. Everyone encounters disturbing experiences and even tragedies, but a well-integrated person recovers quickly.
9. *Self-discipline*. Perhaps no one is perfectly self-disciplined, but the mentally healthy child is usually master of his or her actions, rather than a slave to whim, caprice, or indolence.
10. *Self-reliance*. Although interdependence typifies our complex society, within that framework well-adjusted persons depend on their own resources. They have both stamina and ability to mobilize their resources under stress.
11. *Emotional control*. When the self is frustrated, negative emotions are naturally aroused, but to attain the highest levels of mental health, children must learn to channel these emotions and substitute reasoned conduct.

12. *Confidence in the ability to succeed and enjoyment of success.* No one enjoys failure. Occasional failure is the lot of all, but constant failure is injurious to mental health. Children who believe they can succeed, who do succeed, and who fully appreciate and enjoy their success have valuable ingredients for mental health.

13. *Congeniality.* Whereas happiness is a level of elation that a normal person acquires only occasionally and retains a short period of time, the normal emotional mold or temperament should be cheerful and congenial.

14. *Perception of humor.* Normal children learn that some things in life are incongruous or funny. From these they get an enjoyable experience whether their laughter is a response to frustration or a feeling of superiority because they see the unusual aspects of the situation. Humor is an excellent buffer for the rigors of life. To achieve the highest expression of humor in terms of mental health, children should learn to laugh at themselves. People who can look at themselves objectively have the antidote for inherent egocentricity.

15. *Sincere interest in other people.* Basic to good social adjustment is an active, sincere interest in other people. A child who likes other people is not likely to experience self-consciousness, embarrassment, or loneliness. Alter centricity (self-gratification through interest in others) is the key to successful social adjustment because an interest in people telegraphs itself. A sincere liking for people is an acquired attribute one that makes conversation easier and enhances one's social activities.

SUMMARY

From the human perspective the most important thing in the universe is life, and the most important human life is one's own. Human beings have great adaptive capacity. They have a remarkable ability to bend nature to their will, but frequently they find that solving one problem actually creates another.

This is the essence of learning and living. Our ongoing effort is to improve the quality of life and health and postpone premature death by effectively solving life's daily problems. It's humbling to remember that we do not always succeed.

Each person relies on the collective efforts of the community to aid in this effort. For young people, the school, along with family, constitutes their community. To aid this process, it is important for all involved to accept individual differences as part of a range of normal and accept normality as an evolving concept.

Adaptability, the foundation of all health, implies that people actually move within an accepted range of normal. For example, on some days students or teachers may not be totally healthy and therefore are "not normal" but will return to "normal." Acceptance, understanding, and support speeds this process.

The maintenance of health presents a challenge to all parts of a community. Preventing disease through primary prevention depends as much on the school janitor as on the superintendent, just as secondary prevention and early detection are as much the work of an observant cafeteria worker as a registered nurse. Any community must remember that children are not miniature adults. Therefore their range of behavior may stretch the concept of normal further than adult behavior does. Knowing the signs of health among children assists this understanding.

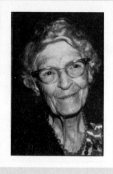

Sally Lucas Jean

BORN   June 18, 1878, Towson, Maryland
DIED   July 7, 1971, New York, New York
EDUCATION   Maryland State Normal School, 1895; Maryland Homeopathic Hospital Training School for Nurses, 1898

Sally Lucas Jean was one of the pioneers in the health education profession. Her educational preparation combined work at Maryland State Normal School with nursing training at Maryland Homeopathic Hospital. However, her experiences as a nurse in the Spanish-American War (1898), as a school nurse for all schools in Baltimore (1911-1913), and as a social health worker at Locust Point, Maryland (1914-1917), and at the People's Institute in New York (1917) were equally important in shaping her life's work. More and more her work moved into the area that is now known as health education. Cofounder and director of the Child Health Organization (1918-1923), she is credited with creating the term *health education*, which was officially adopted in 1918.

As her concept of the meaning of health broadened, so did her concept of the people to be served by this new educational program. She served in Belgium as health education consultant in 1919, and in 1924 was a consultant on health education in the Republic of Panama, Panama Canal Zone. From 1924 to 1941 she held the post of secretary, Health Section, World Federation of Teaching Associations. In 1929 she was a health education consultant in the Philippines, China, and Japan and served in that capacity in the Virgin Islands in 1933. She was supervisor of health education to the Indian Service in 1934 and 1935.

From 1943 to 1951 she held the position of director of educational service, National Foundation for Infantile Paralysis. She was a fellow and life member of the American Public Health Association and life member of the National Education Association and Progressive Education. Her worldwide concern for health education was recognized when she was awarded the William A. Howe Award by the American School Health Association and the Elizabeth S. Prentiss National Award in Health Education. In 1956 she was presented with the Great Medal of Honor of the Union at the close of the Third Conference of the International Union for Health Education of the Public.

STUDY QUESTIONS

1. Is it sound educational policy to treat a child with a defect just as one treats other children?
2. In your judgment, which is of greater importance to school children: their education or their health? What is the basis for your conclusion?
3. Of what significance is the health of the teacher?
4. Why is it important that all teachers have a basic knowledge of health?
5. What would you regard as the best single index of normal mental health?
6. What is normal in one situation may not be normal in another situation. How do you interpret this statement?
7. When a teacher has reason to believe that a certain student under his or her supervision does not have normal health, who should the teacher contact?
8. How will the physical health of a pupil affect his or her mental health?
9. "The most difficult task in health education is to develop an appreciation of health in a child who already has good health." How does a teacher deal with this situation?
10. What is the responsibility of the school in understanding the present health of the child?
11. How is it that a child can be outside the bounds of normal as described in this chapter but still be healthy?
12. In terms of health, what does "normal" mean?
13. If health is a dynamic state, how is it most commonly measured?
14. Differentiate among primary, secondary, and tertiary prevention and describe an example to illustrate these differences.
15. Why are most screening programs not classified as primary prevention?
16. Identify possible agents, hosts, and environmental issues in cancer, mental illness, and accidents.

REFERENCES

Better health for our children: a national strategy, vol. 1, Major findings and recommendations—report of the Select Panel for the Promotion of Child Health to the United States Congress and the Secretary of Health and Human Services, Washington, D.C., 1981, U.S. Department of Health and Human Services, Public Health Service.

Dagg, N.V.: Primary prevention: health promotion and specific protection. In Wold, S.J., editor: School nursing: a framework for practice, St. Louis, 1981, The C.V. Mosby Co.

Dubos, R.: Mirage of health, Garden City, N.Y., 1961, Anchor Books.

Dunn, H.L.: High levels of wellness, Arlington, Va., 1961, R.W. Beatty Co.

Health, United States, 1981, DHHS Pub. No. (PHS) 82-1232, Hyattsville, Md., 1981, U.S. Department of Health and Human Services, Public Health Service, U.S. Government Printing Office.

Healthy people: the Surgeon General's report on health promotion and disease prevention, DHEW Pub. No. (PHS) 79-55071, Washington, D.C., 1979, U.S. Department of Health and Human Services, Public Health Service, U.S. Government Printing Office.

Leavell, R.M., and Clark, F.G.: Preventive medicine for the doctor and his community: an epidemiological approach, New York, 1965, McGraw-Hill, Inc.

McBride, L.G.: Teaching about body image: a technique for improving body satisfaction, J. Sch. Health **56**:76, 1986.

McKeown, T., and Lowe, C.R.: An introduction to social medicine, Oxford, England, 1974, Blackwell Scientific Publications, Ltd.

Wold, S.J.: Secondary prevention and ethical issues In Wold, S.J., editor: School nursing: a framework for practice, St. Louis, 1981a, The C.V. Mosby Co.

Wold, S.J.: Tertiary prevention: mainstreaming handicapped children. In Wold, S.J., editor: School nursing: a framework for practice, St. Louis, 1981b, The C.V. Mosby Co.

4 Physical Growth and Development

OVERVIEW   This chapter provides a general understanding of growth and development from the intrauterine period through the adolescent stage. Some effects of heredity, environment, and nutrition on growth and development are discussed, together with the importance of health care during these various stages. A distinction between growth and development is made in order to emphasize the wide variation that occurs in normal, healthy growth. Characteristics of healthy growth and development at the various stages are discussed. Characteristics of the growth and development of girls and boys are examined in regard to the issue of whether girls should compete with boys in sports and athletics. Recently developed national standards for height, weight, skinfold-thickness measure of body fat for age, sex, and race are presented. Such measures help to characterize healthy growth and development, enabling the school to carry out its role of disease prevention and health promotion.

OBJECTIVES   **After reading this chapter, the student should be able to:**

1. Make a distinction between the terms *growth, development,* and *nutrition*
2. Explain how development or maturation is most accurately and scientifically determined
3. Explain why today's youths are or are not nearing their maximal growth potential
4. Describe prenatal conditions that may result in low birth weight
5. Identify growth and developmental characteristics of children that have important implications for their health and education
6. Explain why comparing an individual child's height and weight with those of peers may not be a good indication of that person's health status
7. Describe how differing maturation levels of children can be of major importance in the planning of school programs
8. Explain what is meant by the expression "adolescent growth spurt" and how this phenomenon is related to adolescent development
9. Explain on the basis of growth and developmental characteristics why athletic competition between the sexes is an acceptable or unacceptable activity

The school deals in futures. How the child develops into the mature adult is a concern of the school. Physical growth and development are no less important than other phases of the evolving youngster. Physical growth and development represent a special phase in the maturing process but are entwined in the total pattern of maturation. Understanding physiologic change and the rate of change enables the teacher to understand each youngster in terms of his or her own particular development and relationship to the normal pattern. It is fascinating to watch the development of a child. It is most fascinating when one has an understanding of the developmental process.

Growth and development are individual matters, each child being distinctive. However, there are typical or recognized ranges of growth into which most children fall. A conscientious teacher is eager to understand each child in terms of individual patterns of growth and development. Perhaps the teacher should think of the child as a "human becoming." After all, human beings require one third of their life span to reach maturity, and the school deals in that future.

GROWTH—CELLULAR AND INTERCELLULAR

Growth occurs at the cellular level in three ways: (1) increase in the size of the cells, (2) increase in the number of cells by cell division or multiplication, and (3) increase of the substance between the cells (intercellular).

This cellular growth consists in the addition of proteins, carbohydrates, fat, water, and minerals to the cell substance. Although vitamins are not directly involved, their regulatory function is also necessary. At least 45 nutrients are needed for healthy growth. However, recent research has led to the conclusion that the most important elements required are proteins and calories. Growth is work, and calories are the units providing the fuel for the energy needed to grow.

Calories are needed for cell multiplication, whereas protein is related primarily to increase in the size of cells. Elements of the major food groups, including carbohydrates, fats, and proteins, can be oxidized and used for energy. However, food must also provide the necessary raw materials for the growth and replacement of cells and cell products. All the molecules of the body must either be obtained directly from the food that is eaten or must be synthesized from other compounds in the diet.

Some molecules are needed in great numbers because they form the structural material making up the tissues of muscle, bone, and cell membranes. Other molecules, such as vitamins, are required in lesser amounts because they are involved in the activities of the enzymes of the body. Although enzymes control chemical reactions, they are not used up in the reaction but can be used repeatedly.

Intercellular growth consists in the addition of organic and inorganic materials between cells. Fat, calcium, phosphate, or other substances retained between cells, though having a relation to the cells, must be considered a part of body growth if they are added to the total mass. Intercellular calcium is the principal constituent of bone growth. The non-cellular part of tissue undergoes considerable increase in mass during the stage of physical growth of life.

DEVELOPMENT

Development, or maturation, is an increase in the complexity and effectiveness of bodily functions, whereas growth usually refers to an increase in size. For example, there is relatively little difference in the physical size of the head of a 3-month-old infant and that of a 16-year-old adolescent. But obviously, the changes that have occurred over this period in the nature and complexity of the brain and its capacity to function are enormous.

In a comparison of the maturational differences between infancy and childhood, a comparatively shorter period of time, the 3-month-old infant is still a bundle of reflexes dominated by the need for food, warmth, and rest, whereas the child of 5 years, about to enter school, has already developed a wide range of abilities and skills.

As Krogman (1972) expresses it, "The postnatal growth period of twenty years is like a race: we all run it, but some run it fast and some run it slow." Thus at any point in time during this period some are biologically ahead and some are behind.

An individual's pattern of growth and development is unique. Because of this uniqueness of individual development, the concept of biologic age has come into use. Standards have now been established for determining an individual's maturity by using x-ray examinations of the wrist or knee joints. Experimental investigations using standards of skeletal age are able to establish the degree of maturity quite accurately. Skeletal age is determined by the number of ossification centers and the amount of cartilage material separating those centers from the main body of bony structure in the extremity. Separation means that the epiphysis is open and that the limb or bone is still growing. Gradually these bony centers grow together, converting the cartilaginous material into bone and concluding growth in adult maturity.

Fig. 4-1, which is based on x-ray films taken by J. Roswell Gallagher, M.D., former Chief of Adolescent Medicine of Children's Hospital in Boston, illustrates the growth matu-

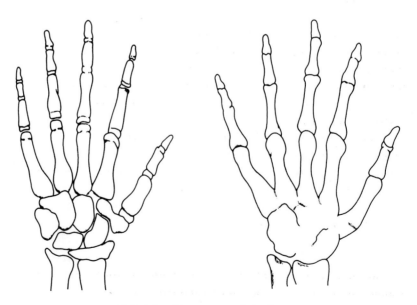

FIG. 4-1. Variations in skeletal age.

rity of skeletal-age differences between two adolescent boys who are of the same chronologic age, 14 years and 11 months. The illustration on the left reveals a skeletal-age rating of 13 years and 6 months, whereas the bone development pictured on the right is considered to be 16 years and 10 months. This represents a maturational difference of nearly 3½ years, thus demonstrating the necessity for school officials to consider more than chronologic age when classifying students for athletic competition or evaluating age-group performances. Tables portraying averages in growth and development are useful, but so-called normal development encompasses a very wide range of differences.

In addition to these differences in growth patterns of normal children, there are variations caused by calorie and protein deprivation. Such malnourished children may never attain their normal complement of cells. Lack of protein in the diet will cause their cell growth to be limited, resulting in smaller stature throughout their growth period and into adulthood.

Since the various systems of the body develop at differing rates, it is desirable that a teacher have an understanding of the patterns of maturation of the various systems. Their separate as well as composite developmental patterns can be the avenue through which the teacher may better understand each child and thus better serve his or her interests.

BIOLOGIC DETERMINATION

Potential biologic growth and development are determined at fertilization. The genetic combinations at that moment set the biologic potential and limit for both.

Inheritance

Growth and development are governed or regulated primarily by the hormones of the body, and a child's genetic endocrine endowment is the principal asset for both growth and development. General body size depends on the output of *somatotropin*, the principal growth hormone, which is produced by the anterior pituitary gland. Carbohydrate, fat, and water balance are affected by other secretions from this gland. Thyroxin from the thyroid gland governs the growth of long bones, the rate at which energy is used, and the rate at which the body matures. Sex hormones affect maturation as well as determine secondary sex characteristics. *Cortin*, the principal secretion of the adrenal cortex, which is located at the tip of the kidneys, greatly affects the rate of maturation. An overactive adrenal cortex produces precocious children.

Considering hormones alone, geneticists calculate at least 40 million possible patterns of genetic endocrine endowment. The particular combination of factors that a child inherits appears to be a matter of mere chance. Once fertilization takes place, nothing can be done to change the inherited characteristics. Therefore a teacher who understands that there are many possible genetic combinations will be more likely to have a better understanding and appreciation of each child in the class.

ENVIRONMENTAL FACTORS

No one attains the absolute genetic maximum in growth and development because environmental factors retard or obstruct normal processes. If it were possible to provide the perfect environment for all life processes, the individual would develop more rapidly than he or she presently does and would attain greater growth. This would entail a better internal bodily environment through scientifically perfected nutrition and respiration, as well as freedom from infection, and an external environment of temperature, humidity, and other factors that best permits processes to function.

A study of growth trends over the past century provides information on the effects of improved health care, improved nutrition, and a more healthful environment on the growth and development of the young. Data collected throughout this period have shown an increasingly earlier age of maturation and an increasing size with each succeeding generation. According to health officials, this universal trend among the young of the Western world has served as a good biologic index of the effects of the environment. Although it is not likely that the perfect environment will ever be created to enable the individual to reach maximum genetic growth potential, there are indications that humankind may be nearing this growth ceiling. For example, after observing several generations of Harvard youth, Damon (1968) has concluded that the growth trend has stabilized. The average heights of Harvard students are no longer increasing and, in fact, have leveled off and are now remaining at a consistent average height.

Damon's findings have been confirmed by an analysis of growth trends conducted by the National Center for Health Statistics (NCHS) (1976). A comparative analysis of the growth measurements taken from representative samples of children and youth from 2 to 18 years of age in the early 1960s shows that the average heights are essentially the same as those taken in the 1970s. It would seem that the average heights of children and youth have stabilized over the past 20 years. However, children in the lower end of the distribution of heights provide an exception. Those of the 5th and 10th percentile levels have continued to show slight increases in heights, whereas the heights of children at the 25th percentile level and above have stabilized. A possible explanation of this fact is that more children from lower socioeconomic backgrounds constitute the 5th and 10th percentile levels of height. Therefore it would follow that these children have not had the full benefits of good nutrition and health care and would have a greater potential for improvement in health. A resulting increase in their heights would be more likely than would an increase in height in children from the upper socioeconomic levels.

Children from disadvantaged backgrounds become a special concern to the school. Although the school represents only a part of their total environmental influences, it can play a vital role in their healthy development. The school health services can protect and supervise the child's healthy growth by promoting the child's health through effective nutrition and health education. As expressed in the NCHS report, "When the stragglers will finally achieve their genetic potential to full stature can probably be better predicted by economic and social factors than by biologic ones."

FULL-TERM INFANT

If the normal gestation period is estimated at 280 days after the beginning of the last menstruation, it is interesting to note that 35% of all births occur within 1 week on either side of this estimate and 65% of births occur within 2 weeks of it. A child who is born at 37 weeks of gestation (within 3 weeks of the 280 days) is considered a full-term infant.

Medical research has revealed that the early stages of pregnancy, between the second and tenth weeks, constitute the most important growth period of life. During this time cell differentiation takes place, and the special tissues of the limbs, eyes, ears, and vital organs are formed. Special emphasis should be given to protecting the mother's health during this period because an illness or adverse condition may affect the intrauterine environment and damage the developing tissues of the fetus. For example, many childhood defects of hearing, vision, and vital function have been traced to an incident of German measles contracted by the mother during this first trimester.

Antibodies passing from the mother through the placenta to the developing fetus give the child an infantile immunity until about 6 months of age. The immunity may be against diphtheria, smallpox, tetanus, measles, and poliomyelitis. This does not give the child the ability to produce antibodies. Thus, when the antibodies received from the mother disintegrate, the immunity ceases unless the child in the meantime has been immunized by other means.

Although usually smaller at birth, girls are about 1 month in advance of boys according to bone development or skeletal-age measures. Girls entering school continue to be more mature in terms of skeletal age than boys are. (This advantage increases progressively to 12 years of age.)

PREMATURITY AND GROWTH RETARDATION

Until recently all infants weighing less than 5½ pounds (2.5 kg) were classified as premature. However, results from medical research have shown that low birth weight may be caused by two distinct conditions: (1) prematurity or (2) growth retardation. *Prematurity* means that such infants are born before completing the normal period of intrauterine life (37 weeks). Therefore premature infants weigh less because they have not had enough time to grow and develop fully. On the other hand, *growth-retarded infants* may have been born after a full-term pregnancy of 40 weeks but still be far below average weight at birth. As many as one third to one half of the incidents of low birth weight are believed to be caused by conditions that retard normal growth. Among the factors believed to be responsible are inadequate placental development, insufficient blood supply to the uterus, genetic defects, the mother's health, and other environmental conditions.

Several techniques are employed to distinguish between the premature and the growth-retarded infant. The ultrasonic sound device is used to measure fetal size, and a precise measure of the duration of pregnancy can be obtained by amniocentesis. Standards describing the various neuromuscular reflexes typical of the neurologic behavior of the different stages of development are used. For example, the growth-retarded infant would be expected to demonstrate behavior patterns similar to those of the full-term infant with normal swallowing and sucking reflexes, whereas the premature infant would not display fully developed reflexes. In general, the premature infant would be expected to be behind the full-term infant in development.

At this time no one has been able to determine precisely what the long-term effects of low birth weight are on the individual. With proper medical care and supervision the premature infant may be expected to reach the developmental level of the full-term infant. However, research on identical twins shows that the smaller individual rarely reaches the same size as the other sibling.

CHARACTERISTICS OF THE PRESCHOOL CHILD

The period from infancy to the school years is a critical one for the child's growth and development. Recently worldwide attention has been focused on the health and nutrition of very young children and the dramatic effects brought about by extreme malnutrition. Pictures of children from underdeveloped countries of the world suffering from marasmus or kwashiorkor stir a sense of concern and compassion in the viewer. But malnutrition is not restricted to distant lands. Actually the breast-fed infant from an underdeveloped country may be better nourished than an infant from the United States who is not breast fed and fails to get an adequate diet from bottle feedings. It is after weaning that the infant from an underdeveloped nation suffers from malnutrition and diarrheal infection from unhygienically prepared food. As a result, these children suffer the severe effects of kwashiorkor, which retards their growth and leaves them dull and listless with the possibility of permanent brain damage. Research has shown that nutritionally deprived children may have brain cell counts 20% lower than those of normal children.

Surveys of child nutrition in the United States show that malnutrition exists in this country to a far greater extent than had been realized, and it is not restricted to poor children who do not get enough food or suffer from dietary deficiencies. Malnutrition also refers to the state of "overnutrition" that can be found in many children from financially stable families. They may suffer from a form of malnutrition that involves taking in too many calories. Overfed children may develop into obese children and adults. Some researchers believe that the consumption of too many calories causes the body to develop an excess of fat cells, thus predisposing the individual to a lifelong tendency to obesity and perhaps to the chronic diseases associated with that condition.

The preschool period marks a transition from the very rapid growth of infancy to the slower but steady, continuous growth of childhood. By the time children reach 5 months of age they will have doubled their birth weight. Moreover, their bodies will have changed from the rounded, plump appearance of infancy to the longer-limbed body type characteristic of childhood.

During this preschool period certain normal growth characteristics predispose children to upper respiratory tract illnesses. Tonsils and adenoidal tissue grow very rapidly, reaching full adult size by the time the child is 5 years old. This large growth of tissue in the relatively small nose and throat area of the child often encourages an infection in the middle ear. Since the child of this age has a shorter eustachian tube leading from the throat to the middle ear, bacterial infections often invade the middle ear. Such infections should receive prompt treatment in order to avoid a possible hearing loss. Teachers and parents should be alert to identify those children with hearing difficulty and a pattern of mouth breathing. Such a condition may indicate the presence of infection.

During the first 2½ years of the child's life, the cerebellum portion of the brain influences to a large extent the child's posture, coordination, and ability to perform certain movements. Efforts to teach neuromotor skills such as those that are involved in walking or in toilet training will be of no avail until such time as the child is "ready" developmentally, that is, until the neural pathways have been established. After a child has attained sufficient physical maturity, it has been demonstrated that preschool programs have a significant and positive effect on the child's development.

Among so-called normal children, there is a variation in physical, social, and intellectual maturity. Some lag behind, some are on schedule, and some race ahead. In a group of preschoolers a variation in maturation of 6 months is not unusual (Fig. 4-2). This seemingly short period of time can represent, however, the equivalent of nearly one fourth of a young child's life span. Children whose birthdays occur in late summer or early fall may be as much as 10 to 11 months behind, developmentally. Such children may not be ready for school simply because of this lack of maturation. Pushing them ahead can lead to difficulty.

THE ELEMENTARY SCHOOL-AGED CHILD

Technically the elementary school growth period includes the time span from kindergarten up to and including the preadolescent growth spurt of puberty. However, since the timing of the growth spurt varies widely and often extends well into the middle or junior high school years, pubertal growth will be discussed with adolescence.

The growth stage of the early elementary school years has often been described as undramatic, as compared to the rapid growth changes that characterize both the earlier and later growth periods. The gradual and steady rate of growth that began in preschool continues well into the elementary school years. Children tend to become heavier in relation to their height. The tendency toward lower back curvature, or lordosis, ends, creating a more erect posture. During this period children lose all their primary teeth, except for the second and third molars, while acquiring their permanent teeth. These children may continue to have problems because of the abundance of lymphatic tissue that makes up the tonsils and adenoids.

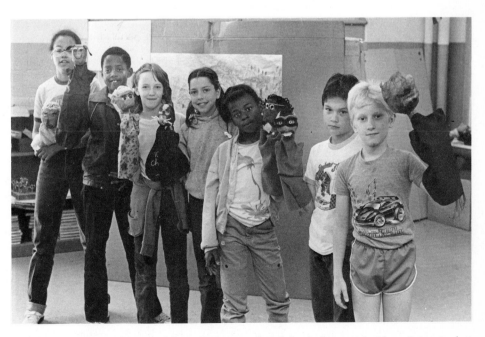

FIG. 4-2.   Children of the same chronologic age and grade level often reveal wide variations in their patterns and rates of growth and development.
(Copyright 1983 by David Riecks.)

The preschool child usually is farsighted, which he or she does not outgrow until about the sixth year of age. At this time both the involuntary and voluntary muscles of accommodation mature to give the child the visual apparatus necessary for reading. At the 6-year level of visual maturity, a child can read large type (12 point) but not without sustained effort.

If a child is nearsighted, the condition usually appears early.

Eyestrain in school is not necessarily a deficiency in visual acuity but may be a tendency of the relatively immature muscles of accommodation to fatigue very easily.

The normal eye reaches its maximum growth and acuity at 12 years of age. It is the first organ to mature.

At 7 years of age children tend to become daring, adventuresome, boisterous, and vigorous in their play. Running, chasing, skating, jumping rope, bicycle riding, and swimming appeal to them. Joy, as an expression of self, motivates the child to master a skill that actually becomes a means to an end.

Manipulative skills begin to improve greatly at 8 years of age. The child normally becomes progressively stronger and sturdier. Legs lengthen rather rapidly, but the rate of general body growth is slower. Considerable variation in muscular development and coordination occurs. The child fatigues quite easily but recovers just as readily. At 8 years of age, the smaller muscles begin to be used, though not too skillfully. Rapid improvement in manipulative skill and eye-hand coordination results in a surprisingly high level of dexterity.

By 11 years of age rapid muscular growth has begun, particularly in the girl. At 12 years of age a child attains a near-adult level of perfection in control of the shoulder, arm, and wrist muscles. Finger control is slower. Development of large muscle skills first and then small muscle skills is a sound practice.

Handedness becomes noticeable by the time a child enters school. Neurologically most persons are right-handed or left-handed. This preference is inherited; right-handedness is a dominant trait, and left-handedness is a simple recessive trait. About 7% of all males and 6% of all females are strongly left-handed. About 20% of the members of both sexes are mixed handed and can use either hand about equally well. The hand that is used more depends on training. These persons can be truly ambidextrous.

These early years of the schoolchild's life, coming between two periods of rapid change, are often termed the healthiest period of the entire human growth span. Children at this age have the lowest death rates and the lowest rates of serious illness of the entire society.

But children of this age group do have health problems. Their leading cause of death is accidents. A common example is the tendency to dash suddenly across the street. Certain forms of cancer, principally leukemia, constitute a major cause of death. The most common illnesses are episodes of infection causing respiratory illness and digestive upsets. Vaccines have been developed for many of the so-called childhood diseases, such as measles, mumps, and German measles, and have brought them under control.

In recent years health authorities have become concerned over the increasing use of cigarettes and marijuana by elementary school children. The community and social pressures to smoke have persisted despite major efforts to inform children about the hazards of smoking. The tendency of children to experiment with drug usage and alcoholic beverages has caused many school systems to strengthen and extend health education in the schools.

Although the emphasis of this chapter is on the child's physical growth and development, many emotional health problems have a direct and important effect on physical development and well-being. The child's adjustment to school, his or her fear of separation from mother, the effect of broken homes or incomplete families, and the tendency to become too involved and stimulated in academic, athletic, and social activities are often the sources of difficulties that affect both health and school progress.

PUBERTY AND ADOLESCENCE

With the exception of the growth period of infancy, the pubertal growth spurt, which precedes adolescence, is perhaps the most dramatic stage of human development. It is widely discussed, but a great deal of misunderstanding still continues about this phase of growth. *Puberty* marks the time in life when a person is first capable of sexual reproduction, whereas *adolescence* is designated as that period of transition between puberty and maturity. Researchers designate *pubescence* as the period extending from the first evidence of sexual maturation (breast development in girls and changes in the genitals of boys) to the onset of menstruation in girls and the production of spermatozoa in boys. Adolescence is defined as the period in a person's life extending from menstruation or spermatogenesis to the time of physical growth maturity. *Maturity* in this sense means the culmination of linear growth when the epiphyses have closed and the person has reached maximum height.

To appreciate the magnitude of the growth change that takes place during puberty, one should compare the amount of growth during this time with that of other periods. Fig. 4-3 depicts the velocity curves (amount of gain in height at various age levels) from infancy to puberty. The amount of gain, though steady, gradually declines until the sharp upsurge takes place at puberty. This spurt of growth occurs at approximately 12 years of age for girls and 14 years for boys. Extensive study and research of the pubertal growth phenomena have revealed that more is involved than simply an abrupt change in linear growth. Instead, puberty consists in a complex sequence of interrelated events. The mechanisms, which are not yet fully understood, involve an orchestration of interrelationships between the endocrine gland system and the various other body systems.

The research by Dr. Li at the University of California (NIH, 1972) has helped to explain the role of the endocrine glands in growth. His studies have provided more information about the pituitary gland and its production of the human growth hormone (HGH), which causes an increase in size. In addition to the growth-promoting qualities of HGH, it also serves an important regulatory function in many metabolic processes. For example, the pituitary gland is believed to initiate the secretion of *gonadotropins*, after which the gonads or sex glands begin to secrete sex hormones. These sex hormones, in turn, promote such effects as protein synthesis, muscle development, bone growth, and the development of secondary sex characteristics (Fig. 4-4).

The female sex hormones *estrogen* and *progesterone* are responsible for inducing the menarche. According to Tanner (1973), the male sex hormone, testosterone, which is also stimulated by a hormone from the anterior pituitary gland, is responsible for much of the

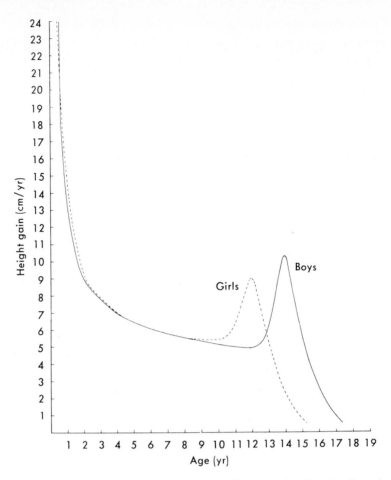

FIG. 4-3. Typical individual velocity curves for supine length or height in boys and girls. These curves represent the velocity of the typical boy and girl at any given instant.
(From Tanner, J.M., Whitehouse, R.H., and Takaishi, M.: Arch. Dis. Child. 41:455, 1966.)

adolescent growth spurt in boys. The presence of testosterone leads to the development of the male reproduction cell spermatozoa in the testes. This event of sexual maturation or spermatogenesis in the male usually occurs some 2 to 3 years after the onset of puberty.

Charts developed by Tanner (1966) (Figs. 4-5 and 4-6) from the Institute of Child Health in London illustrate the sequence of major events occurring at puberty for boys and girls. The symbols on the charts represent the typical ages at which these changes occur. The timing and coordination of these various events, which include height gain, breast development, and menarche in girls and changes in the sex organs along with height gain in boys, demonstrate the interrelationship of growth and glandular functions discussed in Li's research.

Based on several longitudinal studies, researchers at the Harvard School of Public Health describe the variations in physical growth patterns as characteristic of "early" and "late" maturers. In Fig. 4-7 the concept of velocity curves (yearly increments in growth) is

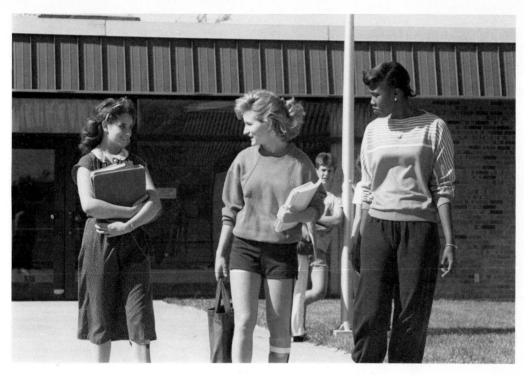

FIG. 4-4. The influence of the endocrine glands can be seen in the adolescent girl's development of secondary sex characteristics,
(Copyright 1985, Creswell Productions/American Heart Association.)

again used to illustrate the differences in the timing of the growth spurt among girls and boys. Although this dramatic increase usually occurs at 12 and 14 years of age, respectively, individual growth patterns may vary greatly from these norms. Tanner speaks of these variations as the individual's "tempo of growth." Variations are present at all ages; however, these differences are more dramatic during adolescence. For example, the range of chronologic ages within which menarche may normally fall is approximately 10 to 16½ years of age. For boys, differences in the chronologic age when the growth of the penis begins may also vary widely, from 10½ to 14½ years of age. This means that some boys and girls have finished their pubescent growth before others of their same chronologic age have started.

Because of these variations, growth authorities recommend the use of other measures in addition to chronologic age in order to make a more accurate assessment of maturity. Bone growth or skeletal age correlates much more closely with growth changes. In this regard, Tanner has developed a technique for the assessment of bone age or maturity (Fig. 4-8) that employs the use of x-ray pictures of the bones of the hand and wrist. Successive changes in the shape and density of the margins of each of the ossification centers are illustrated. In Fig. 4-8, *b* to *h* illustrate the various stages of maturation of the first metatarsal bone of the hand. Bone development is traced from a tiny speck of calcium at stage *b* to the adult state of development or maturity at stage *h*.

Standard percentile curves have been developed so that a boy's or girl's bone age or

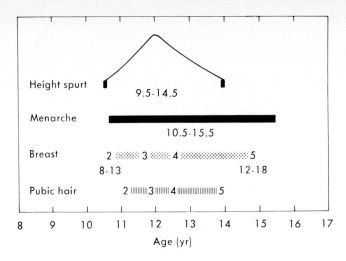

FIG. 4-5. Sequence of events of puberty in girls at various ages is diagramed for the average child. The hump in the bar labeled "height spurt" represents the peak velocity of the spurt. The bars represent the beginning and completion of the events of puberty. Although the adolescent growth spurt for girls typically begins at 10.5 years of age and ends at 14 years, it can start as early as 9.5 years of age and end as late as 15 years. Similarly, menarche (the onset of menstruation) can come at any time between 10 and 16.5 years of age and tends to be a late event of puberty. Some girls begin to show breast development as early as 8 years of age and have completed it by 13 years; others may not begin it until 13 years and complete it at 18 years. First pubic hair appears after the beginning of breast development in two thirds of all girls.

(From Tanner, J.M. In Forfar, J.O., and Arneil, G.C., editors: Textbook of paediatrics, Edinburgh, 1962, Churchill Livingstone.)

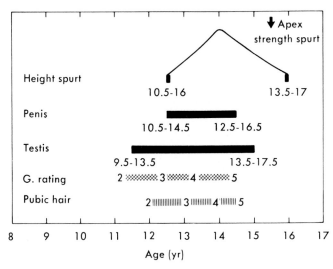

FIG. 4-6. Sequence of events of puberty in boys is also shown at various ages for the average child. The adolescent growth spurt of boys can begin as early as 10.5 years of age or as late as 16 years and can end anywhere from 13.5 years of age to 17.5 years. Elongation of the penis can begin from 10.5 to 14.5 years of age and can end from 12.5 to 16.5 years. Growth of the testes can begin as early as 9.5 years of age or as late as 13.5 years and end at any time between 13.5 and 17 years of age.

(From Tanner, J.M. In Forfar, J.O., and Arneil, G.C., editors: Textbook of paediatrics, Edinburgh, 1962, Churchill Livingstone.)

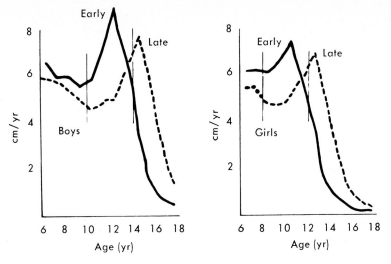

FIG. 4-7. Annual increments in height of early and late maturing boys and girls (means of 20 in each group).
(From Valadian, I.: Proceedings of the National Nutrition Conference, U.S. Department of Agriculture, Nov. 1971.)

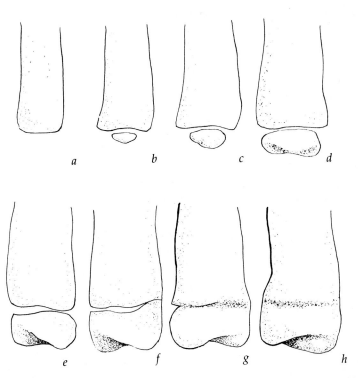

FIG. 4-8. X-ray technique showing successive stages in the maturation of the first metatarsal bone. At stage *a* the calcium is not yet discernible. Beginning at stage *b* the successive stages show a gradual development of the bone to full maturity at stage *h*. Standards of bone development have been established showing stage of bone maturity or development.
(Artwork by William H. Creswell III.)

degree of maturity can be determined by comparison of bone age with chronologic age (Marshall, 1977).

BONE-GROWTH PROBLEMS

Promoting healthy growth and development of children and youth calls for a special awareness of the bone-growth characteristics of this age group. As illustrated in Fig. 4-8, bone growth proceeds from the centers of ossification forming the shafts of the long bones and ultimately fusing with the secondary centers of ossification at the ends of the long bones. However, this area between the two centers of ossification where new bone growth is occurring presents the greatest potential for injury. The epiphyseal, or growth plate, area is composed of growing cartilage cells that are nourished by a network of blood vessels. Injury to the blood vessels and growth plate can interfere with nourishment of these cells, resulting in osteoporosis, a disturbance of the normal growth process.

During this period of rapid growth the potential for handicapping injuries caused by stresses arising from vigorous physical activity or sports participation is a special concern of medical authorities. Without the aid of x-ray films it is very difficult to determine an individual's state of skeletal development and to know when a youngster may be at special risk of injury.

Medical authorities have distinguished between two types of trauma that can occur to the epiphyses, or growth plate area: (1) a traction type of injury or (2) a pressure type of injury. An example of the traction type of injury is Osgood-Schlatter disease, which affects the tibial tuberosity, or the bony projection just below the kneecap (patella). This is the location where the large thigh muscles (quadriceps) attach through the patellar tendon to the lower limb. This injury causes the tibial tuberosity to become very tender and irritated. This condition usually occurs between 9 and 14 years of age. Although the danger of permanent growth injury may not be great, the person can suffer considerable pain and discomfort. Proper care may require special protective padding and restriction from all vigorous activity. Under conditions of excessive strain to the leg, a traumatic separation of the tibial tuberosity may occur.

Scheuermann's disease is an example of the pressure or weight-bearing type of injury to the growth plate. This condition also occurs during the adolescent growth spurt between 12 and 17 years of age. In this instance pressure may cause a wedgelike deformity to one or more vertebrae of the spine, resulting in a rounding of the upper back, or kyphosis of the spine.

Two other conditions that are of special interest to school officials include Legg-Calvé-Perthes disease, a deformity of the hip joint area, and an injury that has become known as "little leaguer's elbow." Fig. 4-9 illustrates an epiphyseal separation occurring on the inner side of the elbow, or the medial epicondyle. The muscles to the lower arm are attached here. The separation is caused by a violent contraction of this muscle group during the act of throwing. Efforts to protect children from such injuries have led to modifications in the rules governing little league baseball such as restricting the amount of pitching and the throwing of curve balls by these young players (Larson, 1973).

Evidently the physiologic processes controlling the ossification and growth of bones are also rather closely related to the other events that occur during this spurt of growth.

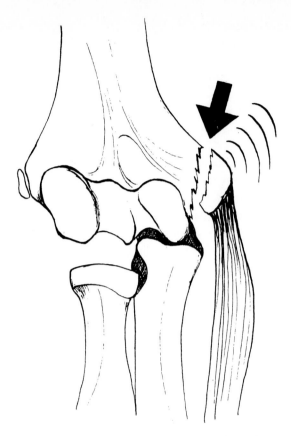

FIG. 4-9. Elbow joint in an adolescent. The violent contraction of the flexor-pronator group of muscles to the forearm in the act of throwing causes a strain in the growth plate of the medial epicondylar epiphysis of the humerus, arrow. This is a traction epiphysis.
(From Larson, R.L.: Physical activity and the growth and development of bones and joint structures. In Rarick, G., editor: Physical activity: human growth and development, New York, 1973, Academic Press, Inc.)

Early-maturing girls start the growth spurt at 9 years of age, whereas late-maturing girls start at 11 years. Early-maturing boys start at 11 years of age and late-maturing boys at 13 years. In addition to the difference between early and late maturers of both sexes, there is also a difference in the amount of incremental gain or height increases. In each instance those entering the growth spurt earliest also achieved the greatest amount of gain. This would seem to indicate that those who enter this growth cycle first not only have an early advantage but also maintain their height advantage in later life. However, this is not always the case. Some late-maturing boys may have a longer growing period and eventually catch up with and in some instances achieve greater height than their age mates.

Because individual growth characteristics loom so important to the adolescent and his or her self-image, the condition of early or late maturity can have lasting personality effects. Since girls begin their growth spurt first, they may suddenly find themselves taller than boys in the same classroom and become very concerned about being "too tall." Boys, on the other hand, especially the late maturing, are greatly concerned about their lack of height and size.

Boys are said to be at greater risk than girls, since their changes in strength and size are correspondingly greater. Teachers need to understand the effects of these changes on students. Patterns of growth should be explained, as should the differences between male and female growth rates. Physicians and counselors can help to allay what, in most instances, is an unnecessary concern about growth. For those relatively few adolescents who have medically diagnosed growth problems, medical science has made great strides in treating growth abnormalities, so that even these boys and girls may be able to grow to heights similar to those of their peers.

Girls begin to taper off in motor performance at 15 years of age. Boys taper off at about 18 years of age. Although both will develop further skills after these ages, the rate of improvement will be much slower, and the maximum skill attained will not be appreciably higher. Biologic maturity is a stage at which motor skill approaches the maximum potential. The girl's maximum potential will be attained at about 20 years of age, and the boy's will be attained at about 23 years of age. Girls generally fall far below their potential skill, largely because of inadequate educational programs.

However, with the recent developments in girls' athletics, new records and higher levels of performance from the older, more mature girls and adult women can be expected in the future. In fact, there are several examples of women athletes in their mid- to late twenties competing successfully at world class competition levels in track and skating events.

A question that is often posed today is, Are we becoming bigger and taller than our ancestors? A frequently made observation, though not based on scientific data, is that today's college football and basketball players are much larger and taller than their predecessors. In this respect, the age-height-weight tables of some 25 years ago are now outdated. The scientifically based data that provide an answer to this question are drawn from what are called "secular-trend studies." Tanner (1978) cites such trend studies of English boys in which he compared the heights of boys in the midnineteenth century with those of English boys in 1965. These data indicate that the differences may result from the effects of environment and nutrition. Although today's youth tend to be taller and heavier than their predecessors, this may result from the differences in their rates of development and maturation rather than from true differences in height. For example, records based on nineteenth-century English working boys revealed that they continued their growth in height until well into their middle twenties. By comparison, such boys would be shorter in height during their teens, but because of their continued growth might eventually be as tall as the earlier maturing boys of the twentieth century. At the same time, there is little doubt that the advantages of superior medical care, nutrition, and environmental conditions have contributed to greater average heights and weights among the youth of today. Figs. 4-10 and 4-11 illustrate such secular trend differences in average heights and weights of North American white boys between 1880 and 1960. However, it is of interest to note the narrowing of the height differences at 20 years of age. This may indicate a delayed maturation or slower growth for the 1880 sample and a continuation of height gain that would eventually catch up to the 1960 comparison sample of boys.

Researchers in the fields of growth and development and in early childhood education point to some of the skills and abilities that can be expected of the nursery school child. For example, most of these children will be able to feed and dress themselves, with certain

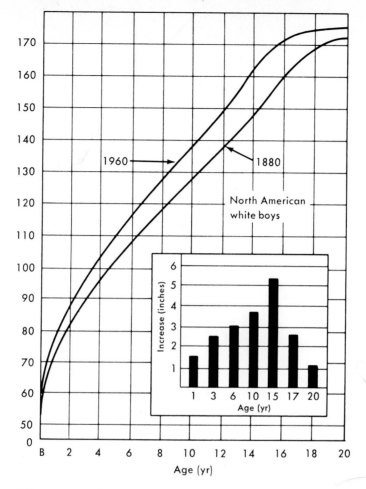

FIG. 4-10. Secular trend in height from 1880 to 1960.
(From Lipsitt, L.P., and Spiker, C.C.: Advances in child development and behavior, vol. 1, New York, 1963, Academic Press, Inc.)

qualifications, of course, as teachers and mothers of children of this age can attest. Tying shoelaces and donning heavy winter clothing present special problems. Most children will have established bowel control by 3 years of age, but bladder control will come later. These behavior patterns respond to emotional pressures, and teachers working with preschool children must be alert to the fact that stresses may cause temporary loss of these controls and regression to previous levels of behavior. The adult's ability to handle these situations with sensitivity and understanding is of paramount importance to the child's satisfactory adjustment and continuing development.

MALE-FEMALE DIFFERENCES

One of the major outcomes of the civil rights movement of the 1960s was legal enforcement of the constitutional right of every person, regardless of race, age, sex, or religious prefer-

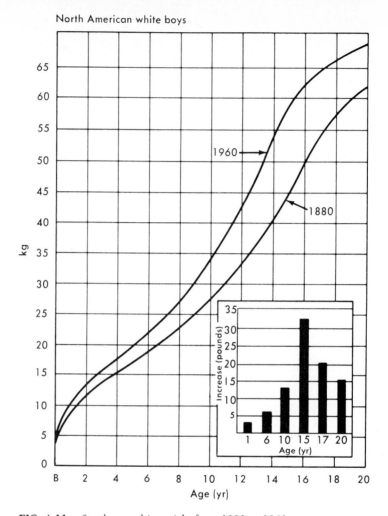

FIG. 4-11. Secular trend in weight from 1880 to 1960.
(From Lipsitt, L.P., and Spiker, C.C.: Advances in child development and behavior, vol. 1, New York, 1963, Academic Press, Inc.)

ence, to receive fair and equal treatment as well as the opportunity to participate fully in all aspects of American life. This has led to major changes in society and in the public school programs. In the past, girls were rarely given the same opportunity as boys to enter certain fields of study, to practice the professions, or to participate in certain activities included in interschool athletics. Many of these restrictions were based on misconceptions and stereo-typed attitudes about female interests, mental and physical capacities, and athletic capabil-ities in particular. Now that these barriers are being removed, many high schools are giving girls an opportunity to participate in school athletics. However, the fact that few secondary schools have the budget, staff, or facilities to provide such an expanded program has, in numerous instances, forced girls to compete with boys "to make the team." Although this effort to give girls opportunities in athletics is commendable, a single, combined sports program for boys and girls cannot be justified. On the basis of their physical growth characteristics, such programs place girls at a distinct disadvantage.

Because girls have a 1- to 2-year maturational advantage over boys that lasts from infancy through childhood, many observers have reached the false conclusion that girls can compete favorably with boys. However, with puberty comes the emergence of the male-female sex differences in height, weight, strength, and speed. Several of these developing characteristics are highly correlated with success in sports activities. For example, boys have the advantage of greater size, both in height and in weight, in addition to having an inherited ?. 1. capacity for speed and endurance. Although the female's maturational advantages during childhood are well known, the fact that boys have a muscle cell advantage over girls is not generally appreciated. Studies have revealed that as early as 3 weeks of age, boys already have a larger complement of muscle cells than girls have. This advantage continues throughout childhood, and adolescent growth increases the difference. By the time a girl has reached 10 years of age, she has undergone a fivefold increase in the number of muscle cells. However, at this stage, the girl's muscle growth has just about reached its maximum. For boys, however, the adolescent growth spurt means an increase in the number of muscle cells, which may increase by as much as 14 times by 18 to 20 years of age.

Other well-known findings have established the fact that females have a greater proportion of fatty tissue to muscle cells than males have. Moreover, adolescent growth causes girls to develop an even greater proportion of fatty tissue.

Until 8 years of age, there is a slight difference between the basal metabolic rate (BMR) of boys of girls. From that age until 20 years, the BMR of both sexes is equal. From 20 years of age onward, a man's basal requirement is 10% greater than a woman's of the same height, weight, and age.

At about 9 years of age a radical change occurs in the rate of growth of boys and girls. This pronounced sex difference in growth is believed to be caused by the male's greater responsiveness to the effects of growth hormone (GH) at the tissue level. Boys evidence a more rapid cell multiplication in muscle tissue and in the epiphyseal plates relating to bone growth (Figs. 4-12 and 4-13). This change in the male is characterized by a remarkable increase in lean body mass as well as a correspondingly greater intake of calories and protein. Although the amount of fat tissue also increases in males during this period, it occurs at a lesser rate than it does for the female. It is believed that the hormone estrogen restricts the stimulating effect of the growth hormone in girls. Also, it is believed that the female responds differently to the effects of insulin, resulting in a greater increase in fat tissue (Fig. 4-14) (Grumbach et al., 1974).

Boys, however, in addition to possessing greater amounts of muscle cells (which determine the development of strength and power) also develop larger hearts and lungs in relation to their size. This means that they develop higher systolic blood pressure and lower resting pulse rate, with a greater capacity for carrying oxygen in the blood. As a result, they have a greater capacity for neutralizing the waste products or lactic acid accumulating from physical exertion. As a consequence, boys enjoy a more rapid recovery from fatigue. The comparatively greater oxygen-carrying capacity of the blood of the male is a result of the greater number of red cells and hemoglobin present in the blood, caused by the presence of the male sex hormone *testosterone*.

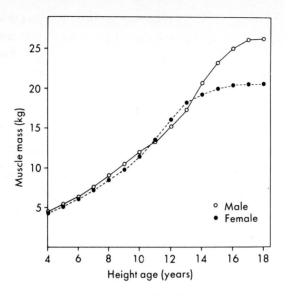

FIG. 4-12. Muscle mass is plotted against height age for boys and girls. Notice that muscle mass doubles in boys from 10 to 17 years of age.
(From Cheek, D.B.: Body composition, hormones, nutrition, and adolescent growth. In Grumbach, M.M., Grave, G.D., and Mayer, F.E., editors: Control of the onset of puberty, copyright 1974, reprinted by permission of John Wiley & Sons, Inc.)

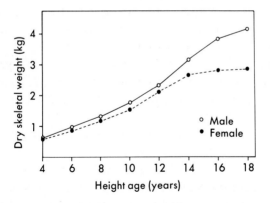

FIG. 4-13. Garn's data (1970) show the growth of skeleton versus height age. Clearly the greater gain in body and muscle of the boy is associated with the greater gain in skeletal mass.
(From Cheek, D.B.: Body composition, hormones, nutrition, and adolescent growth. In Grumbach, M.M., Grave, G.D., and Mayer, F.E., editors: Control of the onset of puberty, copyright 1974, reprinted by permission of John Wiley & Sons, Inc.)

Another difference reported by Tanner (1971) shows that boys develop larger forearms than girls do. This difference is undoubtedly reflected in the greater arm strength of boys.

As a direct result of the anatomic and physiologic differences that develop in the adolescent period, athletic ability increases greatly in boys during this period. Public schools

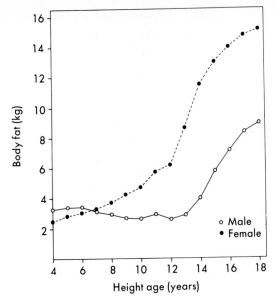

FIG. 4-14. The relationship of fat to body length and the increasing fatness of boys and girls during the adolescent period are shown. The greater increase in fat tissue among girls is also demonstrated. *(From Cheek, D.B.: Body composition, hormones, nutrition, and adolescent growth. In Grumbach, M.M., Grave, G.D., and Mayer, F.E., editors: Control of the onset of puberty, copyright 1974, reprinted by permission of John Wiley & Sons, Inc.)*

have a responsibility to provide a girls' sports program that gives them an equal opportunity to develop to their maximum potential. The unusually gifted girl may be able to compete successfully with boys of her peer group, especially during childhood, but the male-female differences that develop during adolescence necessitate a separate program for average girls in order that they be able to develop athletic skills to their individual level of excellence.

HEIGHT

Teachers have more than an academic interest in the height of their pupils. Besides their personal interest, they will need to help children understand the factors related to growth in height.

Inheritance of stature and size

Height is a multiple factor. The length of the legs, the trunk, the neck, and the head collectively determine the height of a person. Several genes are influential in determining these structures. Genes that affect size also affect other characteristics. The endocrine glands affect both size and other characteristics. Therefore the genes that produce these glands will also have an effect on various other factors.

A child may inherit all the relatively long or short segments of both parents and thus may be taller or shorter than the parents. Because of the many possible combinations, uniformity is hardly to be expected. Tallness is a recessive trait that represents a high output of the growth hormone somatotropin, which comes from the anterior pituitary gland, and of thyroxin, which comes from the thyroid gland. Shortness is a dominant trait. Thus tall parents, having only genes for tallness, will have tall children. Short parents may have tall children if both parents have genes for both shortness and tallness. Parents of medium height tend to have children who vary widely in height. Generally speaking, the prospective tallness shows early in the child, and, as is pointed out later, it is possible to predict in childhood the approximate height a person will be in adulthood.

Dwarfism, an example of abnormal growth, is believed to be caused by a combination of genetic and endocrine factors. In the case of an endocrine disorder, there is an insufficient amount of the growth hormone secreted by the pituitary gland. The shortness is stature results from the premature ossification or closing of the epiphyses of the long bones. When the growth lines ossify early in life instead of at about 20 years of age, the long bones fail to attain their normal length. Short and irregular bones may show some retardation in growth but not to the extent that the long bones are affected.

Simple *gigantism* is an inherited condition that is a chance combination of height-giving genes, abnormal endocrine secretions, and other attributes, which produces an extremely large stature. Gigantism is an anomaly in which the epiphyses do not close, and the eosinophil cells of the anterior pituitary gland secrete excessive amounts of the principal growth hormone. About 90% of all giants are in this category.

Preschool years

The mean for height is not all-important but does serve as a marker of the midstream of height for various age levels. One standard deviation includes 66⅔% of the total, and two standard deviations include 95% of the total.

Children of normal term will be 20 inches (51 cm) long at birth. At 1 year of age they will have added 10 inches (25 cm) to their height and at 4 years of age will be twice their height at birth. More precise figures can be tabulated.

School-aged children

From Table 4-1 it is apparent that up to 10 years of age, school-aged boys gain about 2¼ inches (5.7 cm) per year. The gain drops to 2 inches (5 cm) per year for the next 2 years and then increases to about 3 inches (7.6 cm) per year to 15 years, when the leveling off begins. School-aged girls have a gain of about 2¼ inches (5.7 cm) per year to 11 years of age. The gain steps up to 2½ inches (6.4 cm) for the next 2 years until 12 to 13 years of age, and then it begins to level off. Full height is reached by 16 years of age.

Individual variations from this pattern are to be expected; statistics in Table 4-1 serve merely as an index of the general tendency. Some boys will grow an inch each year for 2 years after the seventeenth birthday. However, the statistics have predictive value. A boy who is 55.2 inches (140 cm) tall at 10 years of age and 57.4 inches (146 cm) tall at 11 years of age will not vary appreciably from 69 inches (175 cm) in height at 17 years of age. The standard deviations can be helpful in charting the likely future growth curve of those children above or below the mean curve.

It is significant that with the onset of biologic maturity, height growth slows down because of the decline in the output of the growth hormone from the anterior pituitary gland. It thus is understandable why persons who mature early have a growth curve that starts to level off sooner than the normal curve.

TABLE 4-1. Height of American children in inches

Age (year)	Boys		Girls	
	Mean	Standard deviation	Mean	Standard deviation
1	29.7	1.1	29.3	1.0
2	34.5	1.2	34.1	1.2
3	37.8	1.3	37.5	1.4
4	40.8	1.9	40.6	1.6
5	43.7	2.0	43.8	1.7
6	46.7	2.07	46.4	2.15
7	49.0	2.13	48.6	2.33
8	51.2	2.33	50.9	2.45
9	53.3	2.64	53.3	2.71
10	55.2	2.67	55.5	2.86
11	57.4	2.75	58.1	3.08
12	59.3	3.35	60.5	2.63
13	61.2	3.39	61.8	2.79
14	64.4	3.40	63.0	2.53
15	66.7	3.13	63.8	2.47
16	68.2	2.68	63.9	2.53
17	69.0	2.78	64.2	2.53

Data for this table are taken from the National Health Examination Survey (HES). Data for children 1 to 5 years of age represent pooled data, USPHS, 1960; data for children 6 to 11 years of age are from Cycle II, 1963-1965; and data for children 12 to 17 years of age are from Cycle III, 1966-1970. NCHS Series II, Numbers 104 and 124, Department of Health, Education and Welfare, Public Health Service.

WEIGHT

From a practical standpoint, for use in the school, weight is not a satisfactory index of growth (Fig. 4-15). Obese children would rate highly if weight were used as the sole index of growth.

Indices of growth

When a child is assessed in terms of a table of mean weights, the constitutional makeup of the child must be taken into consideration if weight is to be of any value as an index to growth. Even then, height must be considered in the assessment.

Inherited factors

Weight is determined by body conformation or proportions as well as by adipose tissue. The person who inherits a conformation of long torso and short legs will tend to weigh above the mean, though he or she appears to be about normal in weight. If a tendency toward obesity is inherited, a sluggish thyroid or pituitary gland may be the inherited factor. Yet if this person reduces food intake, the obesity need not develop. A person is not a helpless victim of heredity. Medical science can help individuals, and they can help themselves.

The misconception that large bones account for excess weight should be dispelled. In two men 6 feet (1.83 m) tall, the skeleton of the one with large bones will not weigh in excess of 3 pounds (1.36 kg) more than that of the one with small bones.

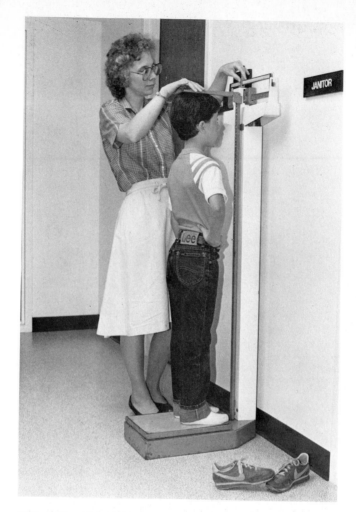

FIG. 4-15. Maintaining accurate records of a child's height and weight during the elementary school years serves as a general index of a child's general growth and development. *(Copyright 1983 by David Riecks.)*

Preschool years

At birth the average boy weighs about 7.6 pounds (3.45 kg) and the average girl weighs about 7.5 pounds (3.3 kg). Blacks are slightly smaller at birth than whites. At 5 months birth weight has doubled, and at 12 months it has trebled. In the next 4 years the child will gain an average of about 5 pounds (2.27 kg) a year.

School-aged children

From Table 4-2 we observe that school-aged boys gradually increase their yearly gain in weight from 6 pounds (2.72 kg) to about 18 pounds (8.17 kg) between 13 and 14 years of age. The annual gain then declines progressively, being only 6 pounds (2.72 kg) between 16 and 17 years of age. Weight gain will continue to 30 years of age. School-aged girls gain from

TABLE 4-2.   Weight of American children in pounds

Age (year)	Boys		Girls	
	Mean	Standard deviation	Mean	Standard deviation
1	23.0	3.0	21.6	3.0
2	28.0	3.0	27.0	3.0
3	32.0	3.0	31.0	4.0
4	37.0	5.0	36.0	5.0
5	42.0	5.0	41.0	5.0
6	48.4	7.65	47.4	8.20
7	54.3	8.94	53.2	9.26
8	61.1	10.68	60.6	12.06
9	68.6	15.00	69.1	15.04
10	74.2	14.58	77.4	17.93
11	84.4	18.51	88.0	20.42
12	91.6	21.16	99.6	20.7
13	100.3	21.5	107.2	22.6
14	118.1	27.2	115.0	21.3
15	130.9	27.9	120.9	20.8
16	140.2	24.7	125.1	21.6
17	146.6	24.1	128.5	26.2

Data for this table are taken from the National Health Examination Survey (HES). Data for children 1 to 5 years of age represent pooled data, USPHS, 1960; data for children 6 to 11 years of age are from Cycle II, 1963-1965; and data for children 12 to 17 years of age are from Cycle III, 1966-1970. NCHS Series II, Numbers 104 and 124, Department of Health, Education and Welfare, Public Health Service.

4 to 8 pounds (1.81 to 3.63 kg) a year until 11 years of age. Then a gain of 11.6 pounds (5.26 kg) is followed by a gradual decline in the increment of gain.

Standard deviations of the magnitude indicated in Table 4-2 indicate a wide range of variation in a group of children. Persons who regularly record the weights of children are surprised at the number of them below the mean. This contrasts with the fallacy that, in terms of the mean, a higher proportion of children are overweight.

NATIONAL STANDARDS FOR GROWTH

The two factors of height and weight in the National Center for Health Statistics (NCHS) charts can be used as a practical growth profile for students. The charts show percentile distribution of boys and girls for height (in centimeters) by age and for weight (in kilograms) by age. These height and weight curves make it possible to compare an individual youth or group with the height and weight of all others in the United States who have the same characteristics (Figs. 4-16 and 4-17). Children should be weighed without shoes and with sweater or jacket removed. Height is also measured with the shoes removed. As a minimum procedure, each child should be measured in September, January, and May. At each measuring period, the point, or child's location, on the chart, is determined by the intersection of two lines formed by a vertical line extended from the base or age line and a horizontal line from the weight or height (stature) portions of the chart. After successive measurements over a period of 2 or 3 years have been recorded, curves of progress can be traced.

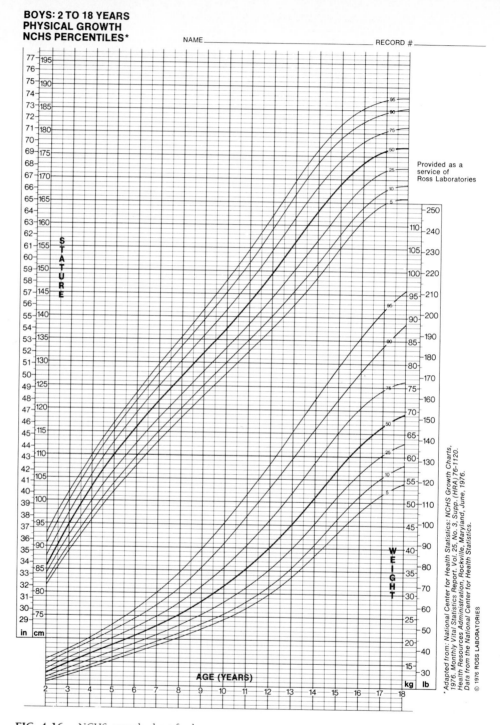

FIG. 4-16. NCHS growth chart for boys.

(Modified from the National Center for Health Statistics: Monthly Vital Statistics Report, vol. 25, no. 3, suppl. [HRA] 76-1120, 1976; courtesy Ross Laboratories, Columbus, Ohio.)

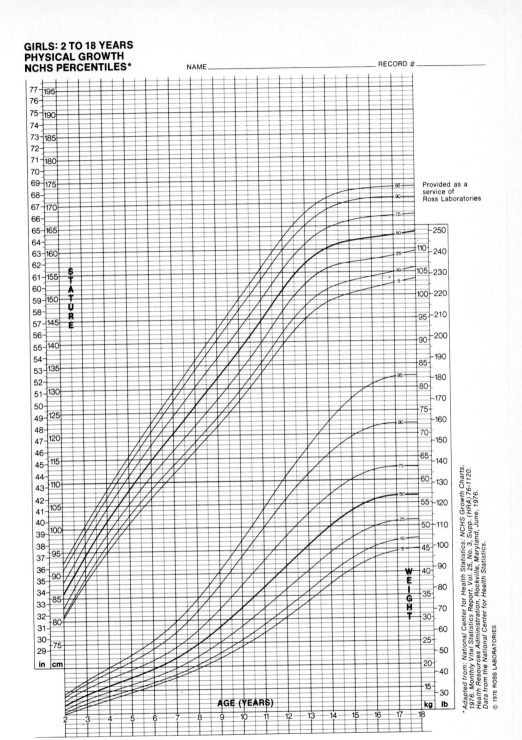

FIG. 4-17. NCHS growth chart for girls.

(Modified from the National Center for Health Statistics: Monthly Vital Statistics Report, vol. 25, no. 3, suppl. [HRA] 76-1120, 1976; courtesy Ross Laboratories, Columbus, Ohio.)

The graphs outline six percentile levels: very tall, moderately tall, average, moderately short, short, and very short. The particular zone in which a child's height point falls indicates his or her position with reference to the heights of other children of the same age and sex. The same principle applies to the location of weight points. The height and weight points of most children fall in corresponding zones; for example, if the weight falls in the average zone (at the 50th percentile level), the height also falls in the average zone for height (at the 50th percentile level). The child is of average size in terms of both height and weight.

When a youngster's weight and height points do not fall in corresponding zones, two possible interpretations may explain the dissimilarity: (1) it may indicate natural slenderness or stockiness, or (2) it may reflect a poor quality of health. Any child with dissimilar height and weight percentile zones may be in need of medical evaluation. Once the child is established in a particular growth zone, there should be a consistent pattern of growth. Any variation from this pattern or zone should be carefully evaluated. It thus is apparent that the physical growth record can indicate possible health deficiencies as well as portray normal growth progress.

Graphs and tables

For practical use in the school it might be well to assess the use of graphs and tables in determining physical growth and development.

Some advantages of growth and developmental graphs and tables are as follows:
1. Implement teacher's observations
2. Aid in understanding a child
3. May indicate the general health level of the child
4. Afford better parental understanding of a child's status
5. Point up abnormalities of growth
6. Help in making comparisons between groups

Some disadvantages of growth and developmental graphs and tables are as follows:
1. May be too complex for everyday use
2. The term "normal" may be misleading
3. Optimums not included
4. Many standards needed
5. Measurement of height and weight may become the end, not a means
6. Not a substitute for personal history and physical examination

When the teacher or some other person in the school has an adequate understanding of a growth index such as the NCHS charts, these instruments can be used to advantage. All children should have their growth evaluated periodically at the time of their general health appraisal by a physician. The school then is governed by the physician's recommendation. The NCHS figures provide representative growth standards for the United States. They may be used in the same manner as the Meredith physical growth record. For example, a 7-year-old boy who is 122 cm (48 inches) tall is of average height, or at the 50th percentile level for his age. If that same boy weighs 20 kg (44 pounds), his relative weight for age is below average or at about the 15th percentile in comparison to other boys of his age. In other words, he is of average height but below average in weight. If he is in good health, as determined by a physician, it may be assumed that he has a naturally slender build. By keeping a record of his growth over a period of years, a much more accurate assessment of his body type can be made, and his ultimate height and weight at maturity can be projected.

SUMMARY

The growth and development process covering the period from prenatal period through adolescence is discussed. At its most elemental level, cellular and intercellular, the quality of growth is dependent on a variety of factors, genetics, environment, and good nutrition. As many as 45 nutrients are involved in healthy growth. A diet composed of the essential proteins are needed for cell multiplication and growth, whereas carbohydrates and fats supply the calories or energy demands of growth. The concepts of growth and development are differentiated. Growth is a quantitative dimension meaning an increase in size, whereas development refers to complexity or maturity. Between infancy and adolescence the child's height, weight, and body will grow and increase greatly in size. However, there is relatively little change in respect to the child's cranium or brain size but a great change in development or complexity of the brain and central nervous system. These concepts are also illustrated with reference to bone growth. During the pubertal growth spurt there is rapid bone growth. However, there may be great variance in the maturation of bones or skeletal age. Skeletal age is determined by the number of ossification centers and the amount of cartilage material between the bony structures. Children of the same age and weight may vary greatly in their skeletal-age maturity. All humans follow a predictable sequence of events in their growth and development. In some respects they are *like all* other human beings, yet in certain aspects they are unique or *unlike* all others.

The pubertal growth spurt, which ushers in the transition from childhood to adolescence and eventual adulthood, is the most dramatic period of growth and development in the life of the school-aged child. Puberty marks the point in life when the human is capable of sexual reproduction. Pubescence, the period leading up to puberty, marks the interval between the first signs of sexual development, which is evident in girls as breast development and in boys as genital development and puberty itself. Typically, girls begin this spurt of growth apparently 2 years earlier than boys, at 12 and 14 years of age respectively.

This period of growth and the varying rates of adolescent development have been the subject of much study. With the advent of interscholastic athletes, competition for girls has raised the question of male and female differences. Although adolescent girls are now establishing physical achievement records far superior to those of the recent past, studies have shown that there are biologic differences in body structure, which means that adolescent boys typically have greater skeletal and muscle mass than girls have, a finding that supports the principle of having separate athletic programs for boys and girls. Charts depicting national standards for height and weight growth for boys and girls covering the ages from 2 to 18 years are presented. Height and weights are graphically portrayed at six different levels for the very tall, moderately tall, average, moderately short, short, and very short.

Once a healthy child's pattern of growth is established he or she should follow a consistent pattern of growth. Any variations from this pattern of growth indicates that the child should be clinically evaluated.

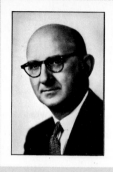

Mayhew Derryberry

BORN   December 25, 1902, Columbia, Tennessee
DIED   December 24, 1979, San Francisco, California
EDUCATION   B.A., University of Tennessee, 1925; M.A.
Teachers College, Columbia University, 1927;
Ph.D., New York University, 1933

Dr. Mayhew "Derry" Derryberry proba-
bly contributed more to the development of the public
health education profession than any other individual.
As chief of health education in the U.S. Public Health
Service from 1941 to 1963, his influence was tremendous. Derryberry's emphasis on the need for strong
state health education programs and for health educators well-versed in the behavioral as well as biologic
sciences, vitalized school health programs and focused
educational activities on behavior change. Derryberry
was also instrumental in the development of schools of
public health.

This emphasis on empirical study, coupled with a
strong interest in behavioral studies, may well reflect
his educational background. Derryberry received his
B.A. in chemistry and mathematics, his M.A. in education and psychology, and his Ph.D. in health and physical education. While completing his Ph.D. program
(1933), Derryberry was made associate director of
research for the American Child Health Association.
Under his guidance the staff of the American Child
Health Association conducted some of the most important research on the evaluation of school health programs ever undertaken. Derryberry was responsible for
organizing and analyzing the statistical data from these
studies, which had been collected over a 10-year period. Publications from this research have produced
wide-ranging and lasting effects on the field.

Derryberry also contributed to publications in the
health education field. His earlier writings dealt primarily with health problems of children and focused
on the assessment of nutritional status, correction of
physical defects, and provision of health services. Later
publications covered general health education topics
such as educational approaches to chronic disease and
educational aspects of family planning.

His expertise was in constant demand internation-
ally. He consulted with health ministries throughout
the world, which included a 3-year assignment in the
mid-1960s as health education advisor to the government of India. He also served as rapporteur to the
World Health Organization's First Expert Committee
on Health Education. The report of this committee
became a basic document in the field of health education.

Derryberry was elected a distinguished fellow and
was a founding member of the Society of Public Health
Education and was one of the few health education
members elected to the National Academy of Physical
Education. He was a 51-year member of the American
Public Health Association and served as chairman of
the Public Health Education Section and as a member
of its governing council.

STUDY QUESTIONS

1. Define the terms *growth* and *development* and give an example of each to show how they differ.
2. Recent growth surveys indicate that certain groups may be nearing their growth potential whereas others apparently have not yet reached their potential. What is the basis for these observations?
3. Explain how the concept of skeletal age is important to the planning of school programs.
4. What is the meaning of the terms *prematurity* and *growth retardation*? How does the physician distinguish between these conditions in the newborn infant?
5. Give an example of a health problem that is related to growth and developmental characteristics among the preschool age group, elementary school youngsters, and the adolescent age group.
6. Explain the sequence of events that takes place during the adolescent growth spurt for both girls and boys.
7. On the basis of growth and developmental characteristics, why should separate athletic programs be provided for boys and girls?
8. Assume that height and weight records kept on John, a 12-year-old boy, during his first 6 years of schooling show that his growth curves for both height and weight have consistently followed the 50th percentile growth level for his age group. On this basis, project his height and weight at age 18.
9. Select a classmate to work with and take the following measurements: (a) height, (b) weight, (c) skinfold thickness, and (d) blood pressure. Also calculate the body mass index (BMI) for both of you. After recording the data, compare the measures with national standards.
10. State some of the principal health implications to be gained from monitoring the growth and development of children and youth: (a) potential for immediate health benefit and (b) potential for long-range health benefit.

REFERENCES

Arteriosclerosis: report of the working group on arteriosclerosis of the National Heart, Lung and Blood Institute, vol. 2, NH Pub. no. 82-2035, Washington, D.C., 1981, Public Health Service, National Institute of Health.

Breckenridge, M.E., and Murphy, M.N.: Growth and development of the young child, ed. 8, Philadelphia, 1969, W.B. Saunders Co.

Damon, A.: Secular trend in height and weight within old American families at Harvard, 1870-1965, Am. J. Phys. Anthropol. **29**(1):45, 1968.

Gallagher, J.R.: Medical care of the adolescent, New York, 1960, Appleton-Century-Crofts.

Gesell, A., Ilg, F.L., and Ames, L.B.: Youth — the years from ten to sixteen, New York, 1956, Harper & Row, Publishers

Grumbach, M.M., Grave, G.D., and Mayer, F.E., editors: Control of the onset of puberty, New York, 1974, John Wiley & Sons.

Height and weight of children in the United States. In Vital and health statistics series, no. 104, National Center for Health Statistics, U.S. Department of Health, Education and Welfare Pub. no. 1000, Washington, D.C., 1970, U.S. Government Printing Office.

Height and weight of youths 12-17 years in the United States. In Vital and health statistics series, no. 124, National Center for Health Statistics, U.S. Department of Health, Education and Welfare Pub. no. (HSM) 73-1606, Washington, D.C., 1973, U.S. Government Printing Office.

How children grow, U.S. Department of Health, Education and Welfare Pub. no. (NIH) 72-166, Bethesda, Md., 1972, General Clinical Research Centers Branch, Division of Research Resources, National Institutes of Health.

Illingworth, R.S.: Development of the infant and young child, ed. 4, Baltimore, 1970, The Williams & Wilkins Co.

Johnson, F., Roche, E.A.F., and Suranne, C., editors: Human physical growth and maturation: methodologies and factors, New York 1980, Plenum Press. (Published in cooperation with NATO Scientific Affairs Bureau.)

Krogman, W.M.: Child growth, Ann Arbor, Mich., 1972, The University of Michigan Press.

Larson, R.L.: Physical activity and the growth and development of bones and joint structures. In Rarick, G., editor: Physical activity: human growth and development, New York, 1973, Academic Press, Inc.

Marshall, W.A.: Human growth and its disorders, New York, 1977, Academic Press, Inc.

McCammon, R.W.: Human growth and development, Springfield, Ill., 1970, Charles C Thomas, Publisher.

National Center for Health Statistics: Blood pressure of youths 12-17 years, United States. Data from the national health survey, Washington, D.C., 1977, series 11, no. 163, U.S. Department of Health, Education and Welfare, Public Health Services, Health Resources Administration.

National Center for Health Statistics: Dietary intake and cardiovascular risk factors. Part 1, Blood pressure correlate, United States 1971-75. Data from the national survey series 11, no. 226, Hyattsville, Md., 1983, U.S. Department of Health, Education, and Welfare, Public Health Service, National Center for Health Statistics.

National Center for Health Statistics growth charts. 1976 monthly vital statistics report, U.S. Department of Health, Education and Welfare (HRA) 76-1120, vol. 25, no. 3 (suppl.), June 22, 1976.

Ojanlatva, A., Hammer, A.M., and Mohr, M.G.: The ultimate rejection: helping the survivors of teen suicide victims, J. Sch. Health **57**(5):181, 1987.

Preventive Medicine, U.S.A.: Theory, practices, and application of prevention in personal health services: quality control and evaluation of preventive health services. Task force reports sponsored by The John E. Forgarty International Center for Advanced Study in Health Sciences, National Institutes of Health, and American Academy of Preventive Medicine, New York, 1976, Prodist, Division of Neale Watson Academic Publications, Inc.

Rarick, G.L., editor: Physical activity: human growth and development, New York, 1973, Academic Press, Inc.

Sinclair, D.: Human growth after birth, ed. 3, London, 1978, Oxford University Press.

Smith, D.W., Bierman, E.L., and Adkinson, N.W., editors: The biologic ages of man: from conception through old age, Philadelphia, 1978, W.B. Saunders Co.

Stott, L.H.: Child development: an individual longitudinal approach, New York, 1968, Holt, Rinehart & Winston.

Stuart, H.C., and Prugh, D.G., editors: The healthy child: his physical, psychological and social development, Cambridge, Mass., 1960, Harvard University Press.

Tanner, J.M.: Sequence, tempo, and individual variation in the growth and development of boys and girls aged twelve to sixteen, Daedalus, Fall 1971; also issued in Proc. Am. Acad. Arts Sci. **100**(4):904, 1971.

Tanner, J.M.: Growing up, Sci. Am. **229**:35, 1973.

Tanner, J.M.: Foetus into man: physical growth from conception to maturity, London, 1978, Open Books Publishing, Ltd.

Valadian, I.: The adolescent — his growth and development. In Proceedings of National Education Conference, November 2-4, 1971, U.S. Department of Agriculture, Miscellaneous Pub. no. 1254, Washington, D.C., 1973, U.S. Government Printing Office.

Watson, E.H., and Lowrey, G.H.: Growth and development of children, ed. 5, Chicago, 1967, Year Book Medical Publishers, Inc.

5 Psychosocial Development

OVERVIEW   *Just as the physical person grows and develops in sequential fashion, so does the psychosocial person. For today's teacher psychosocial development replaces the more simple notion of emotional development. This change acknowledges that the nonphysical development aspects are the products of a person's psychologic makeup and the continuing interaction of that person with society.*

In this chapter the nonphysical aspects of normal growth are discussed from a perspective of a widely accepted theory of personality development and from a perspective of students' evolving sense of right and wrong: their moral development. The interaction of physical and psychosocial aspects of development is acknowledged.

Knowledge about intellectual and physical development as well as psychosocial development is vital to the teacher. Many physiologically mature young people have difficulty adjusting to their social environment. What commonly has been spoken of as mental health is the balance between emotional development, physical development, and the ability to interact with all aspects of the environment—now referred to as psychosocial development.

OBJECTIVES   After reading this chapter, the student should be able to:

1. Recognize various stages of psychosocial development

2. Explain and describe various emotions

3. Outline the physiologic basis of emotions and illustrate how the physical and psychologic characteristics of a person interact

4. Describe a set of developmental tasks that represent psychosocial development among preschool children, school-aged children, and adolescents

5. Identify the role of the autonomic nervous system and the endocrine system in psychosocial development

6. Using Erikson's "stages of man" theory, illustrate the conflicting pressures that young people express

7. Explain how young people develop a sense of right and wrong

8. Explain how peer pressure is an important element in psychosocial development but not necessarily a negative pressure

9. Explain why our knowledge base of psychosocial development is less than our knowledge base of psychologic development

Understanding various levels of psychosocial development enables a teacher to understand each child more fully. The informed teacher not only knows what to expect in emotional responses from children but is also able to interpret unusual social behavior in levels of psychosocial maturity.

PHYSICAL BASIS OF PSYCHOSOCIAL DEVELOPMENT

All overt human conduct arises from a physical source: the protoplasm of the body's cells. Each person possesses a particular constitutional endowment from which emotions arise. When stimuli from the external environment produce an emotional response, virtually all the body is involved, but two systems—the neural and the endocrine—play major roles. These systems function in all coordination and adjustment and are particularly involved in emotional responsiveness. The responses of the neural system are immediate and quick acting, whereas endocrine functions are slower.

A person is conscious of emotional states, which involve the cortex of the brain, where consciousness is located. Original external stimuli reach the cortex of the brain and are relayed to the thalamus, where autonomic impulses originate.

Autonomic nervous system

The autonomic system is particularly important in emotional responses. It is often referred to as the vegetative system, since it maintains functions necessary to sustain life. This involuntary system has two divisions: the *sympathetic nervous system,* which speeds up action, and the *parasympathetic nervous system,* which has the opposite effect. All organs of the thoracic and abdominal cavities have a dual supply of autonomic nerves—sympathetics and parasympathetics—to maintain the balance of function. During emotional states these nerves are stimulated; at times the sympathetics arouse the organs, and at other times the parasympathetics reduce organ activity.

The brain's emotional center is in the thalamus, a large mass of gray matter located toward the center and base of the brain. It also is the area of the pain and temperature-regulating centers. That some people are emotionally highly responsive and others much less so is understandable in biologic terms. Sensitivity may be inherent in the nerve structure and may be further enhanced by particular endocrine influences. However, neither social conditioning nor concious training should be discounted.

Endocrine nature of temperament

Generally temperament is regarded as the emotional mold distinguishing a person. Each person's endocrine endowment greatly affects his or her temperament. Most endocrine influences are rather subtle, but some manifestations are more definite. Irritability, fatigability, apathy, enthusiasm, depression, indifference, and aggressiveness are all understandable in terms of the endocrine system.

The term *endocrine type* presumes a great deal. Persons whose basic makeup is entirely the result of extreme endocrine malfunction are rare, but examples do exist. Persons with an overproduction of thyroxin (hyperthyroidism), in addition to a tendency to lose weight and be thin, are restless, energetic, active, impatient, easily upset, impulsive, and alert. At the other pole are persons with an underproduction of thyroxin (hypothyroidism). For these individuals it is an effort, almost, to live. They maintain a low level of functioning, react slowly, fatigue easily, are usually behind in everything, rarely are enthusiastic about anything, are not easily disturbed or upset, and are usually easygoing and easily pleased.

Most persons represent various intergrades of endocrine balances. Yet a teacher must recognize that students react as they do, partly because of each student's particular biologic makeup. A wise teacher tries to understand students' conduct in terms of their basic constitutional makeup and the environment in which they live.

What motivates human conduct? What gives force and direction to what one does? Why does a person become angry or elated? Through what channels are emotions mediated? These are significant questions to all persons. They are of special importance to teachers, who, to be of the greatest value in guiding children in self-development, must understand why children act as they do (Fig. 5-1).

Human beings are biologically self-centered, self-interested, and selfish. Knowingly and unknowingly they seek self-gratification. These characteristics are principally biologic. Individuals respond physiologically to external threats in terms of survival, meaning to flee or to fight. As social creatures, however, human beings learn to ignore these biologic response patterns. Social learning and biologic urges are to varying degrees at odds, creating a tension often manifest as stress. When persons handle this tension well, it is seen by others

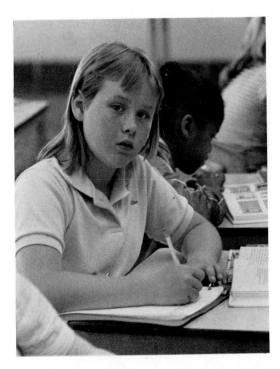

FIG. 5-1. Each student is unique, but each student also shares much in common with peers. The competent teacher will recognize differences and similarities, understand something of the reasons for these differences, and plan classroom activities accordingly.
(Copyright 1983 by David Riecks.)

as a mark of maturity, but even handling tension well can affect physical health as manifested in stress-related diseases.

Children are born with certain physiologic needs, such as hunger, thirst, and pain. The infant's self is gratified by satisfying physiologic needs as hunger and thirst, by relieving pain, by being active, and by eliminating discomfort. If the infant is in pain, hungry, or restrained, he or she responds emotionally by exhibiting emotions of dissatisfaction or fear.

All through life, gratification of these physiologic patterns is a factor in a person's emotional responsiveness. However, as one matures emotionally, emotional control rises accordingly. Although teen-aged children may not cry or show an infant's intense emotional responses, their responses differ when they are hungry from when they are not, or when they are active from when they are inactive.

The basic principles of psychosocial development are less well documented than those of physical development for two reasons. Historically, less attention has been paid to documenting the stages and phases of psychosocial growth than stages of physical growth. Also, psychosocial development is exhibited in behaviors and not the structure of physical growth; therefore it has been more difficult to document and understand.

UNIVERSAL SOCIALLY CONDITIONED MOTIVES

Children become social beings and learn to obtain self-gratification through certain socially conditioned and universally accepted motives. All normal people want attention, affection, approval, praise, and security. They seek mastery, superiority, and achievement.

The exhibition of success and failure varies from person to person. Although all persons have much in common, each is unique, and therefore reactions to similar situations differ. Just as physical health was described earlier in terms of what is normal, so too can behavior based on psychosocial development be compared to a range of normal. Unlike the physical characteristics of health wherein the range of normal is essentially the same for all people, the range of normal behaviors varies greatly. Behaviors considered normal among the people who live in the Kalahari Desert of Africa, for example, may be considered abnormal if carried out in New York City. similarly, some acceptable behaviors in New York City would likely be considered abnormal in an Eskimo village in Alaska.

Although psychosocial development has unique characteristics and is hard to judge in terms of normality, all people share similar experiences. Some groups, however, differ in certain experiences because they belong to different cultures and societies. The French, for example, share much in common with people from Greece, but each national group has certain special experiences because of their cultural heritage. Families in any culture will share some experiences of their heritage, but within this cultural grouping all families will remain unique. Of course, individuals within a family share certain experiences, but every individual in the family experiences events differently. This overlaying of similarities binds people together in cohesive groups, but the experiences make each person unique. The range of normal for psychosocial behavior is broad and is determined largely by the dominant cultural group in any given area (Fig. 5-2).

Although the character of every person is unique, there is basic agreement about important stages of psychosocial development in our society. It is acknowledged that growth of this type is an epigeneric process, that is, a process that builds one stage on another.

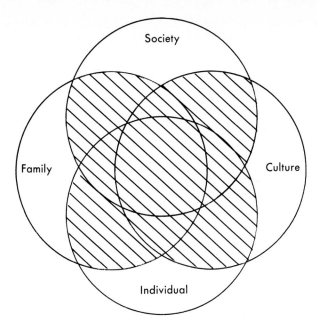

FIG. 5-2. Psychosocial development is influenced by the shared and the unique characteristics of the individual, family, society, and cultural grouping.

Duvall (1971) has described these stages in terms of tasks. Completion of these tasks not only represents health progress, but also is essential to complete subsequent tasks. These development tasks are described here in terms of the preschool child, the school-aged child, and the adolescent.

Preschool child

Developmental tasks of the preschool child include:
1. Settling into a healthful daily routine of rest, activity, and elimination
2. Mastering good eating habits
3. Developing large- and small-muscle coordination and movement skills
4. Becoming a participating member of the family
5. Beginning to master impulses and conform to parental expectations
6. Developing healthy emotional responses for a wide variety of experiences
7. Communicating effectively with others
8. Developing the ability to respond correctly to potentially hazardous situations
9. Using initiative tempered by own conscience
10. Laying the foundation to understand one's place in relation to the physical and spiritual world

Teachers generally expect children to have achieved these tasks before first grade. Preschool and kindergarten can contribute greatly to the mastery of these tasks. Because psychosocial development involves interaction with others, the increased social contact in school can help children achieve these tasks. Social contact alone, however, will not necessarily contribute to the developmental achievement of these tasks. The role of the skilled and understanding teacher is important and, outside the family, represents the most constructive monitor to ensure adequate psychosocial development.

School-aged child

Developmental tasks of the school-aged child include:
1. Mastering basic fundamental skills and a rational approach for problem solving
2. Developing concepts and reasoning abilities for everyday adult living
3. Mastering age-appropriate physical and self-care skills
4. Developing a socially accepted understanding of money: how to get it, how to spend it, and how to save it
5. Assuming an active, responsible, cooperative role within the family
6. Relating effectively to peers and other adults outside the family, that is, making and keeping friends
7. Handling feelings, emotions, and impulses appropriately
8. Learning age-appropriate sex behaviors and adjusting to prepubertal body changes
9. Developing self-respect for one's own behavior and individuality
10. Developing loyalties to religion, culture, moral values, and social institutions
11. Accepting the eternal realities of birth, death, and infinity

Developing skills to master each of these increasingly complex tasks, students grow in emotional, psychosocial maturity. Many of the skills have clear health implications beyond those related to simple psychosocial developmnent. These school-aged tasks compare with many things taught in health classes today. As students gain the ability to respond to others and build a feeling of self-worth, it becomes less difficult to teach young people to value their own bodies. It is then possible to teach students to avoid risky health-related situations such as illicit drug usage, unnecessary risk taking, and promiscuous sex (Fig. 5-3).

Adolescent

Developmental tasks of the adolescent include:
1. Accepting one's changing body and learning to use it effectively
2. Achieving a satisfying and socially accepted masculine or feminine role
3. Finding oneself as a member of one's own generation and establishing mature relations with peers
4. Achieving emotional independence from parents and other adults
5. Selecting and preparing for an occupation and economic independence
6. Preparing for marriage and family life
7. Developing intellectual skills and social sensitivities necessary for civic competence
8. Developing a workable philosophy of life that makes sense in today's world

Adolescence is not a stage bounded by specific age limits. It takes some longer than others, and unless preceded by adequate achievement of earlier developmental tasks, it may be an especially difficult period. Health-related activities for adolescents relate to these tasks in several ways. Education can address the principal public health problems of adolescence, that is, accidents and associated factors of substance abuse and risk-taking behavior; but

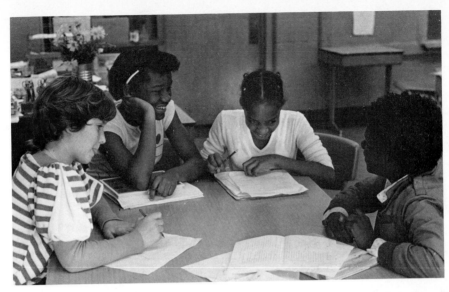

FIG. 5-3. The development of each of a series of developmental tasks is greatly facilitated by the opportunity to interact with others, to learn how they do things, and to personally experiment with a variety of ways of doing things.
(Copyright 1983 by David Riecks.)

unless this learning occurs concomitantly with appropriate psychosocial development, students won't be able to act on the basis of their knowledge. It is very difficult, for example, for a student who lacks an adequate self-concept or a clear sexual identity to deal with social or peer pressures to participate in certain high-risk behaviors.

STAGES OF DEVELOPMENT

A different way to view the psychosocial development of the school-aged child is through the eight stages described by Erikson (1963). These stages are as follows:

1. Trust vs. mistrust
2. Autonomy vs. shame and doubt
3. Initiative vs. guilt
4. Industry vs. inferiority
5. Identity vs. indentity confusion
6. Intimacy vs. isolation
7. Generativity vs. stagnation
8. Integrity vs. despair

Erikson identifies these stages as characteristic of a person's life span. Clearly stages 3 to 5 pertain to school-aged children and youth.

The *initiative vs. guilt* stage is characterized by the tremendous energy, opportunity, and action of childhood contrasted to defeatism, anger, and feeling of responsibility for things he or she can't control. Encouragement, a chance to experiment, and opportunity foster initiative, whereas excessive restrictions or excessive expectations may encourage guilt. Young people, in the early stages of childhood, experience both these pressures. For preschool and early-school children the mastery of this stage occurs at the same time they are moving away from solitary patterns of play toward parallel and cooperative patterns of play. Children are also beginning to realize that there are others, besides the family, who provide models to learn from and imitate. Also occurring at this time is the rapid development of language with all its accompanying advantages. Vocabulary increases from about 90 words at age 3 to 2000 words at age 5, thus providing greatly increased communication power.

Industry vs. *inferiority* represents the focus of energy to solve a particular problem versus a feeling of inferiority, a sense of not doing things well enough or not finishing tasks. Neither of these feelings may bear any resemblance to actual competency. Feelings of inferiority may override actual achievement.

Involvement in constructive activities that can be completed and acknowledged provides clear rewards for the sense of industry and combats feelings of inferiority. This stage occurs as the school becomes an increasingly important part of a young person's life, and there is a distinct change in the nature of family relation. Establishing friends and friendship groups is a way to deal with inferiority and an important step in establishing independence from the family. Friends can assist one another with the difficulties of development. The loner, or the social isolate, finds this time expecially difficult. However, such a person will be obvious to the teacher, who with skill and patience can help the isolated student better cope with inferiority feelings and capitalize on energy available for creative industry.

Identity vs. *identity confusion* is usually a characteristic of adolescence. The onset of adolescence is associated with the physiologic changes that accompany the beginning of sexual maturity. For girls this is initiated by *menarche,* or the onset of menstruation, beginning at about 10 to 11 years of age and developing for about 3 years. For boys development toward sexual maturity begins at about 12 years of age and usually continues for a 4-year period. The beginning of adolescence is marked by physiologic signs, but its ending is less clear.

The rapid growth of adolescents frequently provokes feelings of awkwardness, and new roles often create a sense of identity confusion. Young people respond by trying to emulate different roles, seeking a zone of comfort. Even apparently mature young people may revert to childlike behavior just as they may assume clear adult roles. They may also emulate one adult role and then another. The subsequent reactions of others to these roles and their own desires to be "grown up" leads to a degree of role confusion. Who am I? Why am I different? What do I want to be like? Can I be like I want to be? These are all questions to be dealt with in establishing personal identity.

Conflict with parents is frequent. Parents have a range of expectations, and the role experimentation of adolescents frequently exceeds the range of tolerance established consciously or unconsciously by parents. Young persons seek support and reinforcement in the various roles they try. The degree of reinforcement received encourages the acceptance of one role over another and therefore is an important force in shaping adolescent behavior. Reinforcement comes from many sources — parents, teachers, and peers; and in fact the most appropriate behaviors may not always be reinforced.

MORAL DEVELOPMENT

While physiologic and psychosocial changes are taking place, so too is a developing sense of what is right and what is wrong. Kohlberg (1964) describes moral development as related in part to cognitive development. In the early years, from ages 4 to 10, Kohlberg suggests morality is based on recognition of an action's physical consequences. Right or wrong is defined by punishment. The presence of the threat of punishment indicates a wrong. This is a premoral or preconventional stage of development in Kohlberg's typology.

From about 10 years of age there develops what Kohlberg calls conventional morality. In this stage individuals are pressured to "obey the rules" by the expectations of others and desire to conform out of a sense of duty and respect. This is the level at which the majority of the population operates most of their lives. However, in late adolescence some develop what has been called "postconventional morality."

Postconventional morality operates apart from the pressures to conform to the will of others and represents the development of autonomous moral principles based on an individual's unique experiences. This postconventional morality is linked with the development of cognitive knowledge, past experience, and reasoning ability. Only a small proportion of the population operates at the postconventional level of moral development. They are free of the preconceived constraints of others' expectations and therefore often make significant contributions to society. They dare to break barriers and to lead and experiment, and as a result society often benefits.

In the school years young people break free from the family, develop physiologically, develop a sense of identity, and become moral beings at the same time that they attempt to master the cognitive and affective challenges of schooling. From a psychosocial perspective this is a turbulent period. Many changes take place within each individual and the individual also lives in a changing environment. The family is changing; social conflict within the community is unsettling; and such things as global tensions cannot be forgotten, for each indirectly affects the developing student.

PEER PRESSURE

Peer pressure and how students react to it indicate something about psychosocial development. Similarly, how well a teacher understands peer pressure determines how well he or she can capture some of its energy and use it to positive ends.

Conventional wisdom too frequently suggests that peer pressure is the base of most teen-aged problems and there is little that can be done about it. The concept of peer pressure makes an excellent generic whipping boy to blame for so many failures to "improve" adolescents' behavior.

Peer pressure is not limited to adolescents: it is a phenomenon all people experience. However, for adolescents who are seeking an identity of their own and developing an adequate self-concept, peer pressure is a difficult force to deal with. Young people respond variously to the pressures of others; sometimes they seek to belong and to be like others, but at other times they contradict pressures, seeking to stand alone, testing possible identity roles. Understanding how adolescents interpret and respond to pressures applied by others is critical for teachers who work with young people. The term *peer pressure* oversimplifies a complex process.

Peer pressure is often considered a single force where one youngster is encouraged to do something by others. Careful analysis, however, indicates that this is not the case. Although peer pressure is discussed as a single force, it is in reality a combination of forces. These forces may appear singular in effect, but to consider them as a single entity in planning health education and school health programs overlooks several options. Evans and co-workers (1978), for example, identify peers, media, and parents as the major pressures seen by young people. Parental and media messages present an environmental backdrop against which young people interpret their peers' expectations.

The tendency to see peer pressure as overt acts to coerce one individual to comply with the will of others is only one perspective of this phenomenon. Another perspective is more subtle. It involves pressures presented as others' expectations to which young people respond. All persons, for example, seek recognition; therefore they interpret the expectations of others and act so that they will receive recognition. Adolescents in particular seek to appear "grown up" and to be like adults, and so they emulate adult images and models. Young people also report that there is significant pressure to have fun, but frequently the role of fun overlaps the role of risk-taking behavior, sometimes with unfortunate consequences.

It is important to recognize therefore that peer pressure is in reality a perceptual issue. Peer pressure results from perceptions that others want a person to act in a particular way. Perceptions result from messages received, and like other messages, their meaning is determined by the receiver, not the sender. Adolescents, however, do not have much experience in interpreting these messages. Many adults also inappropriately determine the perception of pressures and have difficulty in dealing with them. In the health area, a critical way to help young people deal with the perceptions of others is to ensure that they have adequate factual knowledge to use in interpreting perceptions. There is good evidence that young people can be significantly helped in this area. For example, Martin and Duryea (1981) report that junior and senior high school students consistently overestimate the proportion of their peers, older adolescents, and teachers who smoke cigarettes. Because adolescents seek to identify a role for themselves and want to be like the majority of people, this misinterpretation encourages them to smoke. The reality is that less than half of the population smokes, and to be like the majority, one need not smoke.

The environment also provides a large number of perceptual cues important to young people passing through adolescence and to which health personnel must be sensitive. For example, mass media, through programs and advertisements, present a variety of messages that imply ways to have fun, establish individuality, establish sex roles, and appear mature, successful, and grown up. Similarly, lax law enforcement presents messages to adolescents; in areas such as alcohol and driving it conveys a message that young people may not be able to interpret adequately.

Role models in person and in discussion are also critically important. If adulthood is not realistically described and presented in the educational process, the idealized images of the mass media may create unrealistic expectations in adolescents.

Because peer pressure is essentially a conforming force, psychosocial development must involve the establishment of an adequate self-concept and the achievement of developmental tasks so that a balance can be struck between the conformity of society and individuals' needs and responsibilities. Later, this text describes educational programs that provide ways for the teacher to help young people in a critical stage of psychosocial development deal with peer pressure in the interest of their personal health.

ADAPTATION

Just as adaptation is a critical component of health, so too is adaptation a critical element in psychosocial well-being. The environment includes physical dimensions, as well as other people, to which individuals need to adapt. At the same time, individuals adapt to the idiosyncratic changes occurring within themselves as developing individuals. The school nurse and health teacher must help students to recognize that although they are unique persons they are also like most others, going through unsettling but predictable changes. However, this should not imply that each student is able to survive these times alone just by knowing others are going through a similar experience. The process of healthy psychosocial development can be greatly facilitated by conscious efforts to adapt the environment, both physical and social. For example, teaching stress-coping skills as a part of physical education or health classes can provide an invaluable skill to use throughout this period. Teachers can coordinate weekly tests so that all are not always given on Fridays. Pleasant work and study environments and judicious use of colors and textures can improve the "spirit" of the school.

The establishment of clear and consistent codes of behavior and discipline clearly delineates expectations and removes one more uncertainty. Within clear discipline guidelines "space" for social experimentation will facilitate adolescents' need to try different roles in establishing self-identity. This means teachers should tolerate change in their students. Unfortunately schools and school personnel sometimes have a tendency to "type" students and unwittingly become insensitive to changes for the better.

Physical health is clearly visible, and any deviations even minor ones, are usually visible to the teacher. Teachers are accustomed to dealing with physical health problems and in the main do an adequate job of handling them. Mental health problems and difficulties in psychosocial development, on the other hand, are less noticeable unless they are extreme.

The fact that suicide and homicide rank third and fourth as causes of adolescent death illustrates the significance of psychosocial issues. Abuse of alcohol and drugs, fatal automobile accidents, and teen-aged pregnancy all are manifestations of difficulty with psychosocial development.

Most schools have the counseling services, but too often the organization of health services within a school indicates a lack of sensitivity to student health as a total concept. One way to assess how well the school has accepted health as a central issue in education is to check the organizational pattern of academic services, health services, and counseling services. Is there provision for a regular review of students who experience educational difficulty by a team of academic personnel, the school nurse, and the school counselor, or are students only referred from one to another of these specialists?

The necessity of interaction between physical health, psychosocial development, and academic performance is clear. A school organization should develop some formal opportunity for records of students with problems to be reviewed by an interdisciplinary team (i.e., teachers, physicians or nurses, and counselors) representing the three initial aspects of education, physical growth, and psychosocial development. The student must be reviewed as a whole to identify how the school can be most effective.

SUMMARY

Physical growth and development are easily observed. Psychosocial development can be determined only by observation of behaviors or the consequences of behavior. The challenge to school personnel is to interpret an ever-changing scene filled with rapidly growing young people and still be able to identify students who may need special assistance.

Psychosocial development is based on physical form and physical health. Frequently problems of psychosocial development can be traced to physical abnormalities. Such problems as low achievement and unruliness may result from undetected vision or hearing problems or even abnormalities in blood chemistry — conditions that can often be easily corrected.

A good school health program exhibits sensitivity to the physical well-being of students. An excellent school health program shows the same sensitivity to the psychosocial needs of its students. This includes knowing the psychosocial skills that are normal for preschool, elementary, intermediate, and adolescent youngsters. All school activities should be geared to helping students develop these psychosocial skills. The challenge is to keep the student's total development in perspective. A math teacher who sees students as junior computers and a coach who emphasizes sports as total commitment are examples of failures to recognize the principles presented in this chapter.

It is important to remember that all development occurs in a social environment, a community. Therefore the psychosocial environment within a school community is important. Developing a supportive environment and helping students understand their place in this environment so that they can develop a sense of self-worth and skills to interact with others is the best that school personnel can do to facilitate psychosocial development.

STUDY QUESTIONS

1. Why is psychosocial development a more appropriate title than mental development?
2. If all behavior has a physiologic basis, what is the difference between the sympathetic and parasympathetic nervous systems and how do they offset behavior?
3. What role does the endocrine system play in behavior?
4. If all behavior is biologically based, what distinguishes the human species from other species?
5. How is it that a person can be said to be part of a social unit yet at the same time be a unique being?
6. Outline the principal developmental tasks that should be achieved by (a) preschool children, (b) school-aged children, and (c) adolescents.
7. Which factor makes it more difficult to define "normal" psychosocial development compared with normal physical development?
8. In which ways are Erikson's stages of development useful in helping school health personnel deal with students?
9. The idea of teaching morals or moral education is an especially controversial topic, but why is it important for teachers to understand how the ability to make moral decisions is related to cognitive development?
10. In which ways can peer pressure be seen as a positive force for school health personnel?
11. Identify some important health problem that may result from poor psychosocial development.
12. How can a health teacher assist students in psychosocial development?

REFERENCES

Capuzzi, C.: Herschi's bond theory, juvenile delinquency and the school nurse, J. Sch. Health **52**:280, 1982.

Crabbs, M.: School mental health services following an environmental disaster, J. Sch. Health **51**:165, 1981.

Erikson, E.: Childhood and society, New York, 1963, W.W. Norton & Co.

Evans, R., et al.: Deterring the onset of smoking in children: knowledge of immediate physiological effects and coping with peer pressure, media pressure, and parent modeling, J. Appl. Soc. Psychol. **8**:126, April-June 1978.

Jerrick, S.: Mental health in schools, J. Sch. Health **48**:559, 1978.

Kohlberg, L.: Development of moral character and moral ideology. In Hoffman, M., and Hoffman, L.: Review of child development research, vol. 1, New York, 1964, Russell Sage Foundation.

Martin, G., and Duryea, E.: The distortion effect in student perception of smoking prevalence, J. Sch. Health **51**:115, 1981.

Moore, R.S., and Moore, D.: When education becomes abuse: a different look at the mental health of children, J. Sch. Health **56**:73, 1986.

Departures from Normal Health, Growth, and Development

OVERVIEW   *Knowledge of departures from normal health is important to teachers so that they can interpret routine information in student files and be sensitive to the daily referral needs of students. Today's philosophies of education and health care mean teachers are almost assured of having students in their classrooms who would previously have been precluded from regular school because of health conditions. Usually major changes are unnecessary to accommodate these children, but the professional teacher will want to know about these conditions to make knowledgeable decisions about classroom activities and individual learning activities.*

In addition, teachers will frequently be the first to notice deviations from normal health or growth and development that are often visible through changes in student performance or student appearance. Teachers are not responsible for diagnosis or treatment, but knowledge of the most common health problems experienced by their students improves their ability to plan and carry out effective learning activities.

OBJECTIVES   After reading this chapter, the student should be able to:

1. Identify and describe the most common medical conditions likely to be found among the student population

2. Recognize and use opportunities to help students understand and accept health conditions among their fellow students

3. Assist students who may need additional care or referral and initiate appropriate referrals with confidence

4. Recognize a teacher's professional role in working with students whose growth, development, or health deviates from normal

Every school can expect to have children who deviate from the normal. Some minor deviations affect the youngster little or not at all. In other instances the deviation may greatly limit the child so that special provisions must be made. Whatever the deviation, there are correct and incorrect ways to deal with the situation. Children with significant disabilities can still reach their optimal levels of health. Handled incorrectly, children with disabilities can be made to feel that they are outsiders, with resulting harm to mental and physical health.

Generally speaking, normal children are eager to accept and assist the child who has some disability. Perhaps nothing in a teacher's experience could be more rewarding than to make a normal or near-normal school life possible for the child who has some departure from the normal. Sometimes the demand on the teacher may be great; at other times it may be small. Whatever the situation, the teacher's present contribution may well benefit the person throughout life.

Teachers are eager to do everything reasonable for children who have a disability or deviation in growth and development but are sometimes hesitant to act because they lack confidence in their knowledge of such conditions. No teacher, whether an elementary classroom teacher or a secondary school health educator, should be considered an expert on any of these conditions, but the teacher should understand their essentials.

Schools do not have a recognized legal responsibility for the correction or improvement of health defects in any child, but schools do have a responsibility to ensure that children receive an adequate education to function well in society. When health problems interfere with learning, the school is obligated to concern itself with these problems. Obviously the sick child cannot learn as well as the healthy child; therefore both the child and society are shortchanged in their investment in education if health problems are overlooked.

Health problems among students interefere with learning in several ways. An illness or health condition that affects a child's rate of learning may attract a disproportionate amount of the teacher's time and energy at the expense of other students. Health problems are often manifest as disciplinary problems, and the resulting class disruption interferes with the entire class's learning. Students with untreated infectious conditions run the risk of infecting others and causing undue absenteeism; they also increase the risks of illness for the teacher.

The responsibility to do everything reasonable for the health and well-being of the schoolchild rests in the basic obligation of the school. This commitment to deal with health issues can be fulfilled in various ways, such as the following:

1. Bringing the child's condition to the parents' attention
2. Following up such a referral
3. Counseling the parents regarding means of obtaining necessary professional services
4. Seeking outside financial assistance to obtain the correct services
5. Carrying out at school certain instructions from the child's physician or other practitioner
6. Adapting the school program to the needs of the specific child

7. Helping the child to help himself or herself in solving health problems that are not directly under the supervision of any practitioner

8. Most important, understanding fully the child's condition and problems and making adjustments in school life to provide a more enjoyable and effective school environment

The role of the teacher is neither diagnostician nor therapist. The teacher needs to know which health conditions can affect the student favorably as well as unfavorably in order to plan in the best interests of the student (Fig. 6-1).

UNDERACHIEVEMENT AND LOW VITALITY

The one condition that is most noticeable to teachers and may not have identifiable health-related causes is underachievement, or low levels of vitality. Underachievement may result from many causes ranging from diagnosed medical conditions to social, psychologic, or other environmental concerns. Heredity, prematurity, lead poisoning, and malnutrition are a few of the conditions that can cause low vitality and underachievement. More common, however, are conditions related to parental support, peer pressure, and family and community problems.

A useful way to consider causes of underachievement is to divide possible contributing

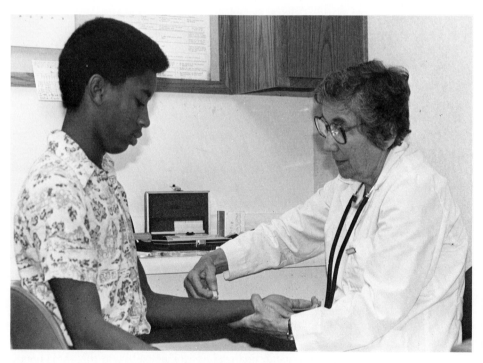

FIG. 6-1. An effective school health program has the potential to aid in the early referral of students with possible health problems. Effective communication between school administrators, local physicians, and health department personnel often facilitates the obtaining of health services for students.
(Copyright 1983 by David Riecks.)

factors into two categories: external and internal. Most causes are external, associated in one way or another with the student's environment rather than actual clinical health. Thus it is not unusual to find children with clear records on both health examinations and health screenings who still exhibit chronic underachievement. However, it is important that children exhibiting low achievement and low vitality be referred for medical examination to ensure that no correctable internal conditions are contributing to the problem.

Students who have a record of underachievement with no clear internal causes for this problem should be examined in terms of inappropriate class placement, family problems, and poor relationships with others. Each of these factors represents an important contribution to understanding and dealing with underachievers.

Inappropriate class placement, for example, can result in a child's boredom with the class content or inability to understand the class content because of failure to master earlier concepts. Personality clashes with teachers are also possible causes, as are many other class-related issues. Families suffering economic hardships, serious illness, marital tension, or recent bereavement may partly explain underachievement. Unrealistic parental expectations and overprotective parents may contribute to this condition. Lack of motivation may result from social messages that do not place a high value on educational achievement and from parents who present models of low achievement and low motivation. Family or community members may be economic and social successes but may not show respect or value for formal education.

Low vitality also results from functional conditions in the environment. Homes that lack any semblance of a regular schedule, in which children get little sleep or sleep irregular hours, are a principal contributing cause. Involvement of children in outside work, as on a farm, may also figure prominently in low vitality in school.

The nature and extent of underachievement from internal causes have not been clearly described. A host of terms has been used to describe conditions related to underachievement and low motivation. These terms include minimal brain dysfunction, learning disability syndrome, and the hyperactive child syndrome. In general, these conditions can be classified as attentional deficiencies and have been grouped in the third edition of the *Diagnostic and Statistical Manual of Mental Disorders* (American Psychiatric Association, 1980) as attentional deficit disorders.

Each of the conditions now grouped under attentional deficit disorders has been described in the past as having some element of attentional dysfunction. The term *minimal brain dysfunction,* for example, implied organic causes or abnormalities, which may not have always been the case. Minimal brain dysfunction correctly covers a group of wide-ranging conditions, and the implication of organic abnormality is unwarranted. *Hyperactivity* is a term that has been used rather loosely and is manifest in schools most prominently as an attentional problem. *Learning disabilities* referred to cognitive deficits, often but not necessarily associated with hyperactivity.

The vagueness of these terms and the likelihood that these conditions are interrelated have led to the more general term of *attentional deficit disorders.* Attentional deficit disorders are separate and distinct from the conditions of mental retardation, sensory disorders, and emotional disorders and can be more objectively identified.

Attentional deficit disorders are more common among boys than among girls. Estimates of prevalence range from 1 per 1000 to 5 or 6 per 100. This discrepancy results from different diagnostic criteria and variation in rates from one population to another.

The *Diagnostic and Statistical Manual of Mental Disorders* (American Psychiatric Association, 1980) defines the diagnostic criteria for attentional deficit disorders as follows:

1. There is excessive general hyperactivity or motor restlessness for the child's age. In preschool and early school years there may be excessive, haphazard, impulsive running, climbing, or crawling. During middle childhood or adolescence, up-and-down activity, an inability to sit still, and fidgeting are characteristic. Activity differs from the norm for the age in both quality and quantity.

2. The child exhibits difficulty in sustaining attention, an inability to complete tasks, or a disorganized approach to tasks. The child frequently "forgets" demands made or tasks assigned and shows poor attention in structured situations or when independent unsupervised performance is required.

3. Impulsive behavior is manifest by at least two of the following:
    a. Sloppy work despite reasonable efforts to perform adequately
    b. Frequent speaking out of turn or making inappropriate sounds in class
    c. Frequent interruption of or intrusion into other children's activities or conversations
    d. Difficulty waiting for one's turn in games or group situations
    e. Poor frustration tolerance
    f. Fighting with children in a fashion indicating low frustration tolerance rather than sadistic or mean intentions

4. The condition lasts at least 1 year.

It is not the teacher's task to diagnose students with any condition, but a review of these conditions should help the teacher who needs to make a referral. Most children with attentional deficit disorders are usually referred for assessment in the first two or three grades of elementary school.

MALNUTRITION

Severe or pronounced malnutrition is relatively uncommon among children in the United States today, but moderate and mild malnutrition are far more prevalent than is commonly known. A teacher easily recognizes pronounced obesity and underweight, but children who lack sufficient protective foods to meet the *recommended dietary allowances* (RDAs) are not readily detectable. Although the general school health program should promote the nutrition of every school child, certain children merit special attention because of recognized or suspected nutritional needs. Teachers should also be aware of nutritional influences of their own school administration's policies and practices. Too often school administrators respond to student and parental pressure to install vending machines that dispense nonnutritional, high-calorie, salt- and additive-laden items. Alert teachers can encourage school administrators to provide nutritious snacks in school vending machines.

The U.S. Center for Disease Control (1973) reports that adolescents between 10 and 16 years old are most likely to have the poorest nutritional status of any age group. Nutritional needs vary with sex and age, with the greatest nutritional need associated with greatest physical growth. The most accelerated growth periods tend to be between 12 and 17 years of age. Among girls, the height and growth spurt begins between 10 and 11 years of age and lasts 2 ½ to 3 years. Among boys this period starts around 12 years and may last to 15 years of age (Heald, 1975). Malnutrition represented by underweight may have both physiologic and social causes (e.g., parental neglect).

Obesity

Children more than 10% overweight for their age are considered obese. In some children overweight by more than 10% may not affect health adversely during childhood, but the long-term effect may lower the level of health. The American Academy of Pediatrics (1981) notes that 15% of adolescent girls and about 7% of adolescent boys are obese. About 80% of obese children become obese adults. Although no physical effect may be discernible, obesity reduces both the effectiveness and enjoyment of living. A child who carries around an excess weight of 15 pounds (6.8 kg) is likely to fatigue easily. Although the added burden may not tax a normal heart, a slightly defective heart may be strained seriously. Obesity handicaps play and muscular reactions. Obese children are frequently taunted and ridiculed and may be considered different by their peers. Being classed out of the normal category is not conducive to the best mental health for a developing child.

Obesity results from eating more calories than one uses. Even when a glandular disorder exists in which organic substances readily turn to fat, the organic compounds come from what a person eats. The remedy for obesity is to eat less or expend more calories or both. Any child who is obese has been eating too much. Long-established family dietary customs may well produce obese children who become conditioned to excessive eating. Once this psychophysiologic pattern is established, obese children find it progressively more difficult to reduce their food intake. Their problem is both physiologic and psychologic.

Hunger is basically physiologic, governed by the glucose (sugar) level of the blood. When the blood glucose level is low, a person experiences sensations of hunger. Immediately after a meal, the blood glucose level is high. This high level affects the output of insulin from the pancreas. Over time insulin converts excess blood glucose to stable glycogen, which is stored in the liver and muscles. This results in a low blood glucose level and hunger. Only limited amounts of glycogen can be stored in the liver and muscles, and the excess is converted to body fat. To meet energy needs and reduce the buildup of fat is the challenge of good nutrition.

About 12% of daily calories in United States diets comes from protein, about 42% from fat and 46% from carbohydrates. Experts suggest that fats be reduced to 30% and the proportion of carbohydrates increased.

Carbohydrates, especially complex carbohydrates (fruits, vegetables, dried peas, beans, cereals, breads, rice, pasta), are the recommended energy source compared to sugars, syrups, and candies, which contribute almost nothing to the diet but calories.

The body metabolizes carbohydrates to provide energy and numerous other benefits. Glycogen helps the liver protect the body against toxins and protein breakdown. Stored glycogen makes available protein for cell repair rather than for energy. Complex carbohydrates also provide needed fiber in the diet.

Obese children who can reduce their caloric intake by 600 calories per day should lose 1 pound (454 g) per week. This is a wholesome weight-reduction rate. Cutting down on portions and increasing the proportion of complex carbohydrates in the diet to allay between-meal hunger are the two points that must be emphasized. If at all possible, dieting should be done under medical supervision. Encouragement from the teacher and cooperation from the family increase the likelihood of controlling.

When there is a combination of underweight and illness, it is the province of the medical profession to find the underlying causes. The observant teacher initiates the chain reaction to bring the child and physician together.

The school correlates its efforts with the home and the family physician. At minimum, the teacher should confer with the parents when concerned about a child's weight. Often parents, too, are concerned and express the wish that something could be done. Proposing a health examination is in order. From the examination may come a recommended program or the identification of the child as healthy and normal in all respects, including weight for his or her particular constitutional type.

It obviously is not the role of teachers to diagnose deficiency diseases. They may suspect that a specific condition results from nutritional deficiency. If, as a health project, each child records the family menus for a week, the teacher's suspicions may receive further support. Yet in the absence of medical diagnosis and direction, the teacher's province is primarily that of education that results in desirable knowledge, attitudes, and practices. A teacher with ingenuity and a sincere interest in the child uses the school lunch, the home, and self-interest to achieve a gradual yet tangible improvement in the student's general condition. A well-thought out plan to assure the child of the necessary quality foods is basic (Fig. 6-2).

EATING DISORDERS
Anorexia nervosa

Anorexia nervosa occurs most frequently among females (10:1). It is seen often among persons 11 to 35 years of age and peaks in prevalence in the late teens. Dally and Gomez (1979) describe anorexia nervosa as a "disorder of puberty." Clinically the dramatic weight loss is associated with (1) refusal to eat and maintain normal weight, (2) a loss of 15% or more of expected body weight, (3) intense fear of becoming obese, and (4) amenorrhea for three consecutive months when menstruation has previously been regular. These conditions appear in the absence of organic disease that would otherwise account for weight loss.

In effect, the anorectic student loses control over eating and out of an extreme fear of being "fat" ceases to eat. The resulting condition interferes with development and produces fatigue, depression, and ultimately a total loss of appetite. Anorexia nervosa is not a 'loss of appetite attributable to nerves' as the name may suggest. Persons with this condition do not actually lose their appetites until a very late stage of their illness.

Bulimia

Bulimia is an eating disorder characterized by periodic binge eating followed by purging. During binges there is a fear of not being able to stop eating. Purging usually includes self-induced vomiting and the use of laxatives and may also include patterns of extreme dieting or exercise to overcome the excessive eating. The clinical definition (DSM-III) indi-

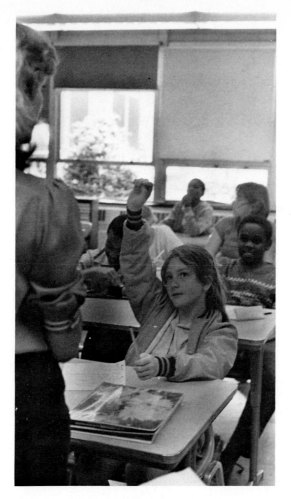

FIG. 6-2. Observations by teachers provide an opportunity for a continuing assessment of student health. Teachers are often the first to notice signs of illness. An effective school health service involves teachers, nurses, parents, physicians, and counselors to ensure students a maximal opportunity to learn.
(Copyright 1983 by David Riecks.)

cates that for confirmed diagnosis of bulimia a person binge eats at least twice a week for at least 3 months.

For the teacher, any evidence of binge eating or discussion of this possibility by a student should be addressed with information about the condition and its consequences. The current trend of "dieting" and the often unrealistic images of the ideal body encourage behavior that can lead to the development of nutritional problems along the continuum of eating disorders. A person may begin to reduce food intake, may begin to believe she can control the process, and, when she feels excessively hungry, may overeat. Guilt follows, and purging is seen as a way to reduce guilt and "get back on the diet." The pattern is established and becomes habitual.

Anorexia nervosa and bulimia are two distinct conditions that result from similar underlying causes: poor self-esteem, insecurity, and the need to be perfect or to control. It is possible for students to exhibit signs of both conditions. To understand the way these two conditions may occur together it is useful to think of them as two ends of a continuum with the area in the middle reflecting some combination of the two.

For the developing adolescent this critical problem needs expert attention. However, in a well-established form, anorexia nervosa and bulimia are not easy to treat, and so referral in the early stages is important. Classes in nutrition, health, and physical education help adolescents understand normal growth and development, and the school staff should facilitate the development of strong and adequate self-concepts and the acceptance of individual differences. Such efforts help prevent anorexia nervosa and bulimia, facilitate early identification and referral, and help others understand and be supportive of those with eating disorders.

Digestive system disturbances

Most digestive disturbances in school-aged children are accompanied by symptoms and signs that warn that something is wrong. The symptoms might include a mild upset from which the child recovers in a relatively short period of time, or they may be chronic in nature, ultimately involving the need for medical service, hospitalization, home care, or special school programs.

Symptoms describe the sensations that the patient experiences. These may include nausea, pain, elevated temperature, irritability, or headache.

Signs describe what can be seen by observation of the patient. These include flushed skin, restlessness, red, watery eyes, or facial grimaces. Mild symptoms and signs do not necessarily denote a mild illness.

Iron deficiency anemia

Anemia literally means 'without blood' (Gr. *an-*, without; *haima*, blood), but in its practical sense anemia is a condition in which the red corpuscle count or the hemoglobin content of the blood is low or both deficiencies are present.

Iron deficiency anemia is more common in girls than in boys. Approximately 5% of adolescent boys have confirmed iron deficiency anemia. Among adolescent girls from affluent homes the prevalence is 12%, and among those from low-income homes the rate is 20% (Faigel, 1973). The reason for the difference in the male and female rates is related to the female body's poorer ability to shepherd iron, to the low level of testosterone (a principally male sex hormone), which stimulates the production of red blood cells, and to the loss of blood associated with menstruation.

The presence of iron deficiency anemia is indicated by low hemoglobin and low hematocrit levels. Hemoglobin is the red pigment of erythrocytes that has the ability to carry oxygen. Hematocrit levels represent the proportion of whole blood volume occupied by cells after centrifuge. Symptoms of iron deficiency are irritability, fatigue, difficulty concentrating, headache, and in females heavy menstrual flow.

Iron deficiency anemia can be corrected relatively easily with an improved diet, including iron-rich foods such as liver, red meats, green vegetables, whole grains, and the prescription of ferrous sulfate. Required diet changes are significant, however, because females need four times more iron than males do.

ENDOCRINE DISTURBANCES
Diabetes mellitus

Although it is generally considered a disease of later life, *diabetes mellitus* does occur among school-aged children and occasionally among preschool children. One child in 1000 is affected by diabetes mellitus, and although this prevalence may seem low, it is the most common chronic endocrine disease among young people between 10 and 19 years of age (Sussman, 1971). Medical authorities point out that for every four known cases, three unrecognized cases of diabetes exist.

Most people who have diabetes can keep well and lead healthful and useful lives. Careful attention to the physician's instructions safeguard the student's health. In this respect the school can be of appreciable service to the diabetic student.

Diabetes mellitus usually results from a deficiency in the insulin output of the islands of Langerhans in the pancreas. It also may be caused by a deficiency of the glycogenic hormone of the anterior pituitary gland. A deficiency of these hormones results in a high level of blood glucose *(hyperglycemia)* and glucose in the urine *(glycosuria)*. Lassitude and weariness result, as well as pronounced thirst after meals and, with the subsequent consumption of water, frequent urination. Increased hunger, a drawn expression, and a loss of weight may occur. The mouth is dry, and the tongue is red and sore. Dry skin, itching, eczema, and boils may occur. The eyes are affected, and neuritis, numbness, and tingling of the hands and feet occur. Pronounced weakness results from the inability of the muscles to use available fuel.

Some diabetic students may be on a restricted diet, often sufficient to control the condition. The physician or parents should inform the school of the prescribed diet and routine for physical activity. The teacher guides the child in adherence to the prescription.

Exercise lowers insulin requirements so that blood glucose levels and insulin dosage levels are also lowered. The American Academy of Pediatrics recommends the following guidelines (1987):

1. During physical activity needed insulin may be 20% to 30% less than other times. Insulin should be injected in muscles not heavily used in the sport or activity.
2. Insulin dosage may need to be adjusted so that peaks do not coincide with high-activity periods.
3. High-carbohydrate foods should be eaten an hour before strenuous exercise. Food with readily available glucose should be available during periods of exercise, and additional food may be needed the day after strenuous exercise to replenish glycogen stores.
4. Coaches and teammates should be taught to recognize and treat insulin reactions.
5. Rapid weight-loss regimes, such as those sometimes unwisely practiced by wrestlers or others, are especially dangerous to diabetics and should be avoided.
6. Medical advice should always be sought and followed.

Children being treated with insulin will probably receive their injection at least 1 hour before coming to school. Occassionally fluctuations of the effect occur, and a low blood glucose level (*hypoglycemia*) may result. In extreme forms the condition is commonly spoken of as *insulin shock,* the early signs of which are trembling, faintness, palpitation, unsteadiness, excessive perspiration, and hunger. Crackers, bread, or juice produces recovery in a few minutes. Some children carry a small supply of crackers or bread and eat them immediately on appearance of symptoms.

Hypoglycemia

Abnormal behavior in children can arise from an unusual body metabolism and, as a consequence, mask the true cause and nature of the illness. *Hypoglycemia* is one of these conditions. The dominant factor is a low level of glucose in the blood, responsible for periods of irritability, confusion, depression, lethargy, complaints of weakness in the extremities, and inability to concentrate. When a physician puts the patient on a selective diet, the patient's behavior improves.

Teachers need to be aware that the signs of hypoglycemia may be mistaken for other behavioral problems. Children who are irritable, confused, or lethargic may be mistaken for being drunk, drugged, or acting out. To overlook the possibility of hypoglycemia or to treat it as a discipline issue can have unfortunate consequences. Teachers who observe these signs should check the student's health records for indications of hypoglycemia or refer the student to the school nurse.

CARDIOVASCULAR DISORDERS

Approximately 1% of schoolchildren in the United States have a diagnosed cardiac disorder. Together, rheumatic fever and its accessory, rheumatic heart disorder, cause more disability than any other disease of childhood. A second important cardiac disorder of childhood is congenital heart defect. In both, the everyday management or supervision of the child is all important. A teacher who knows what should and can be done makes an invaluable contribution to the child's well-being.

Rheumatic fever

Rheumatic fever, an insidious disease, overtakes a child stealthily. Although it undoubtedly is infectious, the causative agent is unknown. However, physicians generally agree that a certain type of infection is the forerunner of rheumatic fever. Group A *beta-hemolytic streptococcus,* which produces a sore throat, is the recognized source of rheumatic fever. From this primary infection two additional phases delineate the evolution of rheumatic fever:
1. Middle (dormant) phase — lasts 2 to 3 weeks after the sore throat during which no visible symptoms appear; child seems completely recovered
2. Final phase (acute rheumatic fever) — lasts from 2 to 3 weeks to several months
Although most afflicted children have a physician's services, some children appear in the classroom without the benefit of medical advice. The teacher who recognizes certain danger signals contributes immeasurably to the child's welfare by bringing the matter to the parents' attention. Early detection may prevent the most serious complication — rheumatic heart disease.

Specific symptoms do not exist in every case of rheumatic fever, but common symptoms include irritability; undue fatigue; nosebleeds; pallor; pain in the joints, arms, and legs; jerky and twitching motions; poor appetite; loss of weight; and a lack of interest in school activities. The teacher makes no mistake in contacting the parents of a child with several of these symptoms because there obviously is something wrong.

Rheumatic fever is not communicable; therefore prevention is directed toward the conditions that precede it. Preventing the spread of throat infections in the school should indirectly reduce the incidence of rheumatic fever. Prompt medical treatment for any throat infection prevents it from becoming the forerunner of rheumatic fever.

Because rheumatic fever tends to run in families, members of the patient's family should be informed of the need for a well-balanced diet, adequate rest, early treatment of respiratory infections, and regular medical supervision. A child with rheumatic fever will receive long-term medication from the physician to prevent repeated attacks.

Rheumatic heart disease

Two out of three patients with rheumatic fever suffer damaged hearts. A single attack may cause minor damage, but recurrence of the disease will likely cause further damage. With regular medical supervision, recurrent attacks can be prevented.

During the acute stage of the infection the heart muscle may be affected. This muscle inflammation (*myocarditis*) may weaken and enlarge the heart. At times the outer heart covering is inflamed (*pericarditis*). As the infection declines, the heart tends to return to normal size. Permanent injury usually results from inflammation of the valves on the left half of the heart. During the healing process scar tissue forms, which prevents the valves from opening or closing properly.

About a third of children with rheumatic fever show no evidence of heart damage; about one third more show signs of cardiac injury but lead practically normal lives.

No limitations should be placed on the child except those advised by the physician. From the physician's advice the teacher makes classroom adaptations. Such adjustments may include permission for the child to be late to school, special transportation, between-meal snacks, rest periods, restricted recess and physical education activity, and a minimum of stair climbing. As much as possible children should be made to feel that they are not abnormal but can, with some exceptions, participate in the regular classroom work.

Congenital heart defects

A child may be born with a defective heart. Some defects are so severe that the child does not survive to school age. With other defects, the child can attend school. Some congenital heart conditions benefit from surgery; others cannot be helped by methods now known. Some congenital heart disorders are so minor that they can essentially be ignored. Others are not serious enough to prevent a child from attending school, yet the child needs everyday supervision and management. From this range, it is apparent that knowledge of these defects enables the teacher to cooperate effectively with the child's physician.

Many cardiac patients can participate in regular classroom activities. Restriction or limitation should not be imposed except on instruction from the child's physician. Many of these children limit their own activity when necessary because of the distress of fatigue. A physician may rule out competitive sports for children because in the excitement of competition they may be oblivious to fatigue. Restrictions imposed by the physician are only those that are necessary because, for children to be mentally healthy, they must live as normal a life as possible. It is essential that children develop a wholesome, positive attitude toward their capacities and abilities. The teacher should emphasize what they can do and give less emphasis to what they cannot do if they are on a restrictive regimen.

Hypertension

High blood pressure is not frequent among children of school age but does occasionally occur. Evidence indicates that young people with elevated blood pressure at two successive annual or biannual examinations are likely to have high blood pressure as adults (National Heart, Lung and Blood Institute, 1982).

Even in a normal person systolic blood pressure may vary considerably, but in *hypertension* the blood pressure consistently will be above 140 mm Hg systolic and 90 mm Hg diastolic. Sometimes the condition is functional, the result of mental and emotional tensions. If tensions are relieved, these persons improve considerably. Sometimes the condition is organic. Certain renal, endocrine, vascular, and cerebral disorders may cause hypertension.

The school should rely on the students' family physicians for guidance in making necessary provisions for students with hypertension.

MENSTRUAL DISORDERS

Menstrual irregularities are common in adolescence and concern the school when they cause absence or prevent full involvement in school activities. The pain of *dysmenorrhea* is usually short and recurring and occurs just above the pelvic bone and in the midabdomen region. Medications can reduce the discomfort, and so referral to a physician is recommended.

DISORDERS OF POSTURE

In the typical school situation, posture is not regarded as an important factor in student health. Although a deviation in posture usually does not produce a serious threat to health, postural defects in children should be a concern.

A child does not stand in a straight line but in four counterbalancing curves — cervical, thoracic, lumbar, and sacral. These vertebral curves are not in perfect compensating alignment but must be supported by the skeletal muscles. Whether a child is standing, walking, or sitting, four criteria can be applied as the index of good posture: (1) head erect, neck back, and chin level; (2) no exaggeration of vertebral curvatures; (3) chest lifted slightly; and (4) shoulders held broadly, without tension.

In standing, the body weight should be over the center of each foot, and the feet should be toeing straight forward. In walking, a rhythmic gait with a free and easy leg swing should be supplemented by a free and easy arm swing. The feet should be nearly parallel. In sitting, the hips, knees, and ankles should point straight ahead and be flat on the floor.

Most poor posture is functional, that is, resulting from careless habits, and a considerable amount results from poor muscle tone. Deformities of the skeleton and joints account for a very small percentage of poor posture.

Does poor posture cause poor health, or vice versa? In many youngsters poor health reflected in poor muscle tone leads to poor posture, which leads to further poor health in a downward spiral. In other youngsters, slovenly habits reflected in poor posture have a deleterious effect on health with a downward spiral of both posture and health.

In recent years school nurses and health instructors have been concerned about scoliosis in junior and senior high school students. *Scoliosis* is a condition in which there is a lateral curvature of the vertebral column. To identify a curvature the student is viewed from behind while standing erect and then as he or she bends forward. Pronounced lateral curvature can be seen easily. The condition often occurs first among junior high students and appears more frequently in girls. Screening procedures for scoliosis are described in Chapter 7. In time scoliosis can interfere with cardiopulmonary function and cause chronic back pain and psychologic problems related to self-image (Shifrin, 1971).

Round shoulders is a concern of both the school health department and the physical education staff, as are *lordosis* (swayback) and *visceroptosis* (abdominal paunch). Whether the corrective program is conducted on a group or individual basis, students with these conditions need to develop muscle tone and participate in physical activity.

Good posture is essential to a vigorous state of health, and it provides an extra dividend of pleasing personal appearance.

DEVIATIONS OF THE RESPIRATORY SYSTEM

Some noninfectious chronic conditions of the respiratory system are of minor consequence. Others are significant in terms of reducing the effectiveness and enjoyment of life. Occasionally, life itself may be threatened.

Nasal congestion

All persons experience some congestion of the nasal passages, but usually it is temporary resulting from an excessive production of mucus associated with respiratory infection. Although temporarily distressing, the accumulation of mucus is not serious, being a natural response to irritation of the mucous tissue. A chronic or permanent congestion may be caused by mucus or a mechanical obstruction such as a stemmed growth (polyp) of mucous tissue. Except for the inconvenience, some congestions are not too serious, whereas others need constant medical care or surgical correction.

Sinusitis

The sinuses of the skull are air cavities lined with the same type of mucous tissue that lines the nasal passages. Two frontal sinuses, one above each eye, and two maxillary sinuses, one in each upper jawbone beneath the eyes, have narrow passageways, or ducts, that empty into the nasal passages. Exhaled and inhaled air passes into the ducts and sinuses. These structures are properly considered part of the respiratory tract. Normally the mucous tissue lining the sinuses secretes a small to moderate amount of mucus. Mechanical or bacterial irritation produces an excessive amount of mucus with resulting congestion. Until the irritation is removed, the overproduction of mucus is likely to continue. Persons with constricted ducts may have painful sinus congestion.

The school should identify children with chronic sinusitis and suggest to parents the need for medical attention.

Deviated septum

At least half the adults in the United States have some degree of deviation of the partition separating the nares, but most deviations are of no particular significance. Deviation can occur without a nasal fracture.

In children, when the deviation is so pronounced that one of the nasal passages is closed, surgery will be advised by the physician. When the condition is obvious, the teacher will observe that, although the youngster has no difficulty in breathing under ordinary conditions, slight exertion requires mouth breathing. Closing the open naris by pressure with the finger and asking the child to exhale forcibly indicates the degree of obstruction in the other passage. Mouth breathing is not necessarily objectionable, but the chronic condition that produces it usually requires correction.

Allergies

Studies have shown that 10% to 28% of the population suffer from major allergic problems (McGovern, 1976). In the United States an estimated 1.6 million young people under 17 years of age have asthma.

Hypersensitivity can affect the respiratory tract in a variety of ways. Hay fever, bronchial asthma, bronchitis, and croup are end products of allergies that affect the respiratory system. Although some of these conditions exist when the child enters school, others do not become evident until the child is a teenager. Sometimes allergies do not appear until adulthood. Because of the factor of inheritance, children with a family history of allergies should be considered to have a possible respiratory allergy if they display chronic respiratory disturbances. Unwittingly some school personnel, suspecting an infectious condition, exclude children from school only to discover that they have an allergy. Had they studied the health records of these students, they might have avoided this problem.

Under medical supervision, children with respiratory allergies usually carry on the normal activities of school life. An asthmatic attack in school may appear dramatic but should not be alarming. Generally the students themselves know what action to take. A sitting position is usually most comfortable. For many children exhalation is the more difficult mechanism, and an attack may leave them near exhaustion. The teacher's poise and assurance often helps the student relax.

DISORDERS OF THE ORAL CAVITY

Disorders of the oral cavity are not an urgent life-and-death matter; yet they play an important role in the quality of health, the length of the prime of life, and life expectation. Thus, early detection and correction are dictated.

Caries and cavities

The process of dental decay is called caries; the result is the cavity. The process is initiated by the *Lactobacillus acidophilus* (LA) organism and can be expressed in the equation:

LA enzyme + Carbohydrate = Acid

Disintegration of the enamel occurs as the acid dissolves it.

Dental cavities occur more frequently than any other disorder of schoolchildren. Yet, of itself, a simple cavity may have no effect on health. However, it may progress to a point at which the tooth is destroyed or must be extracted. Loss of several teeth, without compensating dentures, can affect a person's dietary practices, and more seriously, the oral cavity can become an avenue of invasion for disease-producing organisms that pass, via the pulp cavity, to the apex of the tooth root and produce an abscess.

It is not the province of the teacher to examine children's mouths, but good dental hygiene should be taught to all students.

Abscess

An infection in the gum or at the apex of a tooth root may be painful or virtually painless. Toxins produced at the *abscess* can travel about the body and seriously impair vital tissues. Any gum involvement, including the gum boil, which is an abscess, demands professional attention. Prompt action may save the tooth and prevent injury to the general health.

Pyorrhea

Pyorrhea is an infectious or mechanical irritation of the periodontal membrane, which attaches the tooth to the gum and bone. A red margin of the gum around the neck of the tooth is indicative of this irritation. If permitted to continue, the irritation seriously damages the membrane. Because the periodontal membrane does not have the capacity to rejuvenate itself, the tooth becomes permanently loosened and may have to be extracted.

Gingivitis

Any inflammation of the gum may be termed *gingivitis,* but in its general usage the term designates infection by two known pathogens, *Bacillus fusiformis* and *Borrelia vincentii.* Commonly called trench mouth, or Vincent's disease, it is characterized by inflammation and even ulceration of the gums and other parts of the mouth, bleeding, excess salivation, and considerable soreness.

Gingivitis does not often occur in a healthy child. Malnutrition, poor general health, inadequate rest, and poor mouth care predispose to gingivitis. The infections can be treated successfully by a dentist.

Malocclusion

Pronounced overbite or underbite and poorly aligned teeth create mechanical problems that eventually destroy supporting tissue. For children with these conditions, the services of an orthodontist are a necessity, not a luxury.

DISORDERS OF EYES AND VISION

With a function as complex as vision and a structure as remarkable as the human eye, the wonder is that the incidence of defective vision is not greater. Standard screening tests usually detect children with more pronounced vision disability, and a professional practitioner's examination locates even the slightest disability. Teachers who observe their students closely can detect children whose posturing, squinting, inattention, or poor progress may be caused by their inability to see normally.

Myopia

Myopia, or nearsightedness, is a heritable tendency and is usually caused by elongated eyeballs. The image falls in front of the retina unless the object is close to the eye. Thus close objects can be seen quite clearly, but distant objects are blurred. Concave lenses will compensate for the extra length of the eyeball. Although nearsighted children may be able to read without glasses, they will become less distressed and fatigued with proper eyewear.

Hyperopia

Hyperopia, or farsightedness, is caused by an eyeball so short that the image literally falls behind the retina. With a great deal of effort, a farsighted child can see near objects by overworking the delicate muscles of accommodation though visual fatigue sets in very quickly. A tendency to become cross-eyed is possible. Convex lenses can compensate so that the child can read with a minimum of strain and fatigue.

Astigmatism

Irregularities in the curvature of the cornea and lens prevent a true focus of the eye, and a blurred image with discomfort results. Astigmatism requires carefully prescribed glasses and sometimes frequent renewal of the prescription.

Amblyopia

Vision dimness without known cause can occur in people of all ages. Amblyopia may begin with a central or peripheral spot where there is little vision. The condition may enlarge slowly and will progressively interfere with vision. Visual disturbance will be more pronounced in bright light.

Fortunately, amblyopia in children usually clears up spontaneously, but every child with dimness of vision should be under the supervision of an ophthalmologist for periodic checkups.

Strabismus

Cross-eye, not cross-eyes, is descriptive of strabismus, since only one eye is crossed because of a shortened extrinsic muscle that turns the eye inward. Ophthalmologists can correct many types of strabismus by treatment or surgery or a combination. Early attention is essential. The accommodation or acuity of one or both eyes may be affected in some children if the condition is untreated. Such children exhibit posturing and other signs of difficult vision. The alert teacher calls this difficulty to the attention of the child's parents.

Ptosis

A drooping of one or both upper eyelids, ptosis, is usually an inherited condition in which the nerves that stimulate the elevating muscle do not conduct impulses. Paralysis of the muscle may come on gradually during the school years. If the paralysis is bilateral, children will naturally tilt their heads back in order to see through the small apertures formed by the backward tilt of the head.

Conjunctivitis

Conjunctivitis, or pinkeye, is a highly communicable condition caused most often by pneumococci and staphylococci. Characterized by a mucous discharge in the eyes, a burning and itching sensation, and bright red coloration of the conjunctiva, the disease is easy to detect. Overnight the discharge may seal the eyelids closed. Because of the highly contagious nature of this condition, children with conjunctivitis should be isolated and excluded from school with a suggestion to parents to consult a physician. With medication the condition is quickly managed, but the student should not return to school until the physician's clearance is received. Even at home the child with pinkeye should be careful not to use items such as towels that could be used by others.

HEARING DISABILITIES

Most children who have some hearing loss acquire it gradually. The audiometric test will determine hearing disabilities, but the alert teacher can observe indications that a child has hearing difficulties. Children who cannot hear well will often posture, are inattentive, copy, and make poor progress. Faulty pronunciation and an unnatural voice are hints that the child does not hear well.

Conduction deafness

Almost all hearing loss in children is caused by disturbances of the outer and middle ear that interfere with the conduction of sound. Excessive wax (cerumen), ruptured or rigid tympanic membrane, rigidity of the ligaments of the bones (ossicles) of the middle ear, mucous congestion of the middle ear, and rigidity of the oval window of the spiral shell (cochlea) all interfere with sound conduction. Some conditions of conduction deafness can be corrected, and most are amenable to treatment.

Sensorineural deafness

Sensorineural deafness, or perception deafness, is relatively rare in school-aged children. It may be caused by an injury or disease in the neuron or inner part of the ear. Infected gums or gallbladder can be the primary cause of perception deafness. It also can result from meningitis, influenza, and drugs such as quinine and salicylates. Extremely high body temperature can also cause perception deafness.

• • •

Some types of hearing loss cannot be prevented or corrected. However, hearing aids may compensate for much of the deficiency in persons with impaired hearing. Today prescriptions for hearing aids are written with the same precision as prescriptions for glasses.

NEUROLOGIC DISORDER: EPILEPSY

Epilepsy can cause the uninformed teacher considerable concern. An understanding of the condition and the proper care of afflicted children give teachers the assurance necessary for dealing with an episode of epilepsy.

From its Greek derivation, the word *epilepsy* literally means a seizure. Being merely descriptive of clinical symptoms, the term is not satisfactory, but it usually is employed to designate recurrent seizures and periods of unconsciousness.

Grand mal is the more serious type of epileptic seizure. Essentially it is a convulsive seizure with the following characteristics:

1. Aura, or sensory disturbances (e.g., light or taste), which sometimes precede and warn of the attack
2. Sometimes a shrill and startling cry
3. Sudden loss of consciousness and falling backward
4. Pupils dilated; eyes open at beginning of seizure
5. Tonic spasm — drawing up limbs in rigid, flexed position
6. Clonic spasm — intermittent contraction and relaxation with thrashing about of arms and legs
7. Spasm of respiratory muscles — no breathing and blueness of the face
8. Spasm of jaw muscles — biting the tongue, which results in bloody foam
9. Relaxation, prolonged stupor, and profound sleep

The active convulsion lasts less than 1 minute and terminates in exhaustion. During the seizure attempt to protect the child from injury. It is sometimes possible to catch the person and prevent a fall. Moving the child to a clear space away from hot and sharp objects prevents injury. The seizure should not be resisted. Children who have only two or three grand mal seizures during the school year usually continue school attendance. When seizures become so frequent as to disrupt the class, alternative means of education should be considered. The cause of epilepsy is unknown, but sedatives reduce the severity of seizures and increase the length of time between seizures.

Typical minor attacks (*petit mal*) are characterized by a transitory (3- or 4-second) loss of consciousness without falling and only minor, if any, muscular twitching. These children may attend school without any particular problems. Others however may be classified by teachers as "spacy," "slow," or "inattentive." It is possible to experience as many as 200 *petit mal* attacks per day, and so teachers need to be aware that classroom behavior and deviation from the normal performance may have health-related origins.

With any student whose performance level changes or who repeatedly fails to meet normal expectations, one of the first questions should be, Could this situation be caused by or contributed to by a medical or health problem? In this way school personnel can more responsibly address their mandate to educate by identifying impediments to learning.

SKIN DISORDER: ACNE

Most adolescents suffer from some degree of acne, but about 5% may suffer from severe cases with associated discomfort and embarrassment. Boys are more frequently affected and likely to experience severe cases. For girls, acne problems occur between 14 and 16 years of age and for boys between 16 and 19 years of age. Professional care from a dermatologist minimizes the cosmetic consequences and limits the psychologic stress this condition causes. Teachers can be most effective in correcting some widespread misconceptions about acne. Acne is a natural consequence of the increased flow of androgens associated with puberty and changes in the skin occurring with growth. Acne is not, as often believed, the consequence of diet, and restricting the consumption of chocolate, cola, and candy is not necessary to manage the condition. Scrubbing with soap and water will not necessarily reduce the condition and may produce an irritant dermatitis. Acne is not the consequence of poor personal hygiene, but bacterial soap will limit the spread of the associated bacteria.

CHILD ABUSE

It is estimated that more than a million chidren are abused or neglected each year. The majority of the abuse occurs in the first 6 months of the child's life. Although the incidence of abuse has declined by the time children enter school, the individual consequences are often so evident that they interfere with learning and learning to relate to other people.

Every state now has child protection laws that mandate the reporting of child abuse to the appropriate authorities, and so school personnel can find themselves in a situation where they are required to act as an extension of law enforcement. This creates a difficult situation for schools because it thrusts them directly into the midst of what typically are family problems, usually of long standing, and often sets school personnel in adversarial relationships with parents. Reporting evidence of child abuse also potentially involves teachers in investigative and judicial proceedings, which may result in the state assuming responsibility for the child's custody thus splitting a family.

Despite these consequences, it would be unprofessional, unconscionable, and illegal for a teacher or any other school personnel to overlook evidence of possible chid abuse.

The U.S. Child Abuse Prevention and Treatment Act (PL 93-247) defines abuse and neglect as physical and mental injury, sexual abuse and exploitation, and negligent treatment of any child under 18 years of age by persons who are responsible for their welfare. This would include others besides the child's natural parents.

Physical abuse

Beating, burning, and kicking are the most common forms of physical abuse, but such things as exposure to weather, suffocation, strangulation, and stabbing or cutting have also been identified. Injury results from the hands of the abuser or from whatever item is available to use as a weapon: brooms, bats, electrical cords, hairbrushes, cigarette lighters, coat hangers, cigarettes, flames, hot plates, hot water, or scissors.

Abuse is evident by observation of physical signs and is also suggested by a child's behavior. Signs of physical abuse include:

1. Unusual bruising patterns or bruises in unusual places
2. Bruises that reflect the outline of an instrument
3. Burns
4. Swelling around the mouth and eyes
5. Broken nose
6. Ears torn or injured
7. Unusual skin rashes
8. Lacerations
9. Dental injury or missing teeth
10. Dirty or inadequate clothes

It is not only the existence of these signs but also the fact that they appear with some degree of frequency that indicates child abuse. For the teacher, the school nurse can be an invaluable assistant in identifying abuse. The nurse can examine the child more carefully and keep a record of the youngster's health. School couselors can also be of assistance by noting a child's behavior.

Often abused children also present behavioral patterns that will raise a concern among school staff. Abused children do not look to their parents for assurance, are apprehensive of other children or their parents, do not react under conditions that would normally cause children to cry, are withdrawn, preoccupied and forlorn, and aggressive in their behavior, seek assurances from others in unusual ways such as asking to stay with them, drug abuse, running away, or sexual promiscuity.

Abusive parents also present behavior patterns that can alert the professional teacher, nurse, or administrator. Parents may be overprotective, not allowing their children to participate with other children, give explanations for signs of abuse that are inconsistent with reality, saying, for example, "He fell off a stool" to explain a black eye. Such parents may give vague and evasive answers to direct questions. Parents may blame the child, saying, for example, She's just a klutz, always banging into something. Parents may seek medical help for the consequences of abuse, but it may be from different emergency rooms or distant hospitals or a variety of physicians and nurses so that patterns of abuse cannot be easily detected.

Almost all child abuse occurs at the hand of parents. Child abuse is a family problem sometimes referred to as the "battered child syndrome." Families under stress, lower socio-economic families, single-parent families, parents with limited educations, and poorly housed families cause higher incidences of child abuse. However teachers should not overlook the fact that children from sophisticated families may also suffer child abuse.

Sexual abuse

Sexual abuse is most common in the form of incest between father and daughter. It is the most difficult to identify and deal with. Signs of injury to the external genitalia and anal region with bleeding and swelling would be evident to physicians and nurses but not be detectable to others. Positive tests for sexually transmitted diseases and spermatozoa also may indicate sexual abuse.

Inability to sit still or signs of tenderness when sitting is often a sign of sexual abuse. With careful counseling children may admit to sexual abuse.

Steps to deal with child abuse

Because child abuse reporting initiates a legal action, teachers should act with care.

1. Note possible signs of abuse in some detail in writing. Record date, time, and circumstances the signs were noticed.
2. If a pattern develops or signs are obvious, check with the school nurse for confirmation.
3. Report information to school principal. The principal should initiate the reporting.

4. A decision may or may not be made to contact the parents, but the law in each state mandates reporting to the appropriate authorities.

5. If the primary law enforcement agency does not respond appropriately, contact may be made with other child protective social agencies.

Because child abuse involves families in highly emotional issues, there is sometimes a hesitancy on the part of all authorities to interfere. However, if these conditions exist, the law requires that they be reported.

SUICIDE

According to the Committee on Adolescence of the American Academy of Pediatrics (1981), suicide is the most frequent cause of death among young people 10 to 19 years of age, and there is evidence the prevalence is increasing. Although suicides are not likely to take place at school, gestures for help and attention are. Suicide attempts are more frequent among girls than boys, but boys are more often successful when they do attempt suicide. It is estimated that as many as 100 attempted suicides occur for every recorded suicide. The nature of attempts is so varied that there is no way to assess the extent of the problem. Automobile accidents, drug overdoses, falls, firearm accidents, and drownings may all represent suicide attempts. Gestures likely to be observed in school include depression, daredevil acts, truancy, delinquent behavior, somatic complaints, such as headache, fatigue, and gastrointestinal pain, and behavioral conditions, such as hyperactivity. Outright questions or statements about suicide should not be taken lightly. Because open discussion of this topic does not make it more likely to occur, questions or statements should be discussed. If teachers identify students whom they consider at high risk, they should involve other student personnel in a conference to explore their concern and develop a plan of action. Other teachers and the nurse and counselors usually constitute the primary team, which may then consult the school psychologist for advice.

DEVIATIONS IN MENTAL HEALTH

Numerous behavioral characteristics indicate that a student's mental health or psychosocial development may not be typical. Any of these characteristics taken individually may have little significance, but a complex of factors observed over a period of time gives rise to concern. Major deviations from mental health are relatively obvious, but small differences are difficult to interpret because the accepted range of "normal" is not clearly defined. Accordingly the teacher's first role is to observe a student's behavior carefully and then seek advice and assistance from counselors and other specialists in the school or community.

Behavioral characteristics that may indicate deviations in psychosocial development may include the following:

1. *Undue shyness*. A shy child is a lonesome child and may develop an excessive feeling of inferiority. A teacher with ingenuity will contrive situations in which the child will associate closely with one, two, and then several of the group. If the shyness is to be overcome, it is essential that a child be brought gradually into group activities. It is most helpful for the teacher to express high regard for the child and to point out that the other children in the class feel the same way.

2. *Tendency to be a loner.* Children who seek to be alone or to do everything on their own may never have learned to play or work with others. They may not believe they are equal to the group, or may believe that the group does not accept them.

3. *Restlessness and easy distraction.* A thyroid disorder, malnutrition, or inadequate rest may be the cause of restlessness. Uneasiness may be caused by a feeling of inadequacy.

4. *Excessive daydreaming.* A lack of success, with a resulting escape into fantasy, may be the primary factor.

5. *Chip on the shoulder.* The belligerent, pugnacious, quarrelsome youngster is the defensive youngster. An exaggerated feeling of inferiority, a feeling of rejection, or a defensiveness because of a lack of status may account for this personality mold.

6. *Suspiciousness.* Occasionally a child may be overly suspicious, exhibiting a strong distrust of others, even to the point of suspecting everyone of taking advantage of him or her.

7. *Selfishness.* A youngster who lacks consideration for others and is extremely possessive, particularly in relation to material things, may have acquired a distorted set of values.

8. *Hypochondria.* The child who finds he or she can get attention by having a pain or other physical complaint may resort to this ruse whenever an uncomfortable or trying situation arises. Expression of imaginary pain can be an escape mechanism or an attention-getting device.

Although any one of these conditions may identify a student as different, it does not define a child as sick or in need of medical attention. If the conditions exist in the absence of a medical basis, they may just represent individual differences that we all will learn to live with. For the teacher the task is to assure that small differences in individual students are not masking major problems.

As with communicable illness, people can contribute to the spread of mental illness or the promotion of mental health. Just as a teacher should be free from communicable disease, so too should a teacher be mentally healthy. Introspection may be useful at this point. Certain things can rightfully be expected of teachers in their role as educators:

1. Understanding his or her own behavior
2. Separating personal problems from the classroom and school life
3. Respecting each youngster
4. Understanding individual differences
5. Understanding the cause-and-effect relationship of deviant behavior
6. Maintaining an atmosphere neither too rigid, too severe, nor too permissive
7. Strengthening desirable behavior through recognition and even praise
8. Dealing with behavior problems not serious enough for professional care
9. Substituting acceptable behavior for deviant behavior

In addition, the psychologic or mental health environment of the school should be conducive to good relations among teachers and between teachers and administrators. Teachers should be competent in dealing with students in a guidance and counseling role though they should not usurp the role of the trained counselor. Schools should have an infrastructure of guidance and counseling services, often incorporating community resources to support teachers in their everyday classroom activities.

Skilled teachers with adequate knowledge of deviations from normal growth and development effectively help young people gain the most from their educational experience. The ability carefully to note developmental or health-related irregularities and adapt educational programs accordingly or make appropriate referrals is the mark of a truly professional teacher.

SUMMARY

This chapter reviews a wide range of possible departures from normal. Teachers should have considerable tolerance to allow individuals to develop their own unique characters, but they should also be alert to identify differences that may indicate a larger problem. Developing teachers who are referral agents and keep observers is the desired outcome of this chapter.

STUDY QUESTIONS

1. Indicate some deviations from the normal in children that should be disregarded or even ignored in the school.
2. What is the legal responsibility of the school for the correction of defects in a pupil?
3. What is the professional responsibility of the teacher for the correction of defects in a pupil?
4. What role can a teacher play in aiding the excessively obese child to lose weight?
5. What should be the course of action of the school in dealing with a student who is listless, slow, inactive, disinterested, and chronically late?
6. After a child has had an epileptic seizure while in school, what should the teacher say to the other children in the class?
7. Why can it be said that there is as great a danger for a child with a defect or disorder to underparticipate as there is for that child to overparticipate?
8. What does it mean and what should the teacher do if a child's physician reports, "The child has a functional heart murmur, but it should be disregarded, and she should be treated like any other child."?
9. Explain the statement, "For the growing child with a malocclusion the services of an orthodontist are not a luxury."
10. Which agencies or organizations in your community are interested in helping children with vision and hearing disorders?
11. A schoolchild needs a hearing aid, but the parents do not buy one. What should the school do?
12. What can be done by a teacher for the youngster who does not enter into group activities but always tends to be alone?
13. In terms of its influence on the mental health of the students, what is the most important factor in a classroom?
14. What are some resources a teacher can call on for consultation relating to students with health problems?

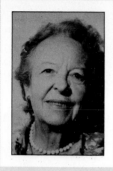

Dorothy Bird Nyswander

BORN   September 29, 1894, Reno, Nevada
EDUCATION   B.A., University of Nevada, 1915; M.A., University of Nevada, 1915; Ph.D.,
University of California at Berkeley, 1926; postdoctoral work, Stanford University

Dr. Nyswander is a pioneer in health education whose contributions have done much to influence the development of health education as a social and behavioral science. One of her earliest professional experiences came as a research assistant for the American Child Health Association. She was involved in some of the first efforts to measure and conduct scientific evaluation of school health programs. Because of this early work in school health, she was invited by the New York City Board of Health and the Board of Education to direct a major school health research project in the Astoria Health District, one of the boroughs of New York City. This study had had a major impact on the nature and function of school health services in the United States. Dr. Nyswander published results of the Astoria Demonstration Study as a textbook entitled *Solving School Health Problems*. One of the most important recommendations from the study has led to a much more effective use of the physician and nursing services in the school health program.

Under her leadership as a professor in the school of public health at the University of California at Berke-ley, a full-fledged department of health education was created. Also, through her influence, the preparation program for health educators at the University of California was broadened to include a strong emphasis on the social and behavioral sciences.

In addition to her major contributions to the fields of school health and public health education, she held several positions at all levels of government in a variety of national and international health programs. These include the Latin American Rockefeller Project on health education and agriculture and the World Health Organization malaria control training projects in Jamaica, New Caledonia, and Turkey. Other assignments include her work with the World Health Organization, the All-India Institute of Public Health and Hygiene, and the United Nations Division of Population in Latin America.

In her honor and to recognize her outstanding contribution to the field of health education, the Dorothy B. Nyswander Lecture on Public Health Education was established in 1957 at the University of California at Berkeley.

REFERENCES

American Academy of Pediatrics: School health: a guide for health professionals, Elk Grove Village, Ill., 1987, the Academy.

American Psychiatric Association: Diagnostic and statistical manual of mental disorders, ed. 3, Washington, D.C., 1980, the Association.

Dale, S.: School mental health problems: a challenge to the health professional, J. Sch. Health **48**:526, 1978.

Dally, P., and Gomez, J.: Anorexia nervosa, London, 1979, William Heinemann Medical Books, Ltd.

Green, P.: Spine deformity screening in Kansas, J. Sch. Health **49**:56, 1979.

Heald, F.: Adolescent nutrition, Med. Clin. North Am. **59**:1329, 1975.

Kempe, R.S., and Kempe, C.H.: Child abuse, Cambridge, Mass., 1978, Harvard University Press.

Lansky, D., and Brownell, K.: Comparison of school-based treatments for adolescent obesity, J. Sch. Health **52**:384, 1982.

Markowitz, M.: Streptococcal infections, rheumatic fever and school health services, J. Sch. Health **49**:202, 1979.

McGovern, J.: Chronic respiratory diseases of school-age children, J. Sch. Health **46**:344, 1976.

McKevitt, R., et al.: Reasons for health office visits in an urban school district, J. Sch. Health **47**:275, 1977.

Meyer, R.: Accepting the challenge of child abuse and neglect: a golden opportunity for school health, J. Sch. Health **49**:480, 1979.

Miller, D., and Lever, C.: Scoliosis screening: an approach used in the school, J. Sch. Health **52**:98, 1982.

National Heart, Lung and Blood Institute: Arteriosclerosis: report of the working group on arteriosclerosis, vol. 2, NIH Pub. no. 82-2025, Washington, D.C., 1982.

Newberger, E.H., and Daniel, J.H.: Knowledge and epidemiology of child abuse: a critical review of concepts, Pediatr. Ann. **5**(3):15, 1976.

Olson, R.: Index of suspicion: screening for child abusers, Am. J. Nursing **76**(1):108, 1976.

Shifrin, L.: Recognizing scoliosis early, Am. Fam. Physician **4**:177, Dec. 1971.

Weiss, G., and Hechtman, L.: The hyperactive child syndrome, Science **205**:1348, 1979.

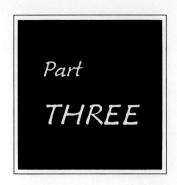

Part

THREE

SCHOOL HEALTH SERVICES

7 Health Appraisal Aspects of School Health Services

OVERVIEW   *Secondary prevention activities involve early detection of possible illness and initiation of treatment. Despite the fact that illness is at its lowest levels among school-aged children, sufficient deviations from normal health go unnoticed to justify regular health examinations and health screening of the school-aged population. This chapter describes the relationships between student health and the school's educational mission. A distinction is made between health examinations and health screenings, and the basic screening techniques are described.*

OBJECTIVES   After reading this chapter, the student should be able to:

1. Describe the relationships between health appraisal activities and the educational objectives of a school
2. Differentiate between a health examination and health screening
3. Describe the advantages and disadvantages of a health screening program
4. Identify possible errors in screening outcomes
5. List the basic methods in health screening for vision, hearing, height and weight, dental care, and scoliosis
6. Illustrate the use of various types of vision screening equipment
7. Describe the sweep test and the threshold test used to determine hearing acuity
8. Identify observable behaviors that indicate possible vision and hearing difficulties
9. Describe the ways height and weight data can be effectively used in health screening
10. State the basic reasons for measuring body fat (adiposity) and describe a means of measuring body fat
11. List basic points of an effective referral follow-up
12. Describe the basic principles governing confidentiality of student health records

Preventive activities that reduce the likelihood of a condition's occurring are preferable to treatment activities designed to overcome illness. This is the fundamental difference between primary prevention and secondary prevention described in Chapter 2. Unfortunately it is not always possible to prevent an illness. The next best option then is secondary prevention: prompt identification of the earliest discernible pathogenesis and initiation of appropriate treatment. The ultimate objective of early detection is the reduction of any illness-related disability and the avoidance of the costs and inconvenience of long-term treatment. For the school and students, the most important immediate cost is absence or distraction from the learning process.

The success of secondary prevention efforts depends on the early detection of disabling conditions. Schools are an excellent place for appraising students' health and detecting early signs of illness. Health appraisal efforts are principally of two types: (1) required physical examinations carried out by physicians at set times during the elementary and secondary school years and (2) health screening activities carried out in school under the supervision of the school nurse or a physician.

Sick and injured students do not learn as well as those who are fit and healthy. Health examination programs and screening programs that identify conditions interfering with learning and aid in the early initiation of treatment improve the school's efforts on behalf of learning. When health conditions reduce a student's ability to learn, the teacher tends to focus special attention on this student and may deprive other students. The recognition that some learning problems are actually health problems can lead to the initiation of treatment and frees the teacher to attend to the whole class.

Unrecognized health problems contribute not only to underachievement but also to inattention, class disruption, absenteeism, tardiness, and disciplinary problems. Early detection of students with communicable diseases, their subsequent removal from the school, and the initiation of treatment reduces the likelihood that other students or the teacher will contract the disease and suffer unnecessary absenteeism.

Health examinations and health screening programs also have educational value. Students' participation in health examinations and screening activities allows students to learn values of personal health, monitor their own health status, and understand the need to seek further diagnosis and initiate special care when appropriate. An effective means for young people to reduce the likelihood of early death from long-term degenerative diseases so common today is to learn skills and responsibilities for early detection and referral to treatment.

HEALTH EXAMINATION

The health examination is a means to an end and potentially a very effective instrument for improving health standards. In keeping with the present-day positive approach the physician's examination of a child is designated a health examination, not a medical or physical examination as it may have been in the past (Fig. 7-1).

The frequency of school children's health examinations is usually set down by law. Where no legal directives exist, the decision must be made by local school and medical officials. The American Academy of Pediatrics (1981) suggests that the order of priority of health examinations should be (1) when children are identified as having special problems,

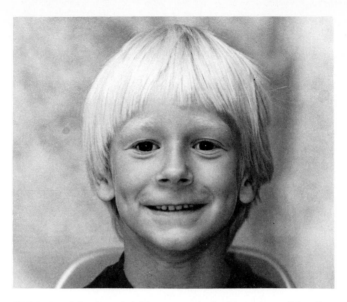

FIG. 7-1.   School-aged children are at the healthiest time of their lives. Careful monitoring of health through regular health examinations and screening programs will guarantee that any problems are treated early to ensure continued good health.
(Copyright 1983 by David Riecks.)

(2) on beginning school, (3) in midschool (grade 6 or 7), and (4) before leaving school (grade 11 or 12). In addition, special health examinations are recommended for students participating in athletic programs.

Students entering school for the first time

Children who are to begin school in the fall should be examined sufficiently early to permit follow-up observation on recommendations of the examining physician. June and July are the most satisfactory months for preschool examinations. Parents are usually asked to complete a health history form for each new student. This form (see box, p. 141) begins the student's health file.

Students new to the school system

If an acceptable health record is received from the student's previous school, a health examination may be unnecessary. If there is no health record or a doubtful health condition exists, health examination requirements should be part of the admission procedures, as should be the completion of a health history form.

Students entering midschool grades

For schools organized on the grade 6-3-3 basis, health examination as a requirement for admission to junior high school is both sound and an easy procedure to administer. Middle schools (5-3-4) should have the examination in the eighth grade. For schools on the 8-4 plan, the requirement should apply for admission to high school.

Sample Health History Form*

1. Name of child_____ Birth date_____

2. **Pregnancy, birth and development**   *Circle one*
   a. Were there any difficulties during pregnancy, labor, or delivery?   Yes   No
   b. If yes, explain:_____
   c. Was this child carried for a full 9 months?   Yes   No
   d. Birth weight was _____lb. _____oz.

   Did this child:
   e. Have any trouble starting to breathe after birth?   Yes   No
   f. Have any problems in the hospital after birth?   Yes   No
   g. Sit alone before 7 months of age?   Yes   No
   h. Walk alone before 15 months of age?   Yes   No
   i. Say words by 1½ years of age?   Yes   No
   j. Check any of the following that have occurred with this child:
      ☐ Sleeping problem   ☐ Eating problem
      ☐ Excessive drooling   ☐ Coordination problem

3. **Illnesses and accidents**
   Has this child:
   a. Had more than one ear infection each year?   Yes   No
   b. Had more than two throat infections each year?   Yes   No
   c. Had a hearing problem?   Yes   No
   d. Had a vision problem?   Yes   No
      If yes, when last fitted for glasses?_____
   e. Had allergy problems, such eczema, hives, wheezing, or asthma?   Yes   No
   f. Had frequent colds, sinus infections, or hay fever?   Yes   No
   g. Received any routine medication?   Yes   No
   h. Had any serious reactions to any medicine or injections?   Yes   No
   i. Had any difficulty passing urine?   Yes   No
   j. Ever had convulsions?   Yes   No
   k. Had a weight problem?   Yes   No
   l. Had any serious accidents?   Yes   No
   m. Been hospitalized for serious illness or accidents?   Yes   No
   Please explain any "yes" answers (use back of sheet if necessary).

4. **Family health**
   Do any other family members have any serious health problems?   Yes   No
   Explain a "yes" answer.

5. **Additional health concerns**
   Please let any additional health concerns or physical limitations of this child.

   _____

   _____

Filled out by_____ Date_____

*To be completed by parent or guardian.

Students participating in vigorous athletic programs

All students participating in interscholastic activities should be examined at the beginning of their particular sports program. Physician certification of the student's fitness to participate will indicate any limitations or restrictions and should be on file in the school before the student is admitted to practice. After an injury, illness, or other incapacity, the student should be admitted to further participation only on recommendation and supervision of a physician. Students participating in various intramural sports should be examined by a physician yearly.

Graduation

Some school districts require health examinations before graduation so that students graduate with an evaluation of both their academic and health status. Some school districts seek the assistance of community service groups and provide examinations as a gift to the graduating seniors. Examinations late in the student's education have little value to the school but serve as an important reminder for routine health examinations throughout life.

Students referred through screening by teacher or nurse

Health screening programs frequently identify conditions requiring medical follow-up observation. When the physician considers the finding of the health screening, he or she also typically provides a thorough health examination. In addition to students referred from organized screening programs, alert teachers and nurses frequently can detect an unhealthy child. Both minor and serious deviations can be recognized by the observant teacher and referred to the school nurse, who will in turn contact the child's parents. Although the teacher may be unsure, it is prudent to err on the side of caution and speak to the nurse or the parents about the advisability of having the child examined by a physician.

Health examination procedures

Most commonly, the student's family physician conducts the health examination. In some cases health department physicians may be used, and in others, physicians may conduct examinations in the school. The student's usual health provider is the most desirable health examiner. The results and their usefulness to the school are greatly enhanced by standardized reporting forms. Information needs vary among school districts and may be dictated by state law. An example of a health examination form is given in the box on p. 143. Notice that this form asks the physician only for information on any immunizations he or she may have given as part of the examination. Most states now require parents to submit a full immunization history when the student enters school (see box, p. 144).

Periodic examinations of healthy schoolchildren rarely reveal major pathologic conditions. Children participating in health examinations are usually healthy, and childhood and adolescence are generally the healthiest periods of life. Nevertheless, there are several values of the periodic health examination.

First, an alert physician may identify an important unrecognized problem. Second, student-physician contact in the absence of a crisis (illness) enhances a healthy physician-student relationship. Third, routine conferences provide opportunities for parents to ask questions that they might not normally ask if they had to initiate a physician visit on their

Sample Physical Examination Form

Dear Parent:

State law requires that each child enrolled in kindergarten and seventh grade present a physical examination report from the family physician. It is extremely important that any physical limitations be discovered at these age levels to prevent more serious difficulties in your child. A physical examination within 6 months of entering kindergarten or seventh grade is acceptable.

Name _____ School _____ Grade _____

Address _____ Zip _____ Age _____ Sex _____

Physical Findings

Height _____ Weight_____   Nose and throat _____

Blood pressure _____ Pulse_____   Heart _____

Urinalysis _____   Lungs _____

Hemoglobin _____   Abdomen _____

Vision report _____   Musculoskeletal:

_____   Spine _____

Audiometric screening: Upper extremities _____

   Method _____   Lower extremities _____

   Results _____   Neurologic: ____No ____Yes

General appearance _____   Evidence of scoliosis: ____No ____Yes

_____   Evidence of hernia: ____No ____Yes

Immunizations given at this time: _____

Significant findings and remarks: _____

_____

Have you any further recommendations to teacher or school nurse for promoting this child's physical and mental health?

_____

Require medication on a daily or episodic routing: _____

_____

Please check classification:

_____ Regular: Student may participate in the regular program of physical education, recreation, intramurals, athletics, or related activities without undue risk or injury.

_____ Adapted: Student has a condition that might risk sustaining injury from participating in the regular program or needs a special adapted program as indicated by the consulting physician. Reexamine each year.

_____ Exempt: Student has a severe handicap that might risk sustaining injury from participating in the regular or adapted program. This student should be reexamined for possible reclassification at the end of the exemption period.

Date _____ Signed _____ (examining physician)

Identification and School Health Data

Name _____ Sex _____ Entry date _____

Grade level   K   1   2   3   4   5   6

Birth _____ Place of birth _____
        Month   Day   Year   City/state
            (Please bring copy of birth certificate.)

Present home address _____ Phone number _____

_____ Zip _____

Parents' names:	Date of birth	Birth place	Nationality	Education	Occupation
(Father)					
(Mother)					
(Guardian)					

Father deceased _____ Mother deceased _____ Parents divorced _____ Parents separated _____

Brothers		*Sisters*	
Name	Birth date	Name	Birth date

Former school attended: _____

Health information: Family physician _____

State law requires all children be immunized against rubella, measles, polio, DPT, and mumps. Please list below the date (month and year) of each dose given. To keep the health record up-to-date, please send dates of immunizations given after this form is sent to school.

1. Immunization against diphtheria, tetanus, and pertussis (combined) (three doses 1 month apart) Dates of doses 1. _____
    2. _____ 3. _____
2. DPT boosters: Date of doses _____
3. Sabin (oral) polio: Dose 1 _____
    Dose 2 _____ Dose 3 _____
4. Sabin polio boosters: Date of doses _____
5. Rubeola (hard measles): Date of dose _____
6. Rubella (German measles): Date of dose _____
7. Mumps: Date of dose _____
8. TB test date: _____ Results: _____

Please list below any medication the child takes on a daily or routine basis.

_____

Please write in date if the child has had any of the following:

Scarlet fever _____ Measles _____ Mumps _____
Other _____
Pneumonia _____ Three-day measles _____ Chickenpox _____
Other _____
Rheumatic fever _____ Poliomyelitis _____ Whooping cough _____
Operations (type and year): _____

Signed (parent or guardian) _____ Date _____

own. Fourth, the opportunity for physicians to tell children and adolescents that they are perfectly normal in their developmental stages is reassuring in times of rapid growth and development.

Health history

The American Academy of Pediatrics (1981) suggests that a medical history or health history may be the most important part of any health examination. Ninety percent of the diagnosis is based on the health history (North, 1974). In addition to a record of past health problems, both physical and emotional, the health history reviews the body systems and seeks information on any special health problems of other family members. A history identifies practices that may influence health such as smoking, exercise, diet, and sleep. Past immunizations and the current use of medication will also be reported (see box, p. 144). Information on emotional problems, parent-child relationships, leisure time activities, school performance, conflicts with authority, and use of drugs, alcohol, or tobacco will also be explored. Because of the wide range of information gathered in a health examination, it is important for parents to be present unless the examination is being conducted on an older adolescent. Some physicians prefer to visit with parents and children separately.

For school health examinations, the physician pays special attention to any conditions requiring modification of the child's current or future school program. Thus parents must understand the importance of providing full information. Reluctance to record such information as epilepsy, mental retardation, or emotional illnesses increases the possibility that the school is unaware of these conditions as well as the likelihood that manifestations of these conditions may be misinterpreted when they occur.

In addition to the health history, a standard health examination usually includes a careful evaluation of the following:
1. General appearance
2. Height and weight
3. Head and neck, nose and throat
4. Vision and hearing
5. Thorax, heart, and lungs
6. Abdomen and genitals
7. Skin
8. Muscular and skeletal systems
9. Posture, gait, and feet
10. Neurologic system

Many schools require parents or guardians to complete a health history for the school's cumulative health record. An example of this form is shown in the box on p. 143.

Dental examination

Most schools require periodic dental examinations when they require physical examinations. Routine annual or semiannual visits to the dentist are relatively common and the prevalence of dental conditions interfering with learning has decreased significantly. The addition of fluoride to the drinking water in many communities has further reduced the prevalence of dental caries among young people.

For the school's purpose it is important to know whether the dentist has identified problems and whether appropriate care has been initiated or completed. The reporting form for dental health examinations given in the box below is relatively simple. Side 1 advises parents of the school's recommendation for regular dental examination, and side 2 provides space for the dentist's report.

Confidentiality of records

The quality of data and usefulness of records of health examinations are greatly increased if all cooperating physicians use standardized forms for reporting results. This not only standardizes procedures in data gathering but also encourages the inclusion of only pertinent information concerning the development of the child's educational program.

Passage of the Family Education Rights and Privacy Act in 1974 meant that all written records from physicians to schools receiving federal funds be open to parental inspection. According to the Family Education Rights and Privacy Act, parents may review their child's educational records on request, challenge the accuracy of any part of the record, and seek deletion or correction.

Dental Referral Card

Dear Parents or Guardians:

The (name of school or health department) recommends that you see your family dentist for regular dental care.

Early and regular care will ensure better dental health throughout life. Only you, as a parent or guardian, can see that your child receives regular dental care. Poor dental health is a menace to general health.

Therefore you are urged to take _____ to your dentist for examination and, if any dental service is required, continue with treatment until all corrections are made. Please have your dentist sign as indicated on other side of card.

_____
(teacher or school nurse)

(over)

THIS SIDE FOR DENTIST'S USE ONLY

I have examined _____

☐ All necessary treatment completed

☐ Patient currently under treatment

☐ No treatment necessary

Date _____ Signed _____ D.D.S.

Because written records are subject to misinterpretation and the potentially destructive effects of labeling are well recognized, schools must develop clear policies on the nature of information recorded and the ways health records are used.

HEALTH SCREENING

In technical terms screening is the "presumptive identification of unrecognized illness or defect by the application of tests, examinations, or other procedures which can be applied rapidly" (Commission on Chronic Illness, 1957). In simple terms screening identifies students who deviate from the average on one or more of a series of tests. Not all deviations indicate health problems, but the presence of a measured deviation indicates the need for a more careful examination.

Health screening can take several forms. Most health screening activities in schools are conducted by the school nurse, teachers, and trained volunteers (often parents) to assess vision, hearing, dental health, tuberculosis (TB), postural problems such as scoliosis, and growth and development. Various screening tests can be conducted separately or, more commonly, as a battery of tests administered in a single screening session, frequently referred to as *multiphasic screening.*

Another type of screening sometimes used in schools is referred to as case finding. *Case finding* is a specific screening activity carried out to identify a specific high-risk or suspicious condition such as head lice (pediculosis capitis). Still another variation is *selective screening,* carried out for portions of the school population who are for various reasons at special risk. Examples of high-risk children may be those of low socioeconomic status, those performing poorly in school, or those who are often absent or exhibit frequent disciplinary problems.

The usefulness of the school's health screening program depends on (1) the quality and care with which the program is carried out and (2) the uses made of the findings. Screening is one way of alerting people of the possible need for special care. The entire value of the screening process depends on how well the results are communicated to the participants and whether parents of students identified "at risk" follow through and seek definitive diagnosis and subsequently cooperate in any recommended treatment regimen.

The value of early detection made possible through a screening program must be constantly assessed against the time and personnel required to carry it out. Similarly, the decision on exactly which problem areas the screening program will assess must be judged against the utility of such a program. The following 10 principles of early disease detection have been suggested by Wilson and Jungner (1968) and apply well to screening program decisions:

1. The condition screened for should be an important health problem.
2. There should be an accepted treatment for persons with the recognized disease.
3. The facilities for subsequent diagnosis and treatment should be available.
4. There should be a recognizable latent or early systematic stage identifiable through screening.
5. There should be a suitable, easily administered screening test.
6. Screening procedures should be acceptable to the population.
7. The natural history of the condition, including the development from latent to declared disease, should be well understood.

8. There should be an agreed-upon policy on who treats patients.
9. The costs of the screening program should be economically balanced against the costs of other case-finding procedures and subsequent medical care.
10. Screening and case finding should be a continuing process. If these conditions are met, screening can be a useful tool contributing to secondary prevention.

Quality of information gathered

The Commission on Chronic Illness (1957) suggests that screening results should be reviewed in terms of (1) validity, (2) reliability, (3) yield, (4) cost, (5) acceptance, and (6) follow-up services.

The *validity* of a screening test is the ability to identify individuals who have the condition. Do the persons identified by the screening test actually have the condition when examined by a physician? Validity is assessed in several ways.

Persons identified at screening as being "at risk" subsequently fall into two groups: those who actually do have the condition and those who do not. Persons identified who are actually diagnosed as having the condition are called *true positives*. Those identified at screening as having the condition but in whom the condition was not confirmed in subsequent diagnosis are called *false positives*.

Similarly, persons not identified in the screening process as having the condition fall into two groups. There is a possibility that those not identified in the screening program do have the condition (*false negatives*), and there is a possibility that those not identified in the screening program actually do *not* have the condition (*true negatives*). A screening test's ability to identify the condition for which the screening is done is referred to as the test *sensitivity*. The ability of a test to identify correctly those who do not have the condition is referred to as the *specificity* of the test. Both sensitivity and specificity are usually expressed as percents.

$$\text{Sensitivity} = \frac{\text{Diseased persons with positive test}}{\text{All persons in population with the condition}}$$

$$\text{Specificity} = \frac{\text{Nondiseased persons with negative test}}{\text{All persons in population with the condition}}$$

Reliability of a screening test refers to the result consistency. Tests are reliable only when the same results are obtained repeatedly over time or when the test is carried out by different people and the same results are presented.

The *yield* of the screening test simply refers to the number of people identified. Screening tests should be reserved for a reasonably common condition to make them worthwhile.

Cost considerations relate both to personnel and to equipment. In the main, school screening programs are carried out with relatively inexpensive equipment that nurses, trained teachers, health aides, or volunteer parents can operate.

Today, *acceptance* of screening programs is seldom a problem. Care should always be taken to inform parents of regular screening activities and allow them to ask questions about procedures.

Follow-up activities ultimately determine the value of the screening endeavor. No matter how carefully the program is conducted, its value depends on communicating the results to parents who must get the necessary medical examinations and follow through on any suggested treatment activities.

Vision screening

Vision screening should be carried out each year of a child's elementary and secondary education and should be required of all students transferring into the school system unless the results of earlier screenings are included in the student's health record. Children with glasses should be checked annually by their health care professional. Eye characteristics change rapidly in childhood and adolescence, and the frequency of vision disorders increases with age. Only 5% of first-grade students have refractive errors (*myopia,* nearsightedness; *hyperopia,* farsightedness; *astigmatism,* irregularities in the curvature of the cornea), but as many as half of the students may have similar problems by high school graduation. *Strabismus* (cross-eye, esotropia) and differences in the visual acuity of the two eyes (*anisometropia*) are found in approximately 5% of children (Fig. 7-2).

Screening for visual acuity is most frequently done with a Snellen or similar test. For some children the illiterate *E* or the STYCAR (Sheridan's test for young children and retardates) is more effective. The illiterate *E* uses the Capital *E,* sometimes called the tumbling *E,* with the arms of the *E* facing at random either left, right, up, or down. Students are asked simply to point the direction of the arms of the E. The STYCAR test uses the letters *H, O, T,* and *V,* and children match letters on the screen chart with the same letters on a card they hold in their laps.

The wall chart for the Snellen test is placed at eye height 20 feet (6 m) from the person to be tested. The chart should be well lit (20 to 30 footcandles) with bright lights, from sources such as windows, eliminated. Both eyes are open during testing; a card covers the eye not being tested. The right eye is tested first, then the left eye, and then both. Children should be able to read at least half the letters and symbols on a given line to "pass" that line. The American Academy of Pediatrics (1981) suggests that "children at the third grade should read the 20/40 line or better with each eye; after third grade they should read the 20/30 line. A child with a difference of two or more lines between the two eyes should be referred." Children who normally wear glasses should be tested wearing their glasses.

Interpretation of the tests is not difficult in most cases. For school purposes 20/20 is normal. A child with 20/30 vision is probably nearsighted, though a definitive diagnosis must be made by the health care professional. A child with 20/10 or 20/15 vision is probably farsighted. However, a deviation from the 20/20 normal standard is simply an indication of a need for retesting and possible referral.

The test for *hyperopia,* a convex or "plus" lens test, can be carried out at the same time. This is an important test because hyperopia may eventually make reading difficult. Generally this test is given only in the early grades.

To test for hyperopia a pair of 2.25-diopter lenses on a frame are placed on the child, over his or her own glasses if necessary. A diopter (D) is a measure of refractive error. The child is asked to read the standard wall chart, described earlier. A child who can identify half or more of the letters or symbols on the 20/20 line in this case may have possible hyperopia of 2 D or more. Because of the concern and expense associated with referral, all students

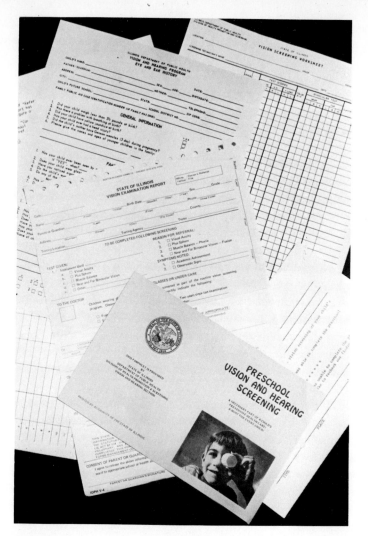

FIG. 7-2. Vision screening records provide a valuable aid for monitoring changes in students' vision and making referrals and follow-up observations. The school nurse, counselors, and teachers can refer to these records to help plan special student learning activities and possibly to help understand unusual behavior.

identified in screening as having a possible need for referral should be retested a second or third time.

Defects in *color vision* are tested for by use of the pseudoisochromatic plates in which a color figure is embedded in a background of another color. Children with normal color discrimination can identify figures and not others. It is estimated that 8% of boys and 4% of girls have color discrimination difficulties.

The possibility of vision problems can often be detected by observation of the student's behavior or appearance. Cross-eye, red, bloodshot eyes, and encrusted or swollen eyes are all signs suggestive of the need for referral or attention. Students' complaints about not being able to see well, dizziness, headaches, and nausea especially after close eye work; and reports of blurred or double vision are also signs of vision problems. Young people's behavior also can indicate the need for eye examinations: rubbing the eyes excessively, shutting or covering one eye, tilting the head, thrusting the head forward in an effort to see, difficulty in reading or other work requiring close eye contact, blinking more than usual, irritability when doing close work, stumbling over small objects, holding books close to the eyes during reading, and poor performance in games requiring distant vision can indicate the need for referral.

Children should be prepared for activities such as vision screening. They should be told in advance what will be done, why it will be done, and how it will be done. In the case of vision screening children can practice using the STYCAR or Snellen chart or illiterate E symbols before the actual tests. The results of screening should be carefully explained, with care being taken that the students do not see screening as a "pass" or "fail" situation and that referral for further testing is a helpful gesture made in the interest of the student's well-being. Only after careful diagnosis will students truly know the status of their eyes and their vision.

Some schools may be fortunate enough to have commercially produced binocular vision screening equipment. Testing effectiveness of this equipment can vary widely. The purchase and maintenance of vision screening equipment should be directed by a cooperating physician or a committee made up of parents and health care professionals. Good equipment, well maintained and correctly used, can enhance the efficiency of vision screening by reducing the space needed, but it does increase the time needed to screen large numbers of students. Some schools establish a policy whereby students not meeting a particular criterion using standard vision screening charts are tested a second time using the commercially produced binocular vision screening equipment. This allows an increased level of specificity in the screening program.

Hearing screening

Hearing loss is frequently so gradual that it is imperceptible to the person concerned. Unconsciously a person adapts to a gradual hearing loss. People with normal hearing do a certain amount of lip reading, but a person whose hearing is declining relies more and more on lip reading. Often a teacher observes behavior symptoms of hearing difficulties, such as posturing, inattention, faulty pronunciation, unnatural voice, poor academic progress, and copying.

However, many children with hearing defects do not show behavior changes, and a hearing screening test is a more reliable device to discover hearing defects than a child's outward behavior.

Many adults with greatly defective hearing could have normal or nearly normal hearing if the defect had been discovered early. Hearing screening will identify the student with possible correctable hearing loss.

Because of the importance of early detection and treatment, the hearing screening should be conducted on a schedule similar to that of vision screening, beginning during the preschool period. Hearing losses are often related to middle ear infections, which occur more frequently among younger children. Screening at this level should be done annually and then every 2 years in secondary school (Fig. 7-3).

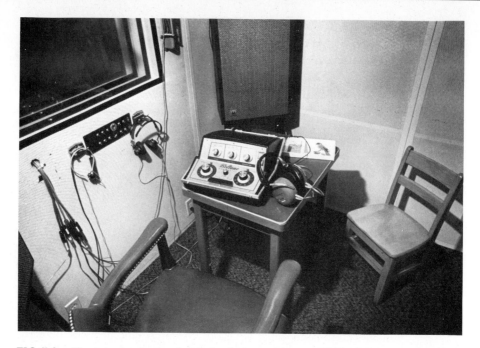

FIG. 7-3. Hearing screening involves a simple noninvasive procedure that can be a useful learning experience for young people. How the equipment works and the procedures followed should always be explained to the person being screened.

The two most common types of hearing loss are *sensorineural* and *conductive*. Sensorineural loss is serious and often irreversible. Causes of sensorineural loss include damage to the auditory nerve and damage to the auditory center of the ear and the temporal lobe of the brain. Viral diseases such as measles and mumps, bacterial infections, prolonged exposure to loud noises from sources such as tractors, rock bands, gunfire, and trauma to the head or ears are known causes of sensorineural hearing loss.

Conductive hearing loss is a more common occurrence among children and results from problems in the external ear, the tympanic membrane, and the middle ear cavity that interfere with the transmission of sound. Causes include wax impaction, foreign objects, otitis media, congenital abnormalities, and ruptured or scarred eardrums. Fortunately, many cases of conductive hearing loss can be treated with either medical or surgical procedures. However, early attention is important to avoid the profound effects on learning that even moderate hearing loss can cause (Fig. 7-4).

An accurate and reliable hearing screening program requires a pure tone audiometer and an audiometrician or trained operator to do the testing. The conventional program involves two stages: a sweep check test and a threshold test. A sweep check test establishes frequencies that can be heard when the volume is constant. The threshold test establishes the lowest volume level at which a child hears tones of a given frequency.

Hearing screening should be carried out in a room that is as quiet as possible, free of background noises such as fluorescent lighting, toilets, music classes, shop classes, cafeterias, and typewriters.

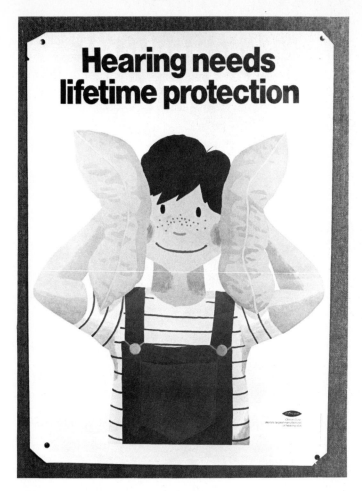

FIG. 7-4.   Often students take their ability to hear for granted. Colorful posters and informational brochures used at screening times and throughout the year are an important reinforcement for a good health education and hearing screening program.

Young people should be prepared by receiving a clear description of the testing process, an equipment demonstration, and instructions for response when they hear sounds in the headphones. Children are usually instructed to raise a hand or signal with a forefinger to acknowledge that they have heard a sound. For actual testing, students should remove glasses and earrings and should not chew gum. Care should be taken that the headphones fit properly and that hair is pulled back from around the ear.

In the sweep-check screening a tone is presented at a consistent 20-decibel (dB) level of intensity, starting with a frequency of 1000 hertz (Hz), or cycles per second, and then sweeping through several different frequencies as follows: 2000, 4000, 500, and 250 Hz. If no response is received from the students at 1000 Hz the tester has the option of proceeding through the other frequencies or increasing the intensity to 25 dB. If a response is received at 25 dB after the sweepthrough of the frequencies at this level, return to the 20 dB.

According to the American Academy of Pediatrics, children who fail to hear 1000 or 2000 Hz at 20 dB or 4000 Hz at 25 dB in one or both ears should be retested after several weeks. Because respiratory tract infections can cause temporary hearing loss, students must be retested after a period of weeks before the final referral decision is made.

The results of a hearing test are recorded on an audiogram as shown in Fig. 7-5.

The second step in hearing screening is the threshold test, which determines the exact decibel level at which a tone can be heard at various frequencies. Each ear is tested at 250, 500, 1000, 2000, and 4000 Hz with the intensity of tone beginning at O dB and increasing to louder levels until a response is obtained. Next the intensity is reduced in steps of 10 dB from the first obtained response level until no response is obtained. Then the tone is presented at 5 dB increments until the child can hear the tone. This procedure is repeated for each frequency. The American Academy of Pediatrics (1981) suggests that a child needs further diagnostic evaluation if the hearing threshold is 25 dB or greater at two or more frequencies in one or both ears or 35 dB or more for a single frequency in either ear.

False-positive hearing tests often occur because the audiometer has not been correctly

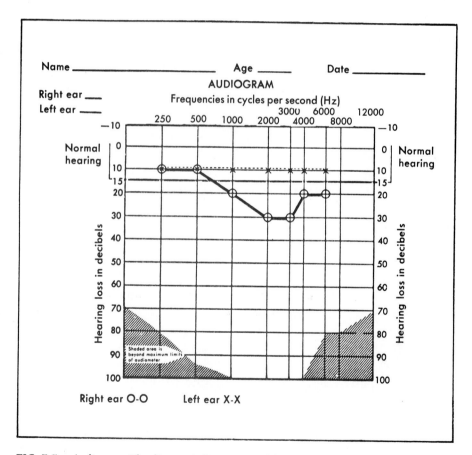

FIG. 7-5. Audiogram. The diagram indicates normal hearing in the left ear, but in the right ear a loss of 20 dB at frequencies of 1000, 4000, and 6000 hertz and a loss of 30 dB at frequencies of 2000 and 3000 hertz.

calibrated. Before any large-scale screening effort is begun, a check should be made of the equipment and the background noise of the room, and if possible an electroacousitic calibration should be carried out to ensure that the equipment is working correctly.

Tympanometry.   New technology now provides some added options in hearing screening. Audiometry provides for the subjective assessment of the threshold of sound. The student provides an indication of when he or she first hears the sound. New equipment designed to check the integrity of the middle ear now also provides an objective measure of sound threshold.

Tympanometry is the measurement of the integrity and sensitivity of the middle ear and combines the resources of miniaturized circuitry, computerized capabilities, and immediate printed test results. Using sound emitted from a hand-held probe, tympanometry compares the emitted sound to sounds reflected by the eardrum. In this way the equipment calculates the ratio of absorbed sound to reflected sound. Infections such as *otitis media* reduce the ear's ability to absorb sound; so if the tympanometer instrument measures a high degree of reflected sound, compared to absorbed sound, there may be a need for further testing and diagnoses.

At the same time this equipment is able to detect the small muscular reflexes associated with the ear's response to sound. Muscular reflexes can be assessed against different sound thresholds, and an objective measure is provided of the ear's ability to actually detect sound. Auditory sensitivity is thereby measured without the subject's subjective assessment of the threshold.

The equipment necessary for tympanometry is widely available at the moment, but it will take time for it to replace the readily available audiometric devices. Several companies are producing tympanometric equipment and are working hard to encourage its adoption and to reduce its cost. Clearly, in the future, audiometric screening in schools will incorporate this new technology and will become significantly more sophisticated.

Dental screening

Even though children are referred to the family dentist for thorough examination before admission to school and at other set times, there is no guarantee that additional dental care will occur.

Dentistry has been especially effective in encouraging good preventive practices and prophylactic care every 6 months, but some parents still believe that first teeth, or deciduous teeth, do not need special care because they will ultimately be replaced by permanent teeth. Dental screening programs provide an excellent opportunity to encourage students to take care of their teeth, eat correctly, and see a dentist frequently.

Absence of clear defects in teeth and the oral cavity at screening does not ensure that no problems exist. Dental caries occurs more frequently than any other disorder among schoolchildren, and until caries reaches an advanced stage, it is likely to cause little pain or concern. Similarly, infected gums may occur painlessly. However, dental screening programs, along with their educational impact, can identify *pyorrhea*, usually indicated by a red margin of the gum around the neck of the tooth, and *gingivitis*, sometimes called trench mouth or Vincent's disease, characterized by inflammation or even ulceration of the gums and other parts of the mouth, bleeding, excessive salivation, and considerable soreness. Gingivitis usually does not occur in healthy children but is associated with malnutrition, poor general health, inadequate rest, and poor personal hygiene. Chronic *halitosis,* or bad breath, may also indicate a problem, especially when it occurs in the presence of an otherwise clean mouth. Changes in the color of a person's teeth also indicate possible problems (Fig. 7-6).

Pronounced overbite or underbite and poorly aligned teeth that will eventually create mechanical and cosmetic problems are also easily detectable. In many cases orthodontists will delay treatment of these conditions until the student reaches a particular growth stage, but the conditions should still be brought to the parents attention. If orthodontic care has been initiated, a note should be made in the student's health record.

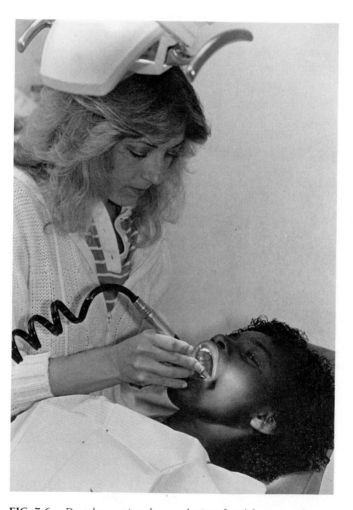

FIG. 7-6.   Dental screening that results in referral for a specific problem will usually result in the student receiving a full dental examination plus prophylactic care and instruction on the care of teeth and gums.
(Copyright 1983 by David Riecks.)

Height and weight measures

The practice of weighing and measuring is perhaps the most firmly established aspect of the school health program. Nevertheless, little evidence supports the value of height and weight data alone as a useful tool in identifying health problems that are not otherwise suspected. However, although growth charts such as those in Chapter 4 are useful in comparing the serial measurements of an individual student's height and weight, they are far from effective in detecting possible nutritional problems such as obesity or growth disorders.

As a health education aid, however, height and weight measurements are invaluable. Emphasis should be placed on interesting children in their own uniqueness, not comparing themselves with the standard table or with other children. In addition to the educational use, height and weight measurements are also useful in the follow-up observation and evaluation of specific nutrition programs such as weight control classes or as useful adjuncts to nutrition surveys, provided that height and weight measures are supplemented with skinfold measures and possible laboratory tests. Eisner and Callahan (1974) also suggest that height and weight measurements may be useful in geographic areas where there are common treatable conditions, such as hookworm and other chronic infections, that retard growth.

Recently the National Child Health Survey (1983) has shown that height and weight measures combined into a body mass index (BMI) and a skinfold measure of body fat tissue (adiposity) are related to blood pressure, both diastolic and systolic. As such, height, weight, and adiposity measures become useful screening devices.

BMI represents a simple extension of height and weight data as described in Chapter 4. The higher the index, the greater is the deviation from normal.

$$BMI = \frac{Weight \ (kg)}{(Height \ [m])^2}$$

Adiposity measures are relatively new in routine school health appraisals. Adiposity, or body fat, is estimated with specially designed calipers that measure body fat under the skin at specific points. This is done by pinching skin between the forefinger and thumb and measuring the thickness with the calipers (Fig. 7-7). The two most commonly used landmarks for screening purposes are (1) the *triceps*, the back of the arm, midway between the elbow and tip of the shoulder with the skinfold parallel to the axis of the arm (Fig. 7-8) and (2) the *subscapular* area, 1 cm below the inner angle of the end of the scapula (shoulderblade) in line with the natural cleavage of the skin (American Alliance of Health, Physical Education, Recreation and Dance, 1980) (Fig. 7-9). Usually the physical education teacher is trained in taking these measurements and can assist with adiposity screening.

Approximately 1 cm of skin is pinched, and the caliper tips are placed 1 cm above the part held by the thumb and forefinger and 1 cm in from the extended edge of the fold. The full pressure of the caliper is gradually released, and the reading is taken within a few seconds. Two or more measures at a given site should be averaged to represent the screening value. Percentile norms for the triceps area for boys and girls are presented in Table 7-1.

Scoliosis

In the typical school situation posture is not regarded as an important factor in the promotion of student health. A deviation in posture usually does not produce a serious health

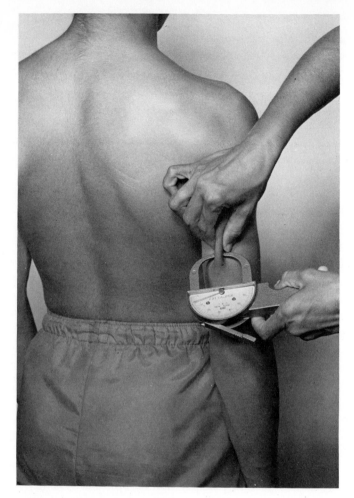

FIG. 7-7. Skinfold measurement is taken in the triceps area approximately midway between the elbow and the head of the humerus.

threat, yet, as with other physical disorders, postural defects are a concern.

Lateral curvature and rotation of the spine, or *scoliosis,* lead to significant disability later in life and are a principal focus for postural screening. It is estimated that 2% of the population has scoliosis, a treatable condition that goes largely undetected, and so the potential for the schools to greatly reduce the prevalence of this disease is significant.

Scoliosis occurs most frequently during the years of rapid growth (10 to 15 years of age); accordingly, screening programs should be arranged to check children in grades 5 through 10 annually.

Scoliosis goes undetected in the early years because many students visit a physician only irregularly and because the condition in its early stages is asymptomatic. Girls more often than boys exhibit the condition, as do those who have close relatives with scoliosis. Linking the school health records of members of an individual family may be a useful administrative practice.

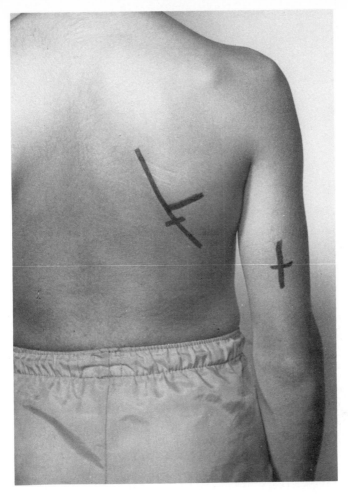

FIG. 7-8.   Landmarks for taking skinfold measurements in triceps and subscapular area.

Scoliosis screening can be carried out by the school nurse, physical education teacher, visiting physical therapist, or health aide who has received special training. Ideally both boys and girls should strip to the waist for screening purposes and should not wear leotards or other physical education clothes. A brassiere will not interfere with the screening of girls. Shoes must be removed so that both feet are level on the floor.

The student stands erect, head up, eyes straight ahead, shoulders back, and arms hanging to the sides. Feet should be together. Five points of perspective of the student's back are examined: (1) shoulders should be the same height, (2) shoulder-blades should appear at the same height, (3) the space between each of the free-hanging arms and the body should be equal, (4) flanks of the hips should be equal, and (5) the alignment of the spinal processes of the spinal cord should be straight (Fig. 7-10).

Standing directly behind the student, the screener asks the student to bend forward to right angles at the hips, head hanging in a relaxed position and the arms dangling relaxed

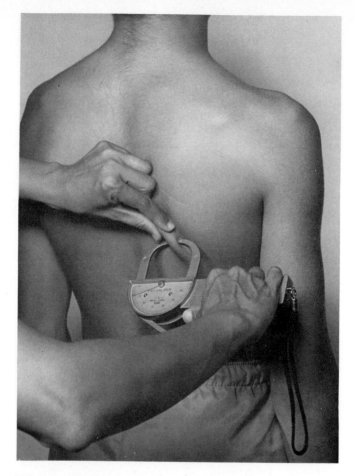

FIG. 7-9. Subscapular skinfold measurement is taken approximately 1 cm below the inner angle of the scapula.

from the shoulders with the palms pressed together and the knees remaining straight (Fig. 7-11). The screener observes the surface of the back at eye level to detect any unevenness. The box on p. 164 identifies points of observation and presents a sample reporting form to record deviations that represent criteria for further referral. Students with noted deviations should be referred to a physician for evaluation.

Blood pressure

The inclusion of blood pressure screening in school health appraisals is relatively new. Although the measurement of blood pressure is a typical part of routine medical care, it has not often been a part of school health programs because the absence of well-established norms for children and adolescents has contributed to this fact. Recognition that high blood pressure is a major heart disease risk factor and that frequently high blood pressure is asymptomatic has led to an increased concern for the early detection of high blood pressure.

Blood pressure is simply the force of the blood pulsing against the arterial wall. Blood

TABLE 7-1. Percentile norms for 6 to 18* years of age for triceps skinfold (mm)

Age (years)	6	7	8	9	10	11	12	13	14	15	16	17
Boys *Percentile*												
5	5	4	4	5	5	5	5	4	4	4	4	4
10	5	5	5	6	6	6	6	5	5	5	5	5
25	6	6	6	7	7	7	7	7	6	6	6	6
50	8	8	8	8	9	10	9	9	8	8	8	8
75	9	10	11	12	12	14	13	13	12	11	11	11
90	12	12	14	16	16	19	20	19	17	16	16	16
95	13	14	17	20	20	22	23	23	21	21	20	20
Girls												
5	6	6	6	6	6	6	6	6	7	7	8	8
10	6	6	6	7	7	7	7	7	8	9	9	10
25	7	8	8	9	9	9	9	9	11	12	12	12
50	9	10	10	11	12	12	12	12	14	15	16	16
75	11	12	14	14	15	15	16	17	18	20	21	20
90	14	16	18	19	20	20	22	23	23	25	26	25
95	16	17	20	22	23	23	25	.26	27	29	30	29

Based on data from Johnston, F., Hamill, D., and Lemeshow, S.: Skinfold thickness of children 6-11 years (Series II, No. 120, 1972) and Skinfold thickness of youth 12-17 years (Series II, No. 132, 1974), Washington, D.C., U.S. National Center for Health Statistics, U.S. Department of Health, Education and Welfare.
*The norms for age 17 may be used for age 18.

pressure is measured with a sphygmomanometer in a simple and painless procedure. Persons deviating from established norms can easily be identified and referred.

Blood pressure should be measured in a quiet area with the student relaxed. Support the student's arm at midchest level and wrap the blood pressure cuff around the upper arm. Blood pressure cuffs come in several sizes, and it is important that the cuff fit snugly and cover at least two thirds of the upper arm. Given the choice of a cuff that is too large or too small, choose the larger cuff. Inflate the cuff to approximately 30 mm Hg above the point where the radial pulse can no longer be heard. Then deflate the cuff while listening to the pulse through a stethoscope placed over the brachial artery. The point at which a clear pulsing sound is heard represents the measure of systolic pressure. The point at which the pulsing sound disappears represents the diastolic pressure.

Routinely, blood pressure should be measured two or three times to overcome the possibility of a single unusually high reading. Repeated deviations of 10% from established norms indicates the need for referral.

As with all screening procedures it must be remembered that deviation from the norm simply warrants further investigation by a medical doctor and does not necessarily indicate the existence of any clinical condition. Students and parents need to be frequently reminded of this point.

Cholesterol

Not yet common in school health screening programs but increasingly available in public screening programs is the measurement of blood cholesterol. Generally agreed to be a major

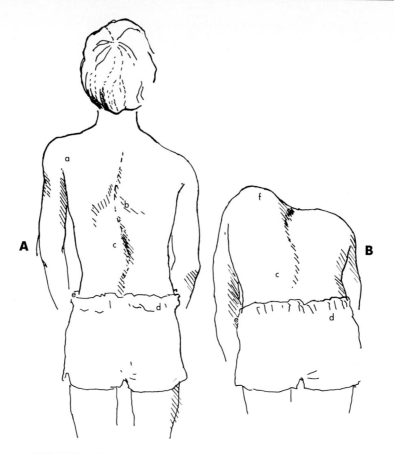

FIG. 7-10. Screening points for scoliosis. **A,** Student standing erect, feet together, arms hanging naturally. **B,** Feet together, hands with palms together, bending forward, arms hanging perpendicular to floor. *a,* Shoulder elevation uneven; *b,* scapula (shoulder-blades) uneven; *c,* misaligned spine; *d,* uneven hip prominence; *e,* unequal arm to body space; *f,* uneven rib prominence.

risk factor for heart disease, cholesterol can now be checked quickly and easily with relatively inexpensive new technology. However, a drop of blood is required for testing. The skin must be punctured, and so usually medical supervision is required.

The identification of elevated cholesterol levels will need medical interpretation. Frequently, however, modifications in the diet,reducing food of animal origin, and increasing fruit, vegetables, and grain products will adequately reduce cholesterol levels. In special cases medication will be prescribed.

Other options.   Cholesterol screening, plus several other screening options, may be suggested for inclusion in school surveillance programs. Diabetes, for example, can be easily screened and is often suggested for screening programs. It is also possible to screen for evidence of the use of several drugs. At this point, however, local philosophy, relative costs, and benefits must be considered.

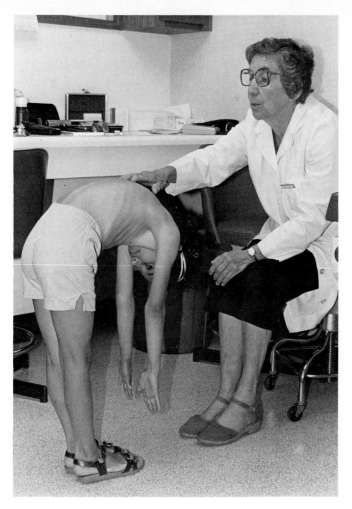

FIG. 7-11. Physician viewing student's back as she bends forward to check for indications of scoliosis. Student should also be viewed from the rear. Notice that this student's hands are not palms together as they should be.
(Copyright 1983 by David Riecks.)

The school exists to facilitate learning. Obviously, the early identification of health problems that interfere with learning is important. But schools are not health care institutions. Screening programs that require technology or specialized personnel or that seek to detect relatively rare conditions may be appropriate to seek the identification of conditions like elevated cholesterol and diabetes through required routine medical examinations conducted by physicians.

In the final analysis, the value and extent of the school's screening program should be the result of local deliberation involving school personnel, parents, and representatives of the medical community. More important, perhaps, than expanding traditional program screening is ensuring the adequte follow-up observation of cases.

Sample Scoliosis Reporting Form

Name _____ Age _____ Date _____ M/F ____

Address _____ School _____ Grade ____

Examiner _____

Back toward examiner and forward bend away from examiner:

1. Head and neck base off center over sacrum? ☐ Yes ☐ No

2. Shoulder elevation uneven? ☐ Yes ☐ No

3. Shoulder-blades uneven? ☐ Yes ☐ No

4. Waist creases uneven? ☐ Yes ☐ No

5. Obvious spinal curvature? ☐ Yes ☐ No

6. Hip prominences unequal? ☐ Yes ☐ No

7. Arm to body space unequal? ☐ Yes ☐ No

Forward bend toward examiner:

8. Ribs prominent on one side? ☐ Yes ☐ No

Side bend toward examiner:

9. Increased round back? ☐ Yes ☐ No

10. Increased swayback? ☐ Yes ☐ No

• • •

Is the student presently under treatment for scoliosis? ☐ Yes ☐ No

Student referred to: ☐ Family physician or orthopedist

☐ Services for handicapped children or other clinic

Follow-up observation

Health appraisal activities actually consist of four phases: (1) planning, (2) conduct of the health appraisal, (3) follow-up observation, and (4) summary and interpretation of the screening results to aid in curriculum development.

Health screening disrupts the normal educational pattern of the school day and poses a different pattern, not necessarily less educational but designed specifically for another purpose. Efficiency is important. Careful planning ensures that classroom disruption is held to a minimum. One can improve efficiency by seeking help in the actual screening activities from local health departments and voluntary health agencies, from volunteer parents, and physical education and speech teachers. All cooperating personnel must be skilled in their tasks, and all equipment must be checked in advance.

Planning should be carried out in detail. The actual screening activities should be carried out in an organized manner with special care to gather accurate information and record it clearly.

For effective follow-up study, screening results must be properly recorded so that they can be clearly understood and interpreted at a later date. Before one confers with parents, other school records should be reviewed to emphasize the importance of suggested follow-up activities in relation to the child's overall school performance.

Follow-up centers around referral. A screening exercise simply identifies a person who needs further careful examination. Care should be taken to avoid unnecessary referrals because of anxiety and expense placed on parents and unnecessary burdens placed on local health care resources.

The simplest referral device is a letter sent directly to parents or guardians with a clear explanation of what was done, the results, and recommended follow-up actions. Care should be taken not to alarm parents or guardians. Include a simple letter or card the health care provider carrying out the suggested follow-up observation can complete, to be returned to the school with referral results. School personnel should establish a time frame for the referral and should state this clearly in the letter. Suggest telephone contact with the school nurse or aide if questions or confusion arises.

If compliance with the referral is not achieved in a set time, a conference with the parents is recommended. Ideally both parents should attend the conference because they may see the problem from different perspectives. Parent conferences may include other school staff such as the nurse or physician, teacher, administrator, or possibly staff members such as the physical education, speech, or special education teacher. Parent conferences serve the purpose of explaining the possible problem and its significance, but just as importantly they should develop a plan of action including suggestions of care sources, means of payment, and limits of the school's responsibilities. The school needs to establish a policy clearly outlining just how far a school will go to ensure parental follow-up observation and just how much of the school's resources will be devoted to such an activity.

Records

A critical element to follow-up relates to interpretation and use of records. Individual student records are confidential documents. Access to these documents is specified in the Family Education Rights and Privacy Act of 1974, Title IV, PL 93-380 (as amended).

A student's individual health record includes health examination results, screening results and records of routine health activities within the school such as accident and illness. This is a confidential document. All members of the school staff should recognize this fact. Health records are also cumulative documents of long standing, and so statements that could damage a student's school career should not be included. Certain entries in the record may be appropriate, but the likelihood of later misinterpretation should always be considered. For example, reference to psychologic care or mental health counseling could be interpreted as evidence of mental illness, and reference to health conditions could possibly interfere with later employment opportunities and insurance eligibility.

Under the terms of the Family Education Rights and Privacy Act all student records must be available to parents and can be subpoenaed as court evidence. Parents, or students who have reached 18 years of age, may review their children's or their own records on request. Further, they have a right to challenge the accuracy of these records and seek corrections or deletions of offending sections. Records cannot be released to a third party without informed consent and only for specified purposes. Summary or aggregated data that do not identify individual students, however, can be compiled for planning purposes without violating the confidentiality of student health records.

The school health examination and routine health screening activities provide a significant opportunity to improve students' health. Early identification of health problems is the next best option to actual primary prevention. Even the healthy child can benefit from participation in a health examination and health screening program.

HEALTH GUIDANCE AND SUPERVISION

Health appraisal information is obviously useful to individual students and their parents. In summary form, these data are also useful to classroom teachers and curriculum planners. Classroom activities should address common health conditions among students. School nurses and counselors can also work with individual students and their parents to help overcome health problems. Individual counseling and direct supervision of a student's educational activities are important follow-up aspects of health appraisals and also form part of the school's educational responsibilities.

Traditionally, schools accept the role of supervising all aspects of a student's activities during the school day. In practice, such supervision at school corresponds to the supervision a conscientious parent exercises in the home. However, inherent in the school's role is more than just the protection and maintenance of the child's health.

Any school health program must be appraised in terms of its effect on individual students' health. No phase of the program has a more direct effect on the student than does the guidance and supervision phase. The effect will be reflected in the student's future well-being and the student's ability to accept responsibility for his or her own health.

Basic concepts

Guidance helps young people plan their own actions, in full light of all facts about themselves and the world in which they live and work.

Health guidance acquaints persons with various ways in which they may discover and use their natural endowments to live as well as possible. Guidance means accepting each pupil as an independent personality. Effective guidance develops the student's ability for self-guidance; if the student continues to lean heavily on the counselor, the guidance has not been effective. As revealed diagrammatically in Fig. 7-12, the counselor should play a diminishing role and the student an increasing role in the process.

Responsibility

In the United States, the school health program and the school general guidance and counseling program experienced parallel growth, since both grew out of the transition to functional education. Both are concerned primarily with students as individuals and with their overall well-being.

Education leaders support the view that all teachers have a role in guidance. These

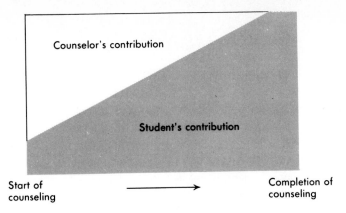

FIG. 7-12. Counselor and student contributions in health counseling. At the outset the counselor makes a considerable contribution but reduces his or her role as students increase their contributions. The final objective is to develop students' abilities to rely on their own resources.

leaders also recognize that school health personnel are in a strategic position to contribute to the school guidance program and consequently to each student's fullest development. Clearly, from a school's perspective, the only issue more important than education is the child's health.

In this context, health education should not be considered exclusively an academic subject. Health instruction is a means to an end, with a goal of the student's fullest possible development. The quality of well-being the student maintains and his or her ability to make necessary decisions relating to personal health reveal the application of health knowledge.

Counseling is a procedure of guidance and a form of mutual deliberation that involves examination of items that will aid a child in comprehending his or her problem and understanding its solution. The school counselor does not make the final decision but aids the student or parent in arriving at a solution. Counseling helps a child see his or her health needs and find the medical or other service required. It may be a matter of working out a pattern of living to attain a maximal level of health. Counseling can also help each child develop a full appreciation of the value of good health and inculcate a determination to promote and protect that asset. Counseling may be an avenue through which a student visualizes future needs and accomplishments.

Primary responsibility for a child's health must always rest with the parents, but the school is in a strategic position to complement and supplement the effort by dealing with expressed and observed health problems. After all, the best and fullest development of each child is the school's cardinal objective. Subject matter is important, but it serves as a means to an end in the development of the student. It is incongruous to teach children about health yet disregard their existing health problems.

The guidance role of the elementary school teacher and the secondary school health educator is to help students understand their problems, to see possible solutions, and to know which professionals and agencies may be of service in helping them solve their problems.

Similarities and Differences Between Counseling and Teaching

Teaching

1. The teacher needs to know pupils so that educational objectives are attained and normal growth processes encouraged.
2. The subject matter outcomes (or objectives) to be attained are known to the teacher.
3. The teacher is responsible for encouraging growth toward objectives partially determined by the social order (citizenship, honesty). The teacher has a responsibility for the welfare of the culture.
4. Teaching starts with a group relationship, and individual contacts grow out of and return to group activities.
5. The teacher is responsible for the welfare of many children at one time.
6. The teacher carries on most work directly with children.
7. The teacher uses skill in group techniques with great frequency, whereas interviewing skills are used less often.
8. The teacher uses tests, records, and inventories to assist the instructional (educational) process.
9. The teacher has many tools (curriculum outlines, books, workbooks, and visual and auditory aids) to increase effectiveness.

Counseling

1. The counselor needs to know pupils in terms of specific problems, frustrations, and plans for the future.
2. The subject matter of the interview is known to the counselor and sometimes unknown to the counselee.
3. The counselor is responsible for helping the counselee resolve personal problems. The counselor has a responsibility for the welfare of the counselee.
4. Counseling starts with an individual relationship and moves to group situations for greater efficiency or to supplement the individual process.
5. The counselor is responsible for only one person at any one time.
6. The counselor works with and through many people. Referral resources and techniques are of considerable importance.
7. The counselor uses interviewing skills as a basic technique.
8. The counselor uses tests, records, and inventories to discover factors relating to a problem. The results are used for problem-solving (therapeutic) purposes.
9. The counselor has no tools that are used with all the counselees. The first task is to help the counselee discover problems and their causes and then the individually appropriate sources of assistance.

Organized health guidance focuses the students' interest on the appraisal of their own health status, making health knowledge personally identifiable and more meaningful.

Teaching and counseling

In many respects teaching and counseling are similar. Many of their objectives are the same. Teaching attempts to obtain these objectives through classroom situations. Counseling seeks these objectives through counseling relationships. The principles developed by the Michigan State University of Counseling, Testing and Guidance illustrate the differences between counseling and teaching (see box above and on p. 169).

Similarities and Differences Between Counseling and Teaching—cont'd

Teaching

10. The teacher needs to increase personal information relating to instructional activities.

11. The teacher has a "compelled" relationship. Children are required to be there.

12. The teacher deals with children, the majority of whose adjustments are happy and satisfying.

13. The teacher is much concerned with the day-to-day growth of pupils and with their general development.

14. The skillful teacher tries to develop many abilities that increase instructional effectiveness.

Counseling

10. The counselor needs information not frequently used by teachers: information about occupations, training institutions, colleges, apprenticeship programs, community occupational opportunities, placement, referral resources, social service agencies, and diagnostic and clinical instruments.

11. The most effective counseling comes from a voluntary association. The counselee must want help and must feel that the counselor can be helpful.

12. The counselor's clients are disturbed by frustrations. They are often characterized by emotional tensions, previous disappointments, and lack of confidence.

13. The counselor is concerned with the counselee's immediate problems and choices but is also interested in helping the counselee develop workable long-term plans.

14. The skillful counselor tries to develop many of the abilities used by a wide variety of highly technical specialists: psychiatrist, clinical psychologist, test technicians, occupational information specialists, social workers, visiting teachers, juvenile deliquency workers, and placement officers.

SUMMARY

Health appraisals seek to identify health conditions that will detract from the general welfare of the student and interfere with learning. This responsibility is shared with the parent, who should report past and present illnesses and handicapping conditions; the physician, who checks the child's health at specific times during his or her school career; and school personnel, who have the opportunity to routinely check a few but important measures of health.

The school screening programs, which identify deviation from the norm, can be dealt with only to the extent that parents and community resources join together to help identify health problems and to provide the means for treatment.

School screening programs are important but limited. They identify students with deviations from a preestablished norm but do not confirm the presence of specific health problems. Screening programs identify the need for further analysis and should clearly be recognized as such. When significant conditions are identified, follow-up observation to ensure that the proper medical opinion is obtained is critical. Similarly, as much effort needs to be devoted to the difficult follow-up observation of many cases as was devoted to the initial screening and subsequent diagnosis.

Equipment and personnel costs and the yield of true-positive results, considered in light of the philosophy of the local school board and community, will dictate the nature and extent of the school's health appraisal practices.

STUDY QUESTIONS

1. Explain the contention that health appraisal is a continuing process.
2. What is the primary objective of the health examination?
3. If certain parents do not arrange to have their children checked by a dentist, what can the school do?
4. Who should have access to the child's health record form?
5. Referral of a child by the school is to the parents, not to the physician. What is the significance of this procedure?
6. Why is it important to start the screening for vision and hearing in preschool?
7. Propose a program to have all elementary school children have at least one dental examination per year.
8. What measures should the school take when a child has been found to have a hearing defect?
9. Why is it unnecessary for all schoolchildren to have a threshold test of their hearing?
10. What is the purpose of a screening examination as opposed to a health examination?
11. What are some of the benefits that can come to students from effective health guidance?
12. What are some common objectives of teaching and counseling?
13. Why should the school administration concern itself with the health of all teachers in the school district?
14. Why is the health of the teacher a significant factor in the school health program?
15. What is the difference between false-positive and false-negative results in a screening test?
16. Distinguish between validity, reliability, and yield in health screening.
17. Why is a federal law needed to govern access to student records?
18. What is the difference between the sensitivity and the specificity of a screening test?
19. List and explain the significance of three common visual defects found in young children.
20. Explain the screening process for scoliosis.
21. Demonstrate the correct way to administer a vision screening test using (a) the Snellen chart, (b) the STYCAR test, (c) the illiterate E, and (d) the test for color vision defects.
22. How do sensorineural and conductive hearing losses differ?
23. How does a threshold test differ from a sweep test?
24. Why is dental screening so important, and what are the basic dental problems that can be detected in a screening program?
25. Describe the limitations of height and weight as a screening device. How do BMIs and measures of adiposity add to the value of height and weight data?
26. What are scoliosis and lordosis?

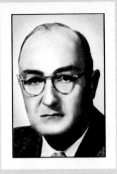

Charles C. Wilson

BORN December 26, 1895, Brooklyn, New York
DIED April 9, 1979, Hamden, Connecticut
EDUCATION B.A., Springfield College; M.D., Yale University

Charles Wilson had a wide range of experience in health, health education, and related fields. He was director of health and physical education in the Evansville, Indiana, public schools from 1928 to 1934 and then held a similar position in Hartford, Connecticut, from 1934 to 1941. From 1941 to 1946 he served as professor of health education and chairman of the Department of Special Education at Teachers College, Columbia University, New York. From 1946 until his retirement in 1965 he was professor of education and public health at the Yale School of Epidemiology and Public Health, a division of the medical school.

Dr. Wilson held many positions of leadership in professional organizations. He was twice elected to 3-year terms on the Governing Council of the American Public Health Association, and he served as secretary, vice-chairman, and chairman of the School Health Section. He was president of the American School Health Association and president of the Health Education Division of the American Association for Health, Physical Education, and Recreation. He acted as chairman of numerous conferences on professional preparation in health education. He was a diplomate of the American Board of Preventive Medicine and Public Health and a fellow of the American Public Health Association and the American Association for Health, Physical Education, and Recreation. From 1933 to 1945 Dr. Wilson was a member of the Joint Committee on Health Problems in Education of the National Education Association and the American Medical Association. He served as chairman of the committee for 6 years and edited three of its major publications, *Health Education, Healthful School Living,* and *School Health Services,* which set standards for school health education programs nationwide.

Dr. Wilson authored numerous articles and wrote a series of health texts for elementary and secondary schools. *The American Health Series* and *Life and Health.* He coauthored, with his wife Dr. Elizabeth Avery Wilson, the *Health for Young America* series.

REFERENCES

American Academy of Pediatrics: School health: a guide for health professionals, Elk Grove Village, Ill., 1987, the Academy.

American Alliance For Health, Physical Education, Recreation and Dance: Lifetime health related physical fitness, Reston, Va., 1980, the Alliance.

Appelboom, T.: A history of vision screening, J. Sch. Health **55**:138, 1985.

Blauvelt, L.: Closing the gaps in school health services, J. Sch. Health **47**:422, 1977.

Blum, R., Pfaffinger, K., and Donald, W.: A school-based comprehensive health clinic for adolescents, J. Sch. Health **52**:486, 1982.

Bonaguro, J.A., McLaughlin, M., and Sussman, K.: An exploration of health counseling and goal attainment scaling in health education programs, J. Sch. Health **54**(10):403, 1984.

Brink, S.G., and Nader, P.R.: Comprehensive health screening in elementary schools: an outcome evaluation, J. Sch. Health **54**(2):75, 1984.

Brown, E.: Multidisciplinary assessment of learning problems — school nurse's role, J. Sch. Health **51**:595, 1981.

Bryan, E.: Administrative concerns and the school's relationship with private practice physicians, J. Sch. Health **49**:157, 1979.

Eisner, V., and Oglesby, A.: Health assessment of school children. III. Vision, J. Sch. Health **41**:408, 1971.

Family Educational Rights and Privacy Act of 1974, Title IV, PL 93-380 (as amended), Fed. Reg. **40**:1208, Jan 6, 1975.

Fox, G., and Harlin, V.: Role and responsibilities of the school physician, J. Sch. Health **44**:369, 1974.

Griffith, B., and Whicker, P.: Teacher-observer of student health problems, J. Sch. Health **51**:428, 1981.

Kaplan, D.L., Rips, J.L., Clark, N.M., et al.: Transferring a clinic-based health education program for children with asthmas to a school setting, J. Sch. Health **56**(7):267, 1986.

Knecht, L.: Consent and confidentiality: legal issues in adolescent health care for the school nurse, J. Sch. Health **51**:606, 1981.

Litwack, J., and Litwack, L.: The school nurse as a health counselor, J. Sch. Health **46**:590, 1976.

Mallick, M.J.: Anorexia nervosa and bulimia: questions and answers for school personnel, J. Sch. Health **54**(8):299, 1984.

National Child Health Survey (NCHS): Dietary intake and cardiovascular risk factors. I. Blood pressure correlate, U.S. 1971-1975. Data from the National Survey Series 11, No. 226, Hyattsville, Md., Feb. 1983, U.S. Department of Health and Human Services, Public Health Services.

Newman, I.: Integrating health services and health education: seeking a balance, J. Sch. Health **52**:488, 1982.

North, A.: Screening in child health care: where are we now and where are we going? Pediatrics **54**:631, 1974.

Northern, J.: Auditory. In Frankenburg, W., and Camp, B.: Pediatric screening tests, Springfield, Ill., 1975, Charles C Thomas, Publisher.

Silver, G.: Redefining school health services: comprehensive child health care as the framework, J. Sch. Health **51**:157, 1981.

Walter, H.J., and Connelly, P.A.: Screening for risk factors as a component of a chronic disease prevention program for youth, J. Sch. Health **55**(5):183, 1985.

Wilson, J., and Jungner, G.: Principles and practices of screening for disease, World Health Organization, Public Health Papers No. 34, Geneva, 1986.

Zanga, J.R., and Oda, D.S.: School health services, J. Sch Health **57**(10):413, 1987.

Preventive Aspects of Health Services
Control of Communicable Diseases

OVERVIEW   *Although communicable diseases are no longer a principal cause of death, they are not eradicated. Only smallpox has been totally eliminated. Thus most other fatal communicable diseases are still present but so infrequent in their occurrence in North America and more developed parts of the world as to be unnoticed by the general public. The continued absence of communicable diseases as a major cause of death rests entirely on society's ability to maintain high standards of personal hygiene, effective sanitary engineering practices (especially the management of sewage and water), good housing, adequate nutrition, and high levels of immunization within the entire population.*

Infectious diseases have always been a scourge of the young, and even today the young are more prone to infections. Because infection depends to a large degree on the close association of many people, the school presents both a great potential to spread infection and a great potential to control infectious diseases. Teachers must understand the dynamics of infection, the principal infectious diseases of school-aged children and the ways to control infection.

OBJECTIVES   **After reading this chapter, the student should be able to:**

1. Identify and describe paths of infection and disinfection
2. Differentiate between types of resistance to communicable disease and different forms of immunity
3. Diagram and describe the course of an infectious respiratory disease
4. Describe the (a) source of infection, (b) mode of transmission, (c) incubation period, and (d) possible school control measures for 12 common infectious conditions of childhood and adolescence
5. Outline various responsibilities for controlling infectious diseases
6. Explain legal and administrative reasons for excluding ill children from school
7. Detail the immunization schedule for school-aged students and explain needs for legal mandate to enforce immunization schedules
8. Recognize the different sexually transmitted diseases and explain why they present a special challenge to school personnel

Today's school is concerned with the prevention of diseases and defects. Yet often the school's main effort focuses on the prevention of communicable disease, though communicable disease rates have declined significantly. Perhaps this decline reflects the school's past efforts.

COMMUNICABLE DISEASE

Disease is a harmful departure from the normal state of health. A *communicable* disease is one transmitted from one person to another or from other animals to humans. It involves parasites that are pathogenic to humans. Most of the organisms are microscopic, though some worms and even mites are visible to the unaided human eye. Microscopic pathogens include bacteria, viruses, fungi, and protozoa.

INFECTION AND DISINFECTION

Infection is the successful invasion by pathogenic organisms under conditions that permit them to multiply and harm the body. The mere presence of organisms in the body, however, does not mean infection. At a given moment many persons harbor pneumococcus bacteria in the lungs without having pneumonia, and many persons have billions of *Streptococcus albus* on the skin without having acne. Bodily harm is usually caused by an organism-produced toxin (biologic poison), though some organisms invade and damage tissues directly. To multiply and thrive, human pathogens require a temperature of about 98.6° F (37° C), moisture, alkalinity, darkness, and nutrients. The human body provides optimal conditions.

The body reacts to infection by increased production of white blood cells, elevated temperature, inflammation, and pain. These body defenses may be sufficient to overcome the infection.

Disinfection kills, removes, or arrests the activity of the pathogens of infection so that the body's defense mechanisms can overcome the invader. Chemical disinfectants are generally used for infections. Tincture of iodine, mild silver protein (Argyrol), gentian violet, mercocresols (Mercresin), nitromersol (Metaphen), thimerosal (Merthiolate), benzalkonium (Zephiran), and alcohol dilutions are examples. A disinfectant must be effective without causing damage to living tissues.

CONTAMINATION AND DECONTAMINATION

Contamination is the presence of human pathogens or nonpathogenic organisms, such as *Escherichia coli* from the alimentary canal, on inanimate objects. Thus one speaks of a *contaminated* handkerchief, glass, water supply, or quart of milk, but one speaks of an *infected* finger, tonsil, or intestine. Water is *contaminated* if it contains *Escherichia coli*. Milk is a good medium for human pathogens, but other inanimate objects are not because pathogens live only seconds in light, dryness, or low temperatures. Inanimate articles, other than milk, water, and solid foods, that harbor pathogenic organisms are called *fomites*.

Decontamination is killing or removing the pathogens and *Escherichia coli* in or on inanimate objects. Several methods can be used, such as burning, heat drying, ultraviolet rays, and highly concentrated chemicals.

CAUSATIVE AGENTS

Knowledge of the classification and nature of disease-causing organisms is essential to understand infectious diseases. Most human pathogens belong to the plant kingdom, as shown in Table 8-1.

CLASSIFICATION OF COMMUNICABLE DISEASES

Different systems have been devised to classify communicable diseases. A simple yet comprehensive classification accepted by many in the health field encompasses four different classes. Each class title describes the diseases in the group and suggests the mode of transmission.

The four classes and some of the more common diseases in each class

Respiratory diseases	*Alvine (intestine) discharge diseases*
Chickenpox	Amebic dysentery
Coryza (head cold)	Bacillary dysentery
Diphtheria	Salmonellosis
German measles (rubeola)	Typhoid fever
Influenza	Serum hepatitis
Measles (rubeola)	Viral hepatitis
Meningococcus meningitis	*Open-lesion diseases*
Mumps (parotitis)	Furunculosis (boils)
Poliomyelitis (infantile paralysis)	Gonorrhea
Rheumatic fever	Impetigo (gym itch)
Scarlet fever	Scabies
Smallpox (variola)	Rabies
Streptococcal throat infection	Syphilis
Tuberculosis	*Insect-borne diseases*
Whooping cough (pertussis)	Malaria
	Rocky Mountain spotted fever
	Tularemia
	Yellow fever

In the normal school situation, respiratory diseases constitute the greatest problem in disease control. Students have more days of restricted activity and school absenteeism because of respiratory conditions than any other condition.

TRANSMISSION OF INFECTIOUS DISEASE

Humans are the greatest reservoir of disease-causing organisms. Although other reservoirs exist the great problem in controlling communicable disease is preventing transmission of organisms from one person to another. The increase in population, travel, and general congestion of people increase the problem of control. Pathogens are transmitted by direct or indirect contact or by an intermediate host.

Direct contact is the most common means to transfer infection. Three conditions are necessary for transfer: the infectious materials must be fresh, the distance traveled must be short, and the lapse time must be brief. Material may be transferred through hand shaking, kissing, coughing, or sneezing. Normal air does not usually contain enough virile pathogens to cause infection by inhalation, but sneezes and coughs may provide a means of transfer. Respiratory diseases are transferred by direct contact, and most are acquired when the

TABLE 8-1. Classification of human pathogens

Plants		Animals	
Bacteria (split fungi)	**Disease**	**Protozoa (one cell)**	**Disease**
Bacillus (rod shaped)	Bacillary dysentery	Ameba	Dysentery
	Brucellosis	Spirochete (spiral)	Syphilis
	Diphtheria	Plasmodium	Malaria
	Tuberculosis		
	Typhoid fever	**Metazoa**	
	Whooping cough (pertussis)	Roundworm	
Coccus (spheric)	Furunculosis (boils)	Tapeworm	
	Gonorrhea	Trichinella	Trichinosis
	Scarlet fever		
	Streptococcal throat infection		
Spirillum (spiral shaped)	Cholera		
	Rat-bite fever		
Rickettsia (small bacteria)	Rocky Mountain spotted fever		
	Typhoid fever		
Virus (ultramicroscopic)	Chickenpox		
	Coryza (head cold)		
	Influenza		
	Measles (rubeola)		
	Mumps (parotitis)		
	Poliomyelitis (infantile paralysis)		
	Rabies		
True fungi			
Mold	Mycosis		
	Tinea (ringworm)		
Yeast	Blastomycosis		
	Dermatophytosis		

organisms are carried to the mouth via the person's own hands. Open-lesion diseases also are transmitted by direct contact.

Indirect contact involves an intermediate vehicle between the reservoir and the new host. The infectious material may be old, the time interval long, and the distance great. Alvine discharge diseases are usually transmitted indirectly via water, milk, or foods. Respiratory diseases may be spread by indirect contact via handkerchiefs, towels, and eating utensils, though the usual method is by direct contact.

An *intermediate host*, the third method of transmission, accounts for the transfer of insect-borne diseases. An insect acquires the organism from an infected person or lower animal and transfers the organism to another person. In some instances the organism spends part of its life cycle in the intermediate host, but in other cases the transmission is a mechanical transfer.

BLOCKING ROUTES OF TRANSMISSION

If one person is the original reservoir of infection and another person is a prospective new host, the organisms must travel by one of several routes between the two. If these routes are blocked, the new host will be protected from contracting the disease. First the organisms must escape from the reservoir. Their ability to travel is limited and, so they must rely on vehicles of transmission. Because conditions outside the human body are decidedly unfavorable to pathogens, the organisms must enter the new host shortly after leaving the reservoir. Several means are available for blocking the routes of transmission of disease.

Early diagnosis is essential to block routes of transmission. Because diseases vary in their mode of transmission, disease identification indicates routes over which the organisms of that disease may travel.

Control of the direct contact route is the most difficult to handle effectively. In a society where citizens enjoy personal freedom, voluntary or compulsory restriction on personal contact is difficult to establish. The control of disease spread by direct contact depends on a willingness to undergo personal inconvenience for the protection of others.

Isolation of persons with diagnosed cases can be an effective means to control direct contact. Also helpful is quarantine of exposed susceptible persons during the period which they might transmit the disease if infected. These are legally enforceable measures though voluntary isolation is the most desirable means of disease control.

Control of the air route is based on the three principal ways by which infection may be spread by aerial contamination: droplets, droplet nuclei, and dust. *Droplets* are the fine drops of moisture composing the spray of coughs and sneezes. Moisture sustains the bacteria for several seconds so that inhalation could carry virile organisms into the respiratory tract of a susceptible host. *Droplet nuclei* are minute particles from the evaporation of droplets, which, being small and light, may float in the air for minutes. *Dust* can become contaminated from droplets and droplet nuclei and thus be a vehicle for the transmission of disease.

Control of the water route is highly effective through community water treatment plants, sewage treatment, and the prevention of stream pollution. The same procedures apply to private and semipublic water supplies. Chlorine added to water effectively controls most waterborne diseases.

Control of the milk route is possible through testing of herds for tuberculosis and brucellosis, milk pasteurization, dairy inspection, and examination of dairy employees.

Control of the solid food route focuses on sustained inspections and sanitary safeguards for food cultivation, production, distribution, and preparation. Foods that are consumed raw, such as fruit and vegetables, are given special attention. Supervision of sanitation in restaurants and other establishments where food is produced or prepared such as canneries and bakeshops, is effective.

Control of the insect route depends on knowledge of the pathogen, the insect, and the disease itself. Control measures are directed toward the destruction of the intermediate host. Elimination of breeding places and insecticide and larvicide use are highly effective direct means. Theoretically, insect-borne diseases can be controlled completely.

RESISTANCE AND IMMUNITY

Resistance is the body's general ability to ward off pathogens. Several body factors act as barriers or defenses against organisms pathogenic to the human being. These mechanisms, nonspecific in their action, attack all foreign organisms with varying degrees of effectiveness.

Human skin is a *mechanical* barrier, and its moderate acidity provides an unfavorable medium for pathogens. *Mucous secretions* of the respiratory tract interfere with pathogens, which are propelled outward by the hairlike cilia of the mucous cells. The *acid* of the stomach and the high alkalinity of the intestines defend against pathogens. *Salinity* of the tears protects the eyes and eyelids against infection. *Fever* is the body's response to invading parasites. Because temperatures above 100° F (38° C) inactivate most pathogens, a fever aids the body's task of destroying organisms.

Perhaps the most important defense mechanism is *phagocytosis,* where microorganisms are enveloped, dissolved, and absorbed. White cells of the blood (leukocytes) and fixed (endothelial) cells of the liver, spleen, and lymph nodes are phagocytes, capable of destroying pathogens.

Immunity, complete resistance to a disease, is specific to a particular disease. Immunity is the result of specific chemical substances (antibodies) that neutralize a particular toxin or cause bacteria to precipitate or stick together.

Active immunity exists when a person's own body produces the antibodies either through an attack of a disease or by inoculation. The time active immunity lasts varies with different diseases. Second attacks are common in the common cold, influenza, and pneumonia and are rare in chickenpox, measles, mumps, poliomyelitis, and scarlet fever. Inoculation during infancy against diphtheria and pertussis may produce lifelong immunity. Artificial active immunization is available for diphtheria, measles, mumps, poliomyelitis, rabies, Rocky Mountain spotted fever, scarlet fever, smallpox, tetanus, typhoid fever, and whooping cough.

Passive immunity occurs when antibodies formed in animals or human beings are infected into another person. Passive immunity is of short duration; the borrowed antibodies tend to exhaust their cycle and disappear as the blood is renewed. An example of passive immunity is the *infantile immunity* of the first 3 to 6 months of life. Antibodies from the mother diffuse through the placenta into the bloodstream of the fetus.

CYCLE OF RESPIRATORY INFECTIOUS DISEASES

Respiratory infectious diseases follow a characteristic cycle of six stages or periods—incubation, prodrome, fastigium, defervescence, convalescence, and defection (Fig. 8-1).

Incubation is initiated by the invasion of pathogens. During the incubation period organisms multiply, but the infected person displays no symptoms. The incubation period varies both from one disease to another and with the same disease. Usually the disease is not communicable during the incubation period, though measles and chickenpox can be transmitted during the last 3 days of the incubation period.

Prodrome is initiated by the first symptoms of illness. Symptoms of the prodromal period, those of the common cold, are the same for all respiratory infections: nasal discharge, watery eyes, mild fever, headache, general ache, irritability, restlessness, digestive disturbances, and perhaps a cough. This period lasts about a day, and a definite diagnosis cannot be made. Since the person often believes the symptoms are mild, he or she may continue a usual mode of life and expose many people during this highly communicable stage. Teachers should be alert to observe prodromal symptoms in children as the signal of impending danger.

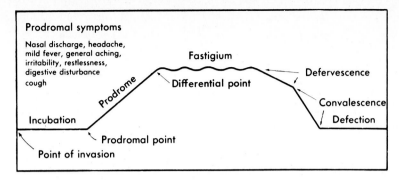

FIG. 8-1. Course of an infectious respiratory disease. All respiratory infections follow the course this graph indicates. In the school the prodrome and convalescence periods pose the greatest problems in disease control because the infected person may be well enough to be up and around, exposing others.

Fastigium represents the height of the disease, initiated by the differential point at which characteristics of the specific disease allow diagnosis. Because the person is now home or hospitalized, not many people are exposed, though this period is highly communicable.

Defervescence is a decline in the severity of the disease. A new disease may produce a *relapse,* but usually the case proceeds to convalescence.

Convalescence, or recuperation, represents a difficult control problem because the disease may still be transmissible.

Defection is casting off organisms and may coincide with convalescence. Recovery from a disease does not imply the end of communicability. Isolation time is based on the length of defection, when the person has cast off all infectious organisms.

INFECTIOUS RESPIRATORY DISEASES

Although the list of known infectious respiratory diseases is extensive, certain ones affect the school population and are of particular interest to the teacher. An understanding of the characteristics, mode of transmission, and control measures for these diseases aid the teacher's efforts to prevent the spread of disease. Although the teacher never attempts to diagnose a particular ailment, knowledge of various diseases gives him or her the necessary confidence to take effective action.

With improved environmental sanitation and the wide acceptance of immunizations, many communicable diseases are no longer common. Teachers should never see advanced cases of these conditions among their students.

Because the early (prodromal) stages of many of these conditions appear similar, teachers should be aware of the guidelines used by nurses and others when deciding to send a student home. Standards may vary, but the presence of any rash warrants a call to parents with a request for the student's removal from school until a physician indicates the condition is not contagious. Students with temperatures 100° F (38° C) or above are usually sent home, as are students with sore throats, swollen glands, clearly inflamed throats, and obvious cold symptoms. Other less specific conditions, such as headache and nausea, must be judged more subjectively. Elevated temperature, but less than 100° F (38° C), along with sore throat, rash, headache, and nausea in some combination clearly indicates exclusion. Ideally the school nurse, aide, or teacher with special training should be responsible for the exclusion decision. Decision guidelines should be developed with the assistance of the local health department, school physician, or school health committee.

Chickenpox. A fairly prevalent, though not serious, disease among schoolchildren, chickenpox can become widespread.
1. *Infectious agent:* unidentified virus
2. *Source of infection:* respiratory discharges; lesions of the skin of infected persons
3. *Mode of transmission:* directly from person to person; indirectly through objects with fresh respiratory discharges from the mucous membranes and skin of infected persons
4. *Incubation period:* 14 to 16 days
5. *Description:* mild constitutional symptoms; slight fever; few eruptions and mostly on covered surfaces; eruption at various stages of development in the same area (Fig. 8-2)
6. *Control measures for the school:* exclusion for minimum of 7 days

Head cold. Typical head colds (coryza) merit more attention than they are usually given. They can be a forerunner of other diseases.
1. *Infectious agents:* unidentified viruses
2. *Source of infection:* nose and mouth secretions of infected person
3. *Mode of transmission:* directly by sneezing and coughing; indirectly from objects with fresh respiratory discharges of infected person
4. *Incubation period:* 1 to 3 days

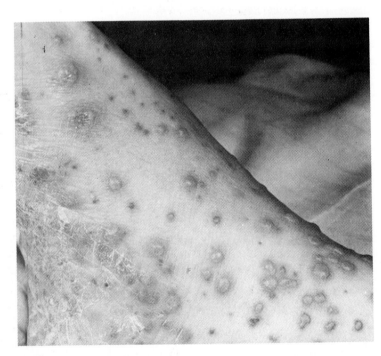

FIG. 8-2. Chickenpox. A severe case of chickenpox with lesions at various stages of development on the foot and ankle area.
(From Centers for Disease Control, Atlanta, Ga.)

5. *Description:* nasal discharge; watery eyes; mild fever; headache; general aches; irritability; cough

6. *Control measures for the school:* exclusion of most severe cases

German measles. Often referred to as 3-day or German measles, rubella is a distinctive disease.

1. *Infectious agent:* unidentified virus

2. *Source of infection:* nose and mouth secretions of infected persons

3. *Mode of transmission:* directly from person to person; indirectly from objects contaminated with fresh discharges from nose and mouth of infected person

4. *Incubation period:* 16 to 18 days

5. *Description:* mild symptoms; slight fever; eruptions varied but often rose pink and small; lymph nodes on neck behind the ear swollen and sensitive

6. *Control measures for the school:* exclusion for sake of infected child

7. *Preventive measure:* immunization

8. *Special caution:* possible damage or deformity of the fetus if women in the first trimester of pregnancy contract German measles; thus immunizations are especially important

Infectious hepatitis. Infectious hepatitis is an acute involvement of the liver that occurs sporadically or epidemically. It occurs most frequently in autumn. Hepatitis can be of two types: infectious or serum. Infectious hepatitis is caused by the virus entering the body through the mouth; serum hepatitis is caused by a similar virus found in blood and tissue and enters the body by contaminated blood transfusions and contaminated needles or syringes. Poor sanitation and overcrowded living conditions appear to increase its spread. An uneventful recovery after a 7 or 8 week illness is usual. Mild symptoms and malfunction of the liver may persist for more than a year. About 12% of patients suffer a relapse, usually because of overactivity or other indiscretions.

1. *Infectious agent:* heat-resistant virus

2. *Source of infection:* usually milk or other food contaminated by fecal discharges of an infected person; feces and blood may be infectious before, during, or after the occurrence of hepatitis

3. *Mode of transmission:* both sporadic and epidemic types usually transmitted from feces of infected person by way of the hands, which come into contact with milk, food, and water; infectious hepatitis spread from direct contact or fomites, and direct fecal contamination of water is possible; serum hepatitis spread by contaminated blood transfusions, medical instruments, or drug-abuse paraphernalia

4. *Incubation period:* 15 to 35 days

5. *Description:* prodromal signs include fever, headache, lassitude, nausea, anorexia, fatigue, and pronounced tenderness and pain in the liver; jaundice appears about the fifth day and then fever subsides (not all patients develop jaundice)

6. *Control measures for the school:* recognition of the disease; exclusion from school until readmitted by attending physician; improved sanitary and hygienic practices in food handling, hand washing, and disposal of sewage; food handlers in school cafeteria should be checked for possible latent infectious hepatitis

Serum hepatitis

1. *Infectious agent:* virus

2. *Source of infection:* blood transfusions, plasma therapy, and inoculations

3. *Mode of transmission:* inoculation or transfusions

4. *Incubation period:* 2 to 4 months

5. *Description:* onset is rather gradual with clinical manifestations and treatments similar to those for infectious hepatitis

6. *Control measures for the school:* because this disease is transmitted by inoculation or transfusion, the school is not directly involved in control; indirectly, drug education can help students understand the risk of using unsterilized needles and paraphernalia; it is apparent that serum hepatitis can be prevented by laboratory blood tests of prospective donors; a history of the donor's health problems can be helpful as a preventive measure, but an accurate assay of the blood is most reliable

Measles. Measles (rubeola) is a highly communicable disease.
1. *Infectious agent:* unidentified virus
2. *Source of infection:* secretions from nose and mouth of infected person
3. *Mode of transmission:* directly by sneezing and coughing from person to person; indirectly from objects contaminated with fresh respiratory discharges of infected person
4. *Incubation period:* 10 to 12 days
5. *Description:* nasal discharge; eyes red and sensitive to light; eyelids swollen; irritability; moderate fever; hacking cough; Koplik's spots on buccal surface of mouth; dusky red skin eruptions that tend to coalesce (Figs. 8-3 and 8-4)
6. *Control measures for the school:* exclusion for not less than 5 days after appearance of rash; exclusion of contacts only if symptoms appear; immunization recommended

Meningococcus meningitis. One of the most feared of the respiratory diseases, meningococcus meningitis can now be treated successfully if discovered early.
1. *Infectious agent:* meningococcus (spheric bacterium)
2. *Source of infection:* nose and throat discharges of carrier or person with active case
3. *Mode of transmission:* directly from person to person; indirectly from objects contaminated with fresh discharges from nose and throat of carrier or person with active case
4. *Incubation period:* 6 to 8 days
5. *Description:* acute onset; intense headache; fever; nausea; stiff neck; irritability
6. *Control measures for the school:* exclusion until recovery, usually minimum of 14 days, or until released by health department after negative laboratory tests; exclusion of contacts in same household for 7 days from last exposure

Mononucleosis. Mononucleosis is an acute infection that may occur in epidemic form among children and youth but more often is sporadic. It usually lasts from 1 to 3 weeks, but involvement of the

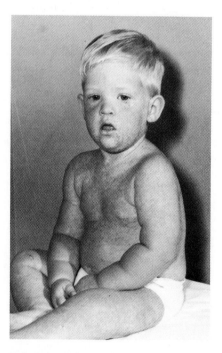

FIG. 8-3. Measles. The characteristic rash occurs 3 to 5 days after onset of symptoms. It begins on the face and neck and spreads to trunk and extremities as it begins to fade on the face. *(From Centers for Disease Control, Atlanta, Ga.)*

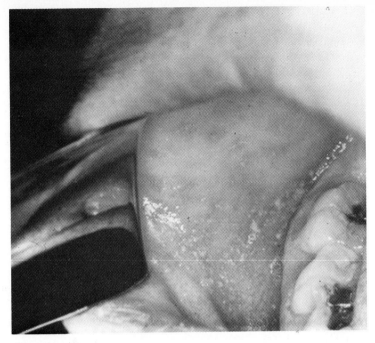

FIG. 8-4. Koplik spots. These red and white pinpoint eruptions on the buccal mucosa are one of the most important signs of measles.
(From Centers for Disease Control, Atlanta, Ga.)

lymph system and general fatigue and weakness may go on for months. Recurrences are frequent but usually short lived.

1. *Infectious agent:* unidentified virus
2. *Source of infection:* probably discharges from nose and throat of infected person
3. *Mode of transmission:* probably by direct contact with infected person
4. *Incubation period:* 5 to 15 days
5. *Description:* fever; sore throat; headache; fatigue; chilliness; malaise; general involvement of lymph systems (white cell count of the blood varies between 10,000 and 20,000); excessive agglutinins present in the blood
6. *Control measures for the school:* recognition of disease; no legal isolation, but patient should not return to school until so advised by attending physician

Mumps. Involving primarily the salivary glands, mumps (parotitis) nevertheless is classified as a respiratory disease.

1. *Infectious agent:* unidentified virus
2. *Source of infection:* saliva of infected person
3. *Mode of transmission:* droplets spread by direct contact; indirectly from objects contaminated with fresh saliva of infected person
4. *Incubation period:* 18 days
5. *Description:* light fever; tenderness and swelling over the jaw and in front of the ear, one side or both sides; involvement of ovaries and testes may occur in persons with mature reproductive systems
6. *Control measures for the school:* exclusion until the disappearance of swelling and tenderness; immunization of 12- to 18-year-old boys recommended
7. *Preventive measure:* immunization

Rheumatic fever. Signs of rheumatic fever may occur 1 to 3 weeks after a sore throat. The associated fever and pain in the joints may not indicate the possible damage done to the heart muscle. Because of these characteristics, rheumatic fever is described as an insidious disease.

1. *Infectious agent:* group A beta-hemolytic streptococcus, producing sore throat
2. *Description:* primary phase—identified as severe sore throat; middle (dormant) phase—no particular symptoms or signs, may last for 4 weeks with apparently complete recovery; final phase—acute rheumatic fever lasting 2 to 3 weeks; without treatment, recurrence of primary phase possible; damage to heart or other organs possible
3. *Control measures for the school:* effective prevention by use of antibiotics at early stage of recognized infection

Scarlet fever and streptococcal throat infection. Scarlet fever and streptococcal throat infection are commonly classed together.

1. *Infectious agent:* hemolytic streptococci
2. *Source of infection:* nose and throat discharges of person with active case or a carrier; articles soiled with discharges
3. *Mode of transmission:* directly by coughing and sneezing from person to person; indirectly via handkerchiefs, clothing, and other objects that reach the mouth; from contaminated milk
4. *Incubation period:* 3 to 5 days
5. *Description:* sore throat; fever; nausea; vomiting; flushing of cheeks; pallor about mouth; if rash occurs, it is on the neck and chest and is a fine scarlet goose-pimple type that blanches when pressure is applied
6. *Control measures for the school:* exclusion for at least 7 days or until all abnormal discharges have disappeared; sore throat is always a signal for exclusion

COMMON SKIN INFECTIONS AND INFESTATIONS

Communicable skin conditions are not a life or death matter but can be a trying problem to the school. Much of the nuisance effect can be reduced by an understanding of the common communicable skin diseases.

A skin *infection* occurs when the pathogen penetrates the skin and causes harm. A skin *infestation* occurs when the parasite remains *on* the skin and causes harm.

Impetigo contagiosa (gym itch). In elementary schools impetigo may spread quite widely from a single unrecognized case; so early recognition is important.

1. *Infectious agent:* streptococci and staphylococci
2. *Source of infection:* skin lesions of infected persons
3. *Mode of transmission:* directly by contact with discharge of skin lesions; indirectly from objects contaminated with such discharges
4. *Incubation period:* 2 to 4 days
5. *Description:* systemic manifestations usually absent except in infants; lesions first appear as pink-red stains that are fluid filled and wet, then fill with pus, and finally form a crust that appears as though it were pasted on; the face (particularly the butterfly area about the mouth) and hands are commonly involved, but other parts of the body may be affected, particularly the scalp; pressure generally releases pus from beneath the oval crusts
6. *Control measures for the school:* exclusion from school until the pustules have healed
7. *Preventive measures:* encourage prompt treatment, which consists in soaking crust until it can be removed and applying 5% ammoniated mercury ointment or sulfonamide ointment to the infected area; some schools have ointments available for the student's own use, and in some instances the parent or student requests the teacher's assistance; a physician's services should be obtained if possible; emphasis on general personal health helps to avoid any wide spread of impetigo

Pediculosis. Pediculosis (lousiness) is a classic example of infestation.

1. *Infesting agent:* head or body louse
2. *Source of infestation:* infested person or his or her personal belongings
3. *Mode of transmission:* directly from infested person; indirectly by contact with clothing of infested person
4. *Incubation period:* ova hatch in 1 week and mature in 2 weeks
5. *Description:* the louse egg (nit), larva, or adult louse on the scalp or other parts of the body or in the clothing; nits attached to the hair shaft; occasionally a severe secondary infection
6. *Control measures for the school:* exclusion until adequate treatment received and proper insecticide applied to scalp, skin, and clothing; inspection of possible contacts and use of effective insecticide for infested pupils
7. *Preventive measure:* emphasis on body cleanliness

Ringworm. The term *athlete's foot* applies to ringworm (tinea) of the feet; however, ringworm can affect all parts of the body. Common dermatophytes are often present on healthy skin and cause disease only when favorable conditions prevail.

1. *Infectious agent:* several types of fungi
2. *Source of infection:* lesions on body of infected persons; objects contaminated by the fungi or their spores
3. *Mode of transmission:* directly by person-to-person contact with lesions; indirectly from objects contaminated by the fungi or their spores
4. *Incubation period:* unknown
5. *Description:* lesions often circular, clear in the center, with vesicular (fluid) borders; not widely distributed; crusting not present, itching common; foot ringworm (athlete's foot) more common in adults; body, face, and head forms more common among children, especially in warm weather
6. *Control measures for the school:* exclusion until treatment initiated, and lesions dry or covered; in foot ringworm, exclusion from privileges of swimming pool and gymnasium
7. *Preventive measures:* personal cleanliness; thorough drying of feet after bathing; gymnasium and shower room cleanliness; regular inspections and treatment; keep feet dry to deny moisture to fungi

Scabies. The common term *7-year-itch* is often used to designate scabies. Both male and female mites live on human skin, but the female burrows into the superficial layer of the skin to deposit eggs. The female can be seen with the unaided eye, but the male, being half her size, is not readily detected. The parasites are short lived, the male dying after mating and the female after she has laid her eggs. Larvae are hatched in 4 to 8 days.

1. *Infectious agent:* Sarcoptes scabiei (itch mite)
2. *Source of infection:* person infected with the mite
3. *Mode of transmission:* directly by contact with infected persons; indirectly from underclothing, bedding, towels, and other objects of the infected person
4. *Incubation period:* 1 to 2 days
5. *Description:* itching of the skin often unbearable; frequent locations: the waist, armpit, and crotch; at times, lesions on the face, scalp, and arms; when infection is mild, systemic symptoms are negligible, but severe infections may result in fever, headache, and discomfort
6. *Control measures for the school:* exclusion from school until successfully treated with an effective miticide
7. *Preventive measure:* personal cleanliness

SEXUALLY TRANSMITTED DISEASES

Among infectious diseases, sexually transmitted diseases (STDs) have always been problematic for school health personnel. The incidence of the most common sexually transmitted diseases is higher than most people realize and has often been described as epidemic. Between 1982 and 1986 in the civilian U.S. population, the annual median reported cases of gonorrhea was 887,936 and of syphilis was 27,947. Gonorrhea is the most widespread reportable sexually transmitted diseases, but syphilis outranks gonorrhea in its potentially damaging effects. Gonorrhea has been difficult to control because evolving strains of gonococcus have developed resistance to medications and because many infected people are essentially asymptomatic.

Because the spread of these conditions involves sexual activity, school personnel have been reluctant to discuss them. In fact, whole communities are reluctant to support discussion of sexuality issues in schools. Because morality is involved, denial often exists. Many parents believe that discussion related to sexuality should be reserved for the home and have openly discouraged school personnel from discussing such matters. Teachers are reluctant to deal with sexuality because they feel ill-prepared. Today, however, public awareness of the prevalence of sexually transmitted diseases, high rates of adolescent pregnancy, and the advent of AIDS have led to a more receptive environment for the schools to teach about and provide services related to sexually transmitted diseases.

Sexually transmitted diseases are transmitted during sexual intercourse, homosexual relations, or other sexual activities. Among the STDs, of most concern to the school are syphilis, gonorrhea, herpes simplex type 2, *Chlamydia,* and AIDS.

Gonorrhea. Gonorrhea is the most widespread sexually transmitted disease

1. *Infectious agent: Neisseria gonorrhoeae*
2. *Source of infection:* sexual activity
3. *Mode of transmission:* contact with infected person
4. *Incubation period:* males, 2 to 4 days; females, 7 to 21 days
5. *Description:* For males the lining of the urethra is usually infected causing a burning sensation on urination and a puslike discharge from the urethra. For females, the first indications include a mild burning sensation in the genital region and possible vaginal discharge. Later the disease may spread to the vagina, uterus, fallopian tubes, and ovaries, causing pain and fever. Women, however, may have no indication that they are infected. Symptoms may disappear with time.
6. *Control measures for the school:* effective education, encouragment of family to communicate behavioral expectations to children, conscious abstinence from sexual activity

Syphilis

1. *Infectious agent: Treponema pallidum* (spirochete)
2. *Source of infection:* skin lesion of infected person
3. *Mode of transmission:* transmitted through mucous membrane or skin abrasions
4. *Incubation period:* 10 to 28 days
5. *Description:* Syphilis enters the body through small skin breaks, usually in the mucous membranes of the genital tract, rectum, or mouth. After incubation, a chancre, or small, moist lump appears at the site of the infection. The chancre is often not visible or is in a location not observable. Without treatment, spirochetes travel in the bloodstream throughout the body. In the second stage, symptoms may appear any time from a few weeks to a year after the disappearance of the chancre. Symptoms include skin rash, small flat sores in moist areas of the skin, whitish patches in the mouth and throat, fever, headaches, and swollen glands. A person with syphilis in this stage is highly infectious. After this secondary stage, all signs and symptoms of the disease disappear. During this latent stage spirochetes invade various body organs, including heart and brain, but it may be as long as 20 years before the patient suffers serious

incapacitating conditions. Pregnant women may transmit the disease to their unborn children. The infection may kill the fetus or produce various malformations.

6. *Control measures for the school:* effective education, encouragement of family to communicate behavioral expectations to children, conscious abstinence from sexual activity

Chlamydial diseases. Trachoma, caused by *Chlamydia,* is sometimes classified as a nonspecific sexually transmitted infection (NSI). The prevalence of nonspecific sexually transmitted infections is unknown because they are not reportable. However, some experts believe that NSI may be more prevalent than gonorrhea. About 80% of NSIs are reported to be caused by *Chlamydia trachomatis.* The second species, *Chlamydia psittaci,* is responsible for the remainder of the chlamydial diseases.

1. *Infectious agent: Chlamydia trachomatis,* a bacteria like a virus that grows only within cells
2. *Source of infection:* direct contact with the infected person
3. *Mode of transmission:* sexual contact
4. *Incubation period:* 7 to 28 days
5. *Description:* Many females experience no symptoms. If symptoms exist, they will include vaginal pain and itching, and in men, pain and itching in the genital area and a urethral discharge. In an advanced stage, the disease can cause pain throughout the pelvic area for women (pelvic inflammatory disease). Because *Chlamydia* often give no symptoms, its detection often follows the testing for other sexually transmitted diseases.
6. *Control measures for the school:* effective education, encouragment of family to communicate behavioral expectations to children, conscious abstinence from sexual activity

Herpes simplex. Once a relatively rare condition it is estimated that between 300,000 and 1 million cases of herpes simplex may occur each year. There is no cure for herpes at this time.

1. *Infectious agent:* herpes virus hominis type 2 (HSV-2)
2. *Source of infection:* direct contact with blisterlike sores of an infected person
3. *Mode of transmission:* sexual contact
4. *Incubation period:* 4 to 7 days
5. *Description:* Blisterlike sores in the genital area that may spread to buttocks and thighs. Sometimes swelling of the legs, difficult urination, watery eyes, and fatigue will result. HSV-2 is cyclic in nature, with the virus retreating to the base of the spine from time to time leaving the patient symptomfree and at low risk to spread the disease. Symptoms recur periodically often in association with sexual activity or stressful life events.
6. *Control measures for the shool:* Avoid sexual contact with an infected person.

Acquired immune deficiency syndrome (AIDS). Although the incidence of AIDS is relatively low, it is increasing, and the fact that no known cure exists means this increase will continue. Some 40,000 adults and 500 children are reported as having AIDS, and many have died. It is estimated that by 1992 some 270,000 persons will have developed AIDS and 180,000 will have died.

For schools the problems caused by AIDS are related to public hysteria and fear of catching AIDS from an infected person. Children infected through blood transfusions are often shunned by the public who demand their exclusion from normal educational activities. The school's challenge is one of community and student education and the development of policies to protect both the public and the infected student at the same time as providing quality education.

1. *Infectious agent:* virus HTLV-3
2. *Source of infection:* infected person or contaminated blood products or contaminated syringes
3. *Mode of transmission:* sexual contact, primarily male homosexual contact, intravenous drug use, and sexual contact with intravenous drug users, transfusion of infected blood or blood products.
4. *Incubation period:* a few months to several years
5. *Description:* No obvious signs during incubation period. Later the victim will develop night sweats, unexpected weight loss, diarrhea, loss of appetite, swollen glands, and fatigue. Later

when the body's defense system is weakened (specifically the helper T-cells), other ordinary diseases develop unchecked. Often the victim suffers from *Pneumocystis carinii* pneumonia and Kaposi's sarcoma, a rare form of skin cancer. Many carriers of the virus have not yet developed symptoms, whereas others develop mild versions of the symptoms referred to as AIDS-related complex (ARC).

6. *Control measures for the school:* Avoid sexual contact with infected person, do not share intravenous drug equipment. There is no clear evidence that casual contact with an infected person actually transmits the disease. Children with AIDS can safely attend school without endangering other students. Some special suspension may, however, be required.

• • •

In the control of infectious disease the teacher need not be limited to specific detailed symptoms. Any time a student has a sore throat, fever, or watery eyes, the teacher should prudently assume that he or she has the beginning of an infectious respiratory disease. Skin eruptions exhibiting inflammation are likely to be infectious as contrasted with noninflamed skin areas such as those occurring in eczema.

A teacher who watches for typical prodromal symptoms quickly identifies the student in the early stages of any usual infectious respiratory diseases. Skin disorders will also be recognized early in their development.

RESPONSIBILITY FOR CONTROL OF COMMUNICABLE DISEASES

Both legal and professional responsibilities must be considered in the control of communicable diseases. Responsibilities written into law or health codes represent the minimal desirable control, usually in terms of restrictions. Beyond these legal responsibilities are the moral or professional responsibilities of individuals and groups.

Public health personnel

Health authority is vested in the police power of the state. *Police power* is the authority of the people vested in government to protect society's health and general welfare. Health departments have police power and promote public welfare by regulating and restraining the use of property and liberty. Police power is based on the concept of the greatest good for the greatest number and may inconvenience some of the interest of the common good.

State legislatures delegate authority to a state board of health to set rules and regulations governing health. Accordingly the health board passes regulations to control communicable diseases. This includes the imposition of isolation and quarantine, milk control, water treatment, and all other measures necessary to disease control. The state code specifies the time and terms of isolation, quarantine, and other control measures. States may also promulgate these standards in law.

The state may delegate many of its powers to subdivisions of local governments. The state grants charters to cities giving them absolute self-rule (home rule) to exercise within their own borders and within specific limits or fields. Police power thus delegated to the municipalities enables them to control communicable diseases within their own geographic borders.

In terms of direct effect on individual citizens the county or city health department is charged with legal responsibility for communicable disease control. Standards may not be lower than those of the state code, but they may be higher. Thus if the state code sets the isolation period for a particular disease as 7 days, the local code may require 9 days but not 6 days. Generally the local code coincides with the state code.

Local health personnel enforce isolation and quarantine, immunization, and such other provisions as pertain to disease control. To fulfill their respective duties concerning children's health, school personnel and health department personnel usually establish some means of liaison.

Private physician

Practicing physicians have always been key figures in communicable disease control. Because they diagnose and supervise each case, they are in the best position to advise the patient.

Practicing physicians advise and perform immunizations as a routine part of family medical care.

Parents

An obvious responsibility of parents is the protection of their children's health. Parents observe their children for symptoms of disease, keep them out of school when symptoms of communicable disease are present, and follow the practices recommended by the school and the physician. Parents have legal responsibilities when isolation has been imposed officially.

School personnel

Promotion of immunization, early recognition of disease symptoms, and effective control of exclusions and readmissions allow the school staff to carry out its communicable disease control responsibilities.

Teachers who recognize early symptoms of communicable disease aid in their control. Early disease detection and early exclusion benefits the affected person as well as the student's classmates. It is relatively simple and highly effective to exclude students and to refuse readmission until all communicability has passed (Fig. 8-5).

Teachers as well as the school nurse can advise students and parents on matters relating to disease control and suggest a desirable course of action.

ISOLATION OF A STUDENT AT SCHOOL

A student with the symptoms of a communicable disease should be segregated from other students. The nurse's office is ideal for a student who appears only slightly ill and may recover in a short time, or who may not have a communicable disease. This student should lie comfortably on a cot in a moderately darkened room and should be kept warm with blankets. Someone should be in attendance or visit the student at intervals.

If the isolated student does not improve in a reasonable time, the parents should be contacted and arrangements made to take the student home. If the student becomes seriously ill and no contact with the parents can be made, the family physician should be called and his or her advice followed.

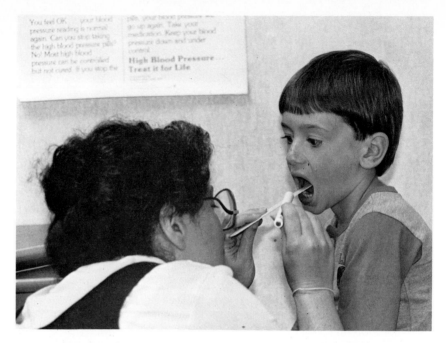

FIG. 8-5. Qualified school health personnel can detect communicable diseases early and develop effective programs to control their spread. In this way school health services help keep as many students in school as many school days as possible so that school personnel can provide a complete education for their students.
(Copyright 1983 by David Riecks.)

EXCLUSIONS

A question of considerable concern to classroom teachers is their responsibility for the exclusion of students who appear to have a communicable disease. Ideally a school nurse makes the decision, but if the teacher must decide, a set of established guidelines should be followed. Teachers readily recognize their professional responsibility to do everything reasonable on behalf of the student's health, but the administrative dimensions often cloud the issue.

Legal aspects

Do teachers have the right to exclude a student they suspect of having a communicable disease? If it develops that the student's condition was not communicable, can teachers be held legally liable for their action? These two vital questions have been answered by the courts. The classic decision was laid down by the court in the case of *Stone v. Probst*, in which parents instituted a civil suit against a public school educator for excluding their child from school because of suspected communicable disease. The key sentence of that decision is this: "Pupils who are suffering, or appear to be suffering, from a communicable disease may menace the well-being of all pupils and therefore should be denied the privilege of school attendance" (Supreme Court of the State of Minnesota, 1925).

It is significant that the court emphasized the mere *appearance* of symptoms of communicable disease as sufficient basis for exclusion. The court did not require proof that the well-being of other pupils was menaced but merely that their well-being *may* be menaced. The court did not assert that the school may exclude the student but that it *should* exclude the student. This decision means that if a teacher has reason to believe a student has a communicable disease that student should be excluded. If it is subsequently found that the student did not have a communicable disease, no jury would ever hold the teacher liable for such reasonable actions.

Administrative procedures

Various situations require different methods, and typical examples illustrate standard procedures:

1. If the student is not well, but doubt exists as to whether the condition is communicable, he or she may be isolated in the nurse's suite or similar area.
2. If no doubt exists that the student is quite ill and very likely has a communicable disease, the student should be sent home. First, the parents should be called, and one of the student's parents should come after him or her. Under no circumstances should the ill student walk home alone. All decisions to exclude a student should be channeled through the principal's office.
3. In a doubtful case when a school nurse or physician is unavailable a group of two or three teachers share their collective judgment. Ultimately the decision rests with the principal.
4. When the ill student must ride home in a school bus, the bus driver should be informed, the student seated near the driver, and the parents notified.

READMISSIONS

The problem of readmission of students does not occur as frequently as the exclusion of students with questionable symptoms. However, school personnel may face this problem. A medically confirmed communicable disease, when no longer communicable, should be so certified in a physician's note sent with the student when he or she returns to school.

Generally, courts hold that it is the parents' responsibility to demonstrate that the student is not in a communicable state and thus should be readmitted to school. This interpretation is expressed in the case of *Martin v. Craig:* "It is the responsibility of the parents to prove otherwise if the child is not to be denied the privilege of school attendance" (Supreme Court of North Dakota, 1919).

When doubt exists as to communicability, the parents must resolve the doubt by obtaining a written clearance from the health department or a practicing physician.

In practice, when a student has been absent for a day or two, the nurse or teacher should attempt to judge whether symptoms such as nasal discharge or rash have abated and indicate that the student can return to school. Review of Table 8-2 shows a set of possible indicators for exclusion or readmission.

Repeated controversy on readmission indicates an inadequate program for educating parents on policies and procedures of disease control. Where parents are well informed and cooperative, students will be kept out of school until there is no doubt that the student should be readmitted.

TABLE 8-2. Communicable disease inspection points for teachers to use in observing students

Inspection	Directions to child	Signs
For respiratory disease		
General condition	"How do you feel?"	Facial expression, listlessness, irritability, sneezing
Eyes	"Move your eyes about."	Watery eyes, inflammation, puffiness, redness
Nose	"Tilt your head back."	Discharge, inflammation, odor
Skin	"Do you feel hot?"	Flushing; hot, cold, or clammy feeling
Forehead	"Raise the hair from your forehead."	Eruptions along hairline
For skin infection		
Chest	"Open your shirt (or dress)."	Eruptions, redness, irritation
Hands and wrists	"Pull up your sleeves and spread your fingers."	Eruptions, redness, irritation

The other side of this issue is the parent who excludes a child from school for even the slightest deviation in health. Although doing no harm to other children, such a parent unduly interferes with the educational process. Here again the school has a professional responsibility to discuss this matter with the parents and explain the school's health care responsibilities, the resources, and the effect of such behavior on a child's education. A school nurse, physician, or counselor may be able to assist in this situation.

EPIDEMICS AND SCHOOL POLICIES

Experience demonstrates that during an epidemic it is better to keep the schools in session unless the epidemic is extreme and all public gatherings are prohibited. This is a decision for the health department. When students remain in school, their contact with others is limited to their peers, and careful observations are possible.

If the health department recommends school closings, prohibiting groups of children in theaters, recreation centers, churches, and other places is also in order. School personnel can assist by appealing to parents and students to follow health department regulations and remain away from public places.

Occasionally a widespread outbreak of influenza or other respiratory disease in a school population may prompt school officials to close the school. If more than half the student body is absent because of influenza, it may be wise to close the school temporarily. Most of the schoolwork for that week would have to be repeated for those who were absent. Although not done to control communicable diseases, it might be profitable academically and economically.

IMMUNIZATION PROGRAM

Even in a well-educated democracy such as the United States it has not been possible to voluntarily maintain immunizations at a high enough level to stop the spread of preventable diseases. Today most states have legislated required immunizations and linked the immunizations with permission for children to enter school.

This situation illustrates a dilemma of public health. When a disease can be prevented or quickly, if not cheaply, controlled and cured, the public quickly forgets the threat and ceases to participate in the measures that reduced the incidence of the disease in the first place. Short-term success in the public health may, in other words, increase the risk of long-term failure. Of course, the most effective educational means of increasing immunization levels would be an epidemic, but it would also be the most costly method.

Among the preventable diseases, immunization levels must be kept around 90% to 95% in the vulnerable population to prevent the spread of these conditions.

Schedule for immunizations

Various immunization schedules have been recommended. The recommendations of the Committee on Infectious Diseases of the American Academy of Pediatrics present perhaps the most widely followed standards; these are shown in Table 8-3. Immunization status is checked on admission to kindergarten or first grade. Parents are usually asked to complete an entry health history that includes questions similar to those shown in the box on p. 194. State law usually allows for exemptions under certain conditions, for example, religious objections. If immunization status is not complete, the school will notify parents to have their children immunized by a specific date. Exemption requests must be reviewed and filed in the student's permanent health record. The box on p. 195 gives a simple form for parents to notify the school of refusal to have a student immunized.

TABLE 8-3. Recommended childhood immunizations

	Immunization schedule* *Recommended schedule for active immunization of* *normal infants and children*	
2 months	DTP[1], OPV[2]	Can be initiated as early as 2 weeks of age in areas of high endemicity or during epidemics
4 months	DTP, OPV	Two-month interval desired for OPV to avoid interference from previous date
6 months	DTP (OPV)	OPV is optional (may be given in areas with increased risk of polio exposure)
15 months	Measles, mumps, rubella (MMR)[3]	MMR preferred to individual vaccines; tuberculin testing may be done
18 months	DTP, OPV	
24 months	HBPV[4]	
4-6 years	DTP, OPV	At or before school entry
14-16 years	TD[5]	Repeat every 10 years throughout life

*Adapted from American Academy of Pediatrics Committee on Infectious Diseases: School health: a guide for health professionals, Elk Grove Village, Ill., 1987, American Academy of Pediatrics.
[1]DTP, Diphtheria and tetanus toxoids with pertussis vaccine.
[2]OPV, Oral poliovirus vaccine contains attenuated poliovirus (types 1, 2, and 3).
[3]MMR, Live measles, mumps, and rubella viruses in a combined vaccine.
[4]Haemophilus b polysaccharide vaccine, which replaces HIB.
[5]TD, Adult tetanus toxoid (full dose) and diphtheria toxoid (reduced dose) in combination.

Sample Section of School-Entry Health History Form

State law requires all children be immunized against rubella, measles, poliomyelitis, DPT, and mumps.

Please list below the date (month, day, and year) of each dose given. To keep the health record up to date, please send dates of immunizations given after this form is sent to school.

1. Immunization against diphtheria, tetanus, and pertussis (combined):
   3 doses 1 month apart. Dates of doses: 1. _____
   2. _____ 3. _____
2. DPT boosters. Dates of doses: _____
3. Sabin (oral) polio. First dose: _____
   Second dose: _____ Third dose: _____
4. Sabin polio boosters. Dates of doses: _____
5. Rubeola (hard measles). Date of dose: _____
6. Rubella (German measles). Date of dose: _____
7. Mumps. Date of dose: _____
8. TB test. Date: _____ Results: _____

Please write in date if the child has had any of the following:

Scarlet fever: _____ Measles: _____ Mumps: _____
Other: _____ Pneumonia: _____
3-day measles: _____ Chickenpox: _____ Other: _____
Rheumatic fever: _____ Poliomyelitis: _____
Whooping cough: _____

Date signed _____ Parent or guardian _____

Special immunization practices

In practice, immunization against certain diseases is not advocated except under certain circumstances. When a disease is peculiar to a special area (endemic), health authorities may recommend immunization of all persons in that area, particularly those who risk exposure.

For mumps, prepuberty immunization protects the body through the critical transition years to adulthood. As a preventive measure for exposed men who lack prior immunity, a special gamma globulin is used to give temporary immunity and thus prevent possible sterility. High school boys exposed to mumps and lacking prior immunity should consult a physician on the advisability of gamma globulin administration.

Because German measles in a mother during the first 3 months of pregnancy can cause the birth of defective infants, it is urgent for all girls to be immunized before 12 years of age.

National immunization objectives

Immunizations represent one of the most effective means of primary prevention. However, without public understanding and cooperation, immunizations will remain an underused

---

Refusal of Immunization

As the parent/guardian of _____

Name   Age   Birth date

_____

School   Grade

I do not wish to have my child receive the following immunizations:

(check disease)

☐ Rubeola (measles)
☐ Rubella (German measles)
☐ Mumps
☐ Poliomyelitis
☐ Diphtheria
☐ Tetanus (lockjaw)
☐ Pertussis (whooping cough)

Comments _____

_____

_____

Signature of parent/guardian   Date

---

resource. Immunization effectiveness is especially clear when differences in morbidity and mortality are compared between the years of their initial development and recent records:

- Diphtheria: approximately 160,000 cases and 10,000 deaths or more annually in the early 1920s; no cases in 1986 and no deaths in 1985 (most recent year for which data are available)
- Whooping cough: approximately 200,000 cases and approximately 5000 deaths annually in the early 1930s; 4162 cases in 1986 and 4 deaths in 1985
- Poliomyelitis: 21,000 cases of paralytic polio in 1952 (epidemic year); 2 cases in 1986 and 3 deaths in 1985
- Mumps: 152,000 cases in 1968; 6807 cases in 1986
- Rubella: 60,000 cases in 1969; 502 cases in 1986
- Measles: 480,000 cases in 1962; 5974 cases in 1986

So strategic are immunizations that specific national goals, the *National Immunization Objectives for 1990*, have been set. If the goals are achieved, these infectious diseases will be almost eliminated.

1. By 1990 reported measles incidence should be reduced to fewer than 500 cases per year—all imported or within two generations of importation.
2. By 1990 reported mumps incidence should be reduced to fewer than 1000 cases per year.

3. By 1990 reported rubella incidence should be reduced to fewer than 1000 cases per year.

4. By 1990 reported congenital rubella syndrome incidence should be reduced to fewer than 10 cases per year.

5. By 1990 reported diphtheria incidence should be reduced to fewer than 50 cases per year.

6. By 1990 reported pertussis incidence should be reduced to fewer than 1000 cases per year.

7. By 1990 reported tetanus incidence should be reduced to fewer than 50 cases per year.

8. By 1990 reported poliomyelitis incidence should be fewer than 10 cases per year.

National goals, however, will be achieved only if individuals use available technology. The technical knowledge for widespread immunization exists, and cost no longer is a barrier for the majority of families. Technology to reduce health risks in the environment also exists, and when communities share the costs, they are not exorbitant. Human behavior at personal, family, and community levels is the critical element of prevention. Education provides the knowledge and skills to affect behavior. Education, especially health education in elementary, middle, and secondary schools, is critical in how individuals accept prevention options, how society devotes resources for prevention, and ultimately how much society benefits in terms of health.

STUDY QUESTIONS

1. Explain the possible paradox that all cases of communicable disease are infectious diseases but not all cases of infectious diseases are communicable.

2. What is each citizen's responsibility for the health of his or her neighbor?

3. "Infectious disease is but the reaction of the host to a parasite." Explain this statement.

4. What are the sources of disease that threaten a school-child?

5. What class of communicable diseases poses the greatest problem for the school, and why are these diseases so difficult to control?

6. What forms of isolation can a school use to prevent communicable disease spread?

7. What are the responsibilities of the county health department in controlling communicable diseases in the schools of a community?

8. Why do health officials contend that teachers are the first line of defense against the spread of communicable disease?

9. Why do epidemiologists maintain that at least 90% of children entering school be immunized against diptheria, smallpox, and poliomyelitis or there could be a major epidemic?

10. Explain why in communicable disease control in the school problems of readmission can be more difficult than those of exclusion.

11. How would parents establish that their child is no longer in a communicable state and should be readmitted to school?

12. Under what circumstances should a school be closed because of an epidemic?

13. List those communicable diseases that a teacher may have and he or she may transmit to students.

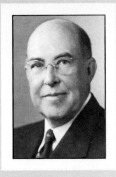

William P. Shepard

BORN   July 6, 1895, Hull, Iowa
DIED   June 26, 1969, Martha's Vineyard,
            Massachusetts
EDUCATION   B.S., M.D., and M.P.H., University of Minnesota

Dr. William Shepard, during his career with the Metropolitan Life Insurance Company, made an outstanding contribution to the health and welfare of the people of the United States and Canada. He received two of medicine's highest honors: the Albert Lasker Award for 1956 and the Knudsen Award for 1959-1960. The citation of the Lasker Award stated that he was honored for "influencing the health of all Americans as a pioneering industrial health physician, health educator, and government advisor."

Dr. Shepard received his education at the University of Minnesota and returned to his native state for the private practice of medicine. In 1924 he accepted a position as a health officer and director of health and development in the Berkeley, California, public schools. In 1926 he joined Metropolitan Life Insurance's Pacific Coast head office staff in San Francisco as assistant secretary and welfare director. In 1944 he was appointed third vice-president, heading health and welfare activities on the West Coast. In 1953 he was transferred to New York, and in 1954 he was named second vice-president, health and welfare. In 1959 he was appointed medical director and then chief medical director, in charge of both the Medical and Health and Welfare Divisions. He held this position until 1961, having worked in the field of public health for over 35 years.

His extensive participation in public health affairs led to presidencies of the American Public Health Association, the National and California Tuberculosis Associations, the Western Association of Industrial Physicians and Surgeons, and the San Francisco Social Hygiene Association. He was founder and diplomate of the American Board of Preventive Medicine and chairman of the Council on Occupational Health of the American Medical Association, a member of the Industrial Hygiene Foundation, and chairman of the committee on professional education of the American Public Health Association.

The Industrial Medical Association, on selecting him to receive the 1959-1960 Knudsen Award, credited him as being "the American doctor whose contributions to the field of industrial medicine are regarded as having exceeded those of any other physician." He was described as "a scholar, a philosopher, a teacher, and administrator, and a doer, who has unselfishly given himself and his time to fostering medical beliefs." The position achieved by industrial medicine in the medical world today is a tribute to Dr. Shepard.

REFERENCES

American Academy of Pediatrics: School health: a guide for health professionals, Elk Grove Village, Ill., 1987, the Academy.

Burnet, F., and White D.: Natural history of infectious disease, ed. 4, London, 1972, Cambridge University Press.

Centers for Disease Control, 1987, Morbidity and Mortality Weekly Report, vol. 35, no. 53, Jan. 9, 1987.

Cockburn, A., editor: Infectious diseases: their evolution and eradication, Springfield, Ill., 1967, Charles C Thomas, Publisher.

The Facts About AIDS, a special guide for NEA members from the health information network; insert in September 1987 issue of NEA Today.

Harvard child study project: Developing a better health care system for children, vol. 3, Cambridge, Mass., 1977, Ballinger Publishing Co.

Herzlich, C., and Graham, D.: Health and illness: a social, psychological analysis, New York, 1974, Academic Press, Inc.

Jolly, H.: Diseases of children, ed. 4, Philadelphia, 1981, J.B. Lippincott Co.

Kendig, E.J., and Chernich, V., editors: Disorders of the respiratory tract in children, ed. 3, Philadelphia, 1977, W.B. Saunders Co.

Krugman, S., Ward, R., and Katz, S.: Infectious diseases of children, ed. 7, St. Louis, 1981, The C.V. Mosby Co.

Melby, C.L., Dunn, P.J., Hyner, G.C., et al.: Correlates of blood pressure in elementary schoolchildren, J. Sch. Health **57**(9):375, 1987.

National Center for Health Statistics: Vital statistics of the United States 1985, vol. 2, Mortality, Part A, Atlanta, 1985, U.S. Department of Health and Human Services, Public Health Service, Centers for Disease Control, NCHS.

National Education Association: Recommended guidelines for dealing with AIDS in the schools from the National Education Association, J. Sch. Health **56**(4):129, 1986.

Price, J.M.: AIDS, the schools, and policy issues, J. Sch. Health **56**(4):137, 1986.

Silver, G.: Child health: America's future, Germantown, Md., 1978, Aspen Systems Corporation.

Supreme Court of North Dakota, April 22, 1919, 42ND213, 173, NW 787, Mand. 81 Schools 157.

Supreme Court of the State of Minnesota, 165 Minn., 1925, 361, 206 NW 642; appeal from the District Court, Hennepin County.

Top, F., and Wehrle, P., editors: Communicable and infectious diseases, ed. 9, St. Louis, 1981, The C.V. Mosby Co.

U.S. Department of Health and Human Services: Promoting health/preventing disease: objectives for the nation, Washington, D.C., Fall 1980, U.S. Government Printing Office.

Update: serologic testing for antibody to human immunodeficiency virus, MMWR **36**(52): Jan. 1988.

Werner, D.: Where there is no doctor, Palo Alto, Calif., 1978, Hesperian Foundation.

Preventive Aspects of Health Services
Safety, Emergency Care, and First Aid

OVERVIEW   *The leading cause of death for school-aged children and youth is accidents. The most frequent type of accident that youths and adults die from is by motor vehicles. Most accidents do not happen by accident as the word incorrectly implies. Most accidents are a repeat of other accidents and have quantifiable contributing factors that can be prevented. The number and rate of accidents in the schools are relatively low when compared with other youth activities. Although the school itself is relatively safe, the school environment presents its own hazards and safety concerns. Children and youth do get injured and die while engaged in school activities. The school requires a system for preventing accidents as well as dealing with them immediately and effectively when they do occur. Because the school is an ideal peer-referenced environment, important opportunities for teaching health and safety education avail. This chapter prepares the responsible teacher and administrator to deal with these areas.*

OBJECTIVES   **After reading this chapter, the student should be able to:**

1. Explain the concept of "injury control" and the factors that contribute to an accident.
2. Explain the terms "external controls" and "internal controls" and how they contribute to the prevention of accidents.
3. Explain why school officials are often taken by surprise when an accident occurs.
4. Interpret the expression, "There hasn't been a new type of accident in 50 years."
5. Identify areas of the school environment that pose a potential threat to students for accidental injury.
6. Explain the concept of negligence and the conditions under which teacher liability may be determined in cases where students are injured.
7. Explain the Community Emergency Medical Services and what the school's role is in the handling of a school emergency.
8. Explain the components of a basic training program for school personnel that enables them to handle a school emergency appropriately.
9. Conduct a comprehensive survey of the school safety environment.
10. Use the findings of their school safety survey as the basis for developing the school's safety education curriculum.

ACCIDENTAL DEATH AND INJURY AND THE ROLE OF THE SCHOOL

The leading cause of death for school-aged children and youth is accidents. The leading causes of death for *all* ages (child to adult) are heart disease, stroke, and cancer, followed by accidents. For 1 to 44 years of age, *accidents* claim the most lives every day. (See Table 9-1.)

Although children and youth between 5 and 18 years of age spend roughly a third of their lives, or most of their waking hours, engaged in school activity, most injuries and deaths do not occur during these hours. The school is a controlled environment, and accidents are generally the result of an uncontrolled behavior occurring in an uncontrolled environment. Most school activities are scripted and take place within prescribed boundaries. That is, if something is going to happen to a student, it is going to happen with a certain room, building, or outside area and be part of a organized activity, whether a health education class, a physical education class, lunch, or recess. Most activities within the school are planned and therefore can be controlled. Knowing when, where, and how a student is to be involved in an activity makes it possible to recognize patterns over time that can lead to accident behaviors. With enough experience, these behaviors can be controlled. Therefore, when accidental injury and death do occur in the school, administration and teachers are really called to question not only because of their legal responsibility for the health and welfare of the students, but also because the accident occurred in a controlled environment during a controlled activity. The actions that led to the injurious behavior should have been predicted and controlled. (See Table 9-2.)

SCHOOL SAFETY PROGRAM

The school deals with accidental injury and death in three ways: by teaching students to avoid or deal with risky situations, by reducing hazards in the school environment, and by teaching skills to cope with accidents and care for accident victims when accidents do occur.

It is apparent that safety in the school does not imply that the physical environment be converted into an accident-proof situation or that children's actions be completely restrained so that an accident cannot possibly happen. Rather, it means pursuit of the normal demands

TABLE 9-1. Percentages of deaths from injury and other causes in the United States by age.

Age	Injuries	Congenital anomalies	Cancer	Pneumonia/ influenza	Heart disease	Liver disease	Stroke	Other
1-4	46%	13%	7%	3%	4%	—	—	27%
5-14	55%	5%	14%	—	3%	—	—	23%
15-24	79%	—	5%	—	3%	—	—	13%
25-34	62%	—	10%	—	6%	3%	—	19%
35-44	31%	—	21%	—	20%	6%	4%	18%
45-64	7%	—	32%	—	36%	4%	5%	16%
65+	2%	—	19%	3%	48%	—	10%	18%

Committee on Trauma Research, Commission on Life Sciences, National Research Council, and the Institute of Medicine: Injury in America, a continuing public health problem, Washington, D.C., 1985, National Academy Press.

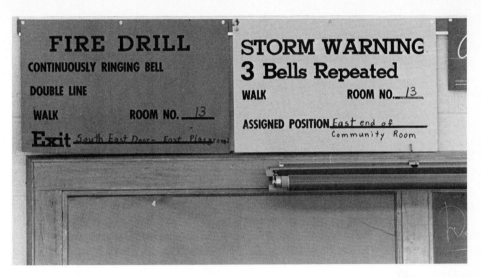

FIG. 9-1. Posted directions and emergency drills reduce the potential risk when real emergencies do occur.
(Copyright 1983 by David Riecks.)

of life in an environment in which hazards are reduced to a practical minimum and the behavior of the pupils is adapted to safe and effective living (Fig. 9-1).

Student rates for accidents occurring in school-related activities give some indication of the relative risks associated with school activities. In terms of days lost per injury, travel to and from school in a motor vehicle is the most dangerous school-related activity. Activities apart from organized athletics and class work but carried out on the school property are the next most costly in terms of lost school days. Among formal school activities, interscholastic activities rank third for girls, and for boys physical education class accounts for the next most frequent loss of school days. The accident death rates decline during the ages 5 to 10 years and then increase dramatically during the teenage years (Tables 9-3 and 9-4 and Fig. 9-2).

TABLE 9-2. Mortality from accidents among youth 5 to 14 years of age (1977-1978)

Cause	Deaths per 100,000 population	
	Girls	**Boys**
Accidents (all types)	11.1	23.2
Motor vehicles	6.4	11.0
Pedestrian accidents	2.3	4.1
Drowning	1.1	4.3
Fire and flames	1.5	1.7
Firearm missile	0.3	0.4
Falls	0.2	0.5
Water transport	0.1	0.4
Other	1.5	3.9

From Report of the division of vital statistics, National Center for Health Statistics, U.S. Public Health Service.
Reproduced in Statistical Bulletin **62:**3, July-Sept. 1981, New York, Metropolitan Life Insurance Co.

TABLE 9-3. Student accident rates by school grade

The table below summarizes more than 7,500 school jurisdiction accidents[a] reported to the National Safety Council for the 1984-85 and 1985-86 school years. The rates are accidents per 100,000 student days. In the "total" column only, a rate of 0.10 is equivalent to about 8000 accidents among the nation's enrollment.

The rates indicate principal accident types and locations within grade groups. Since reporting is voluntary, the experience may not be representative of the national accident picture. These rates are not comparable to rates of previous years because of a decrease in the number of schools included. See footnotes.

Location and type	Total[b]	Kgn.[c]	1-3 Gr.	4-6 Gr.	7-9 Gr.	10-12 Gr.	Days lost per injury
Enrollment reported (000)	720	46	167	153	176	153	
Total school jurisdiction	**5.86**	**4.81**	**4.01**	**6.89**	**8.27**	**6.11**	**1.19**
Shops and labs	**0.24**	**0.00**	**0.00**	**0.01**	**0.63**	**0.40**	**0.87**
Homemaking	0.02	0.00	0.00	0.01	0.07	0.02	0.63
Science	(d)	0.00	0.00	0.00	0.05	0.02	0.82
Vocational ind arts	0.12	0.00	0.00	(d)	0.28	0.25	0.97
Other labs.....................	0.01	0.00	0.00	0.00	0.03	0.04	1.35
Other shops	0.01	0.00	0.00	(d)	0.02	0.03	0.92
Building — general	**1.26**	**1.35**	**0.85**	**1.33**	**2.00**	**1.17**	**1.14**
Auditoriums and classrooms	0.47	0.92	0.45	0.60	0.55	0.37	1.04
Lunchrooms	0.08	0.05	0.07	0.07	0.14	0.07	1.00
Corridors	0.31	0.15	0.19	0.25	0.58	0.30	1.15
Lockers (room and corridor).......	0.05	0.00	(d)	0.03	0.12	0.08	0.87
Stairs and stairways (inside)	0.18	0.02	0.04	0.16	0.36	0.21	1.24
Toilets and washrooms	0.06	0.12	0.08	0.09	0.06	0.02	1.11
Grounds — unorganized activities	**1.16**	**1.93**	**1.99**	**2.40**	**0.32**	**0.22**	**1.17**
Apparatus	0.36	1.18	0.75	0.68	0.01	(d)	1.44
Ball playing....................	0.22	0.24	0.23	0.59	0.12	0.03	1.01
Running	0.20	0.15	0.37	0.39	0.04	0.08	1.14
Grounds — miscellaneous	**0.32**	**0.36**	**0.29**	**0.57**	**0.28**	**0.22**	**1.23**
Fences and walls	0.02	0.02	0.02	0.02	0.02	0.02	1.07
Steps and walks (outside)	0.11	0.15	0.10	0.16	0.17	0.12	1.08
Physical education	**2.14**	**0.82**	**0.66**	**2.28**	**4.02**	**2.36**	**1.12**
Apparatus	0.17	0.51	0.15	0.23	0.22	0.09	1.04
Class games	0.14	0.19	0.09	0.30	0.13	0.10	1.05
Baseball — hardball	0.01	0.00	(d)	(d)	0.01	(d)	1.25
Baseball — softball................	0.11	0.00	0.02	0.13	0.19	0.16	1.15

Source: Reporters to the National Safety Council: Accident Facts 1987, Chicago, 1987, p. 100.

[a]Accidents are those causing the loss of one-half day or more of (1) school time or (2) activity during nonschool time, or any property damage as a result of a school jurisdictional accident.

[b]All totals include data not shown separately.

[c]Adjusted for half day.

[d]Less than 0.005.

ACCIDENTS AND THE INJURY CONTROL MODEL

The word "accident" is a poor and inappropriate descriptor. To the lay person, most accidents happen "by accident," but in reality most injury and death attributable to accidents are a repeat of another accident or injury. In fact, there is a saying in the field of safety education and research that "there hasn't been a new type of accident in 50 years." Motor vehicle accidents are a good example, not only because the number and type of car accidents are repeated virtually every year, but also because of the magnitude of the problem as the leading cause of death for children and youth. A car can run into another car or stationary object in only one of several ways. The number and type of collisions are limited. They include hitting

TABLE 9-3.   Student accident rates by school grade — cont'd

Location and type	Total[b]	Kgn.[c]	1-3 Gr.	4-6 Gr.	7-9 Gr.	10-12 Gr.	Days lost per injury
Physical education — cont'd							
Football — tackle	0.05	0.00	0.00	0.05	0.12	0.05	1.07
Football — touch	0.12	0.00	0.00	0.04	0.21	0.26	0.88
Basketball	0.32	0.00	0.01	0.17	0.67	0.53	0.95
Hockey	0.02	0.00	0.00	0.01	0.04	0.06	1.10
Soccer	0.15	0.00	0.08	0.16	0.26	0.15	1.24
Track and field events	0.12	0.00	0.02	0.17	0.27	0.04	1.07
Volleyball and similar games	0.19	0.00	0.01	0.16	0.38	0.29	0.89
Other organized games	0.17	0.05	0.09	0.21	0.29	0.18	0.95
Swimming......................	0.05	0.00	0.00	0.01	0.12	0.08	0.98
Showers and dressing rooms	0.06	0.00	0.00	0.01	0.17	0.06	0.72
Intramural sports	**0.07**	**0.00**	**0.00**	**0.01**	**0.20**	**0.10**	**1.12**
Football — tackle	0.01	0.00	0.00	0.00	0.02	0.01	0.75
Basketball	0.02	0.00	0.00	(c)	0.04	0.04	1.28
Interscholastic sports	**0.42**	**0.00**	**0.00**	**0.01**	**0.53**	**1.38**	**1.65**
Football — tackle	0.18	0.00	0.00	0.00	0.19	0.64	2.39
Basketball	0.07	0.00	0.00	0.01	0.09	0.22	1.02
Track and field events	0.02	0.00	0.00	(d)	0.03	0.08	1.47
Special activities	**0.06**	**0.05**	**0.03**	**0.06**	**0.08**	**0.08**	**1.23**
Trips or excursions	0.03	0.05	0.02	0.04	0.04	0.02	1.32
Going to and from school (MV) .	**0.11**	**0.24**	**0.10**	**0.08**	**0.13**	**0.16**	**2.60**
School bus	0.08	0.10	0.08	0.06	0.08	0.10	2.99
Other motor veh. — pedestrian	0.02	0.10	0.01	0.01	0.02	0.02	2.19
Other motor veh. — other type	0.01	0.00	0.00	(d)	0.01	0.04	3.00
Going to, from school (not MV)	**0.07**	**0.05**	**0.07**	**0.12**	**0.09**	**0.01**	**1.10**
Bicycle — not motor veh.	0.01	0.00	(d)	0.01	0.01	(d)	0.81
Other street and sidewalk	0.04	0.02	0.04	0.06	0.05	0.01	0.93

another object, fixed or moving, being hit in the front or rear, or, in fewer situations, being hit on the side. After the car impacts, this causes what is known as the "second collision," where the occupants actually impact on the inside of the car. This second collision of the occupants with the inside of the car causes injury and death. This scenario plays itself out many *million* times each year resulting in just under 50,000 deaths every year. All aspects of this type of accident have been quantified over and over, yet they happen over and over, every day of every year. Other factors involved in motor vehicle death also happen over and over. Alcohol consumption, for example, has a strong relationship to motor vehicle accidents.

TABLE 9-4.   Accidental death rates[1] by type of accident, ages 5-22, 1984

About 302 of every 1 million children and young adults ages 5 to 22 died accidentally in 1984 according to the latest detailed information from the National Center for Health Statistics. Death rates generally decline from age 5 to 10, then increase dramatically through the teenage years. The increase is mostly due to motor-vehicle accidents, the leading cause of accidental death for all individual ages shown.

The table below shows the number of deaths per 1,000,000 population.

Age	All accidents	Motor-vehicle	Drown-ing	Fires, burns	Fire-arms	Falls	Poison (solid, liquid)	Mechanical suffo-cation	Poison by gas	Other accident
5 to 22 years	301.9	214.6	24.7	12.0	10.3	5.6	4.9	3.4	2.9	23.5
5 years	128.9	65.5	15.5	27.5	2.6	1.5	0.3	1.8	2.0	12.3
6 years	120.7	66.5	12.3	20.5	2.4	2.1	0.3	3.0	1.8	11.7
7 years	108.4	54.5	15.2	17.6	2.4	1.5	0.3	2.1	0.0	14.9
8 years	115.8	60.5	15.4	15.4	9.0	2.3	0.0	2.3	1.0	10.0
9 years	107.3	61.5	14.4	13.5	4.0	0.9	0.0	3.1	0.9	8.9
10 years	104.1	54.7	13.3	11.4	3.7	3.1	0.3	5.9	0.0	11.7
11 years	114.2	60.6	18.0	10.7	6.1	2.7	0.6	3.0	0.0	12.5
12 years	117.3	65.3	14.4	6.1	11.0	2.6	0.0	5.2	0.9	11.8
13 years	138.5	70.4	18.5	8.4	14.8	1.6	1.3	5.3	1.6	16.6
14 years	171.3	101.2	18.7	7.5	16.3	1.9	3.2	4.0	1.3	17.1
15 years	256.7	167.8	26.9	7.6	18.2	5.7	3.8	3.8	1.4	21.5
16 years	376.0	287.6	27.7	6.9	14.7	6.7	5.0	3.6	2.8	21.1
17 years	463.4	356.0	38.1	8.2	15.0	7.9	5.4	1.1	3.5	28.3
18 years	563.1	441.0	41.1	9.9	12.1	10.7	6.2	3.2	6.7	32.2
19 years	577.2	461.1	34.0	12.0	11.0	7.8	8.3	2.0	5.4	35.7
20 years	567.7	435.2	38.6	9.7	13.0	13.5	12.3	4.3	6.9	34.3
21 years	576.2	422.1	34.1	14.1	12.4	11.4	16.2	4.0	6.7	55.3
22 years	535.1	394.1	34.2	11.3	11.6	10.8	16.7	2.8	6.4	47.2

Based on 1984 National Center for Health Statistics data. Components may not add to totals because of rounding. National Safety Council: Accident Facts 1987, Chicago, 1987.

[1]Death rates = deaths per 1,000,000 population.

The concept of *injury control* is a useful model for school administrators and teachers to use in the prevention and control of accidental injury and death. The model quantifies the accident scenario and makes it possible to control factors that contribute to the accident event. The idea that when an accident happens it happens to a particular person within a particular environment in contact with a particular "tool" (e.g., a car, a jungle gym, a floor, a big piece of meat in the case of a choking) during a particular activity makes it possible to observe and control either the environment, the activity, the person, or any combination of these to control the possibility of an accident event from happening. It is possible to quantify all factors related to environment, tool, and person engaged in the activity and then effectively control these factors. The injury-control model takes advantage of the fact that contributing factors of a particular accident type can be found within three categories, the person, the tool, and the environment. These categories can be factored out and effective controls can be implemented.

Once these factors are known, they can be removed or "controlled" to lessen the possibility of accident. Controls that relate to the environment or tool are called *external controls*. Controls relating to the person involved in the performance of the activity are called *internal controls*. External controls involve changing the environment or creation of rules or

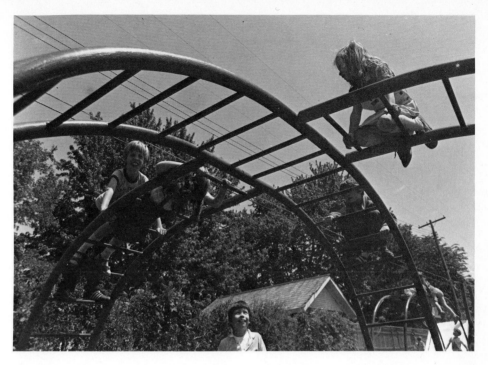

FIG. 9-2. It is not the school's responsibility to remove all potential hazards from a student's environment, but school personnel do have a responsibility to teach students how to use equipment safely and to be prepared in case accidents do occur.
(Copyright 1983 by David Riecks.)

regulations for the behavior. Speed limits and grooved highways are examples of external controls. Internal controls involve modifying the behavior of the actor involved in the unsafe behavior. A person recognizing the hazards involved with driving around a curve at high speed and slowing down is an example of an internal control. Education programs are in effect designed to promote internal control, control of the person or actor. Many individual behaviors that contribute to accidental death are played out among students in the school setting, and the health educator and school administrator can capitalize on these real-world teaching moments. Internal control of injurious behavior can be promulgated through effective health and safety education programs, which capitalize on utilizing peer-referenced learning.

As logical as the injury approach may seem, the incorrect assumption that accidents occur accidentally and cannot be controlled pervades society and the accident rates in certain categories are still high. The school administrator and health education teacher can take advantage of the injury control model and quantify factors in the school setting that have a history of contributing to accidents.

Prevention of accidents in school

Not all accidents can be anticipated, and one cannot foresee all situations that cause accidents. Yet most hazardous conditions can be recognized and unsafe practices detected if the school has a well-organized safety program. Safety programs, financially speaking, are not costly. What they demand is vision, organization, leadership, and cooperation. They should be programs that are put into action, not just programs on paper. A well-planned program evaluates the conditions and practices in the school in terms of safety and then undertakes to modify those that are not adequate.

A necessary first step in the prevention of school accidents is to make a survey to detect all potentially hazardous conditions. The survey form given in the box on pp. 208 and 209 is one that from experience has proved highly satisfactory and that any school can adapt to its use.

Legal aspects

Although the number of injury-producing accidents that happen in and around the school is low when compared with other exposures that children and youth have, children and youth *do* die or get injured at school and the potential for accidental death and injury is always present. Because the school is a controlled environment (i.e., most activities are well defined and take place within a defined space), as we have seen, it is possible to quantify and control specific behaviors that could lead to injury. From a legal point of view, because the environment is controlled and most accidents can only be repeats of former ones, it would be reasonable to assume that the school would have an effective injury-control program.

Emergency health needs always involve trauma. Trauma is experienced by the victim, and to a lesser degree trauma is experienced by the teacher or other school personnel who have to tend to the victim of an accident or medical emergency. To lessen this trauma teachers should be skilled in emergency health care procedures and be aware of their legal responsibilities.

Teachers and other school personnel are responsible to provide basic emergency care. In more technical terms this means they can apply nonmedical and nonsurgical procedures of an immediate and temporary nature until a physician or medical emergency personnel are available. This means that efforts can be made to stem excessive bleeding but that neither an aspirin may be administered nor possibly a sliver removed from a finger.

Teachers and other school employees run the risk of a lawsuit from injured students because of alleged negligence unless they are careful in emergency situations.

In general, *negligence* is any conduct below the legally established standard for the protection of others against unreasonable risk of harm. Two basic types follow:

1. An act that a person of ordinary prudence or judgment would realize involves unreasonable risk to others
2. Failure to act for the protection of another

Thus negligence can be acts of commission or omission. The specific details of each case determine whether there has been negligent behavior.

The following set of guidelines (Harper, 1938) illustrates a variety of possible negligent actions:

1. Failure to employ or properly carry out appropriate care
2. Creating undue risk by the circumstances under which care is provided
3. Actions involving an unreasonable risk of direct and immediate harm to others
4. Creating a situation that is unreasonably dangerous to others because of the action of a third person

5. Entrusting dangerous devices or instruments to persons incompetent to use or care for them properly
6. Failure to employ due care to give adequate warning
7. Failure to exercise the proper care in looking out for persons whom one has reason to believe may be in the danger zone
8. Failure to employ appropriate skill to perform acts undertaken
9. Failure to make adequate preparation to avoid harm to others
10. Failure to inspect and repair devices to be used in emergencies
11. Preventing a third person from assisting in an emergency

Liability for negligent conduct is affected by the nature of both the act and its results. Carelessness is a relative term. In general, a person is considered to be careless or negligent when actions are not those of a person of ordinary prudence. If a pupil is injured because a teacher's actions were not those of a prudent person or the teacher failed to act, a lawsuit may be instituted by the parents and the teacher held liable. Each teacher is responsible for his or her negligence that results in physical harm to others. A teacher's administrative superior will be held liable when he or she directs the teacher to do some dangerous act resulting in injury to a pupil or fails to correct a hazardous situation that has been reported by a teacher. The teacher must have tangible evidence that the administrator was notified of the hazard.

School boards are not usually held liable for negligence, but several state supreme courts have removed this immunity by making it possible to sue the school board as well as the teacher.

Teachers are not often defendants in lawsuits that allege negligence resulting in an injury to a pupil. Teachers tend to be conservative, and their conduct usually is prudent. Courts recognize the problem of close supervision of 35 to 40 children at a given moment, and only when the teacher has displayed deplorably poor judgment does the court tend to hold him or her liable. The low premiums for liability insurance for teachers attest to the small likelihood that a teacher will be a defendant in a lawsuit resulting from injury to a pupil.

The best safeguard against such a lawsuit is a well-planned functioning program for the prevention of accidents to pupils. Such a program will also be assurance to the parents that the school has taken definite steps to reduce student injuries to a minimum. The safety of the students is the first consideration, but here, as usual, student and faculty interests are at one.

EMERGENCY CARE

In any situation in which relatively large numbers of young people are assembled, emergencies occur despite the best precautions. Wisdom dictates preparation for such emergencies. Experience indicates that such preparation need not be elaborate but must be well organized.

When students visit the school nurse's office, the reason is most likely for an emergency. The emergency may in reality be minor, but to the student or the referring teacher the condition is important enough to warrant interruption of classroom activity. Of course, students also visit the nurse or aide for routine matters such as health screening, but the majority of visits are for special causes. A review of the patterns of use of the nurse's office

Survey of Conditions and Practices Affecting Safety in the School Environment

Reporting of accidents

1. Are accident report cards or forms available?
2. Is a complete written report on file for every accident that results in an injury?
3. Is a special study made of the causes of each accident?
4. Is an adequate constructive follow-up study made after accident analysis to prevent recurrence of the accident?
5. Is a regular inspection (weekly) made of the building and grounds?
6. Are adequate first aid equipment and personnel available at all times?

Fire protection

1. Are vacant rooms, basements, and attics free from flammable material?
2. Is there proper insulation between heating equipment and flammable material?
3. Are there two or more exits from every floor with doors swinging outward?
4. Are there adequate fire escapes on buildings of two or more stories?
5. Are fire extinguishers of an approved type provided for every 2000 square feet of floor space?
6. Are fire extinguishers tested regularly?
7. Do the older pupils know how to use the fire extinguishers?
8. Are fire alarms centrally located?
9. Are fire drills so proficient that the building can be emptied in an orderly manner in less than 3 minutes?
10. Are student organization and lines of exit well established (Fig. 9-1)?

Gymnasium, pool, and locker rooms

1. Is equipment in good condition?
2. Are all exposed projections covered?
3. Is the floor treated to prevent its being too slippery?
4. Are doors of a safe type?
5. Are fountains in a safe location?
6. Are definite rules for the use of the gymnasium and pool posted and practiced?
7. Are students properly dressed for gymnasium activities?
8. Is horseplay prohibited?
9. Is unsupervised use of the gymnasium and pool prohibited?
10. Are pool users classified according to skill?

Halls and stairs

1. Are all obstructions removed?
2. Are the floors and stairs treated to prevent them from being slippery?
3. Are worn or broken stairs replaced?
4. Are railings provided so that every person using the stairs can hold a railing?
5. Is undue congestion of hall traffic prevented by changing routes, practices, and schedules?
6. Are horseplay and running in the halls prohibited?

Shops, laboratories, and home economics rooms

1. Is all equipment in good repair and regularly inspected?
2. Are all possible safety devices and attachments available and in working order?
3. Are good housekeeping practices followed?
4. Are lighting and space adequate?
5. Are machines stopped for oiling and adjustment?
6. Are safety rules posted and practiced?
7. Are students properly instructed in the use of equipment?
8. Are horseplay and running prohibited?

Survey of Conditions and Practices Affecting Safety in the School Environment — cont'd

9. Is the unsupervised use of the shop, laboratory, or home economics rooms prohibited?
10. Is protective clothing and eyewear worn?
11. Are first aid supplies immediately available?

Classrooms and auditoriums

1. Are all obstructions removed?
2. Are exposed projections covered?
3. Are sharp objects placed in protected places?
4. Are radiators and electric fixtures properly protected?
5. Are dropped objects picked up immediately?
6. Is an orderly routine followed, with running and pushing prohibited?

Playground

1. Is the playground space allocated in terms of safety?
2. Is apparatus in safe condition and checked regularly?
3. Are children taught the proper use of each piece of apparatus?
4. Is supervision always provided when the playground is used?
5. Do new students in kindergarten and first grade receive special instruction and supervision?
6. Are horseplay and stunting prohibited?
7. Are caution and courtesy stressed at all times?
8. Do the children assume cooperative responsibility for playground safety?
9. Is the playing surface in good repair and nonslippery?

Athletics

1. Is the playing area constructed in terms of safety?
2. Are all hazardous obstructions removed?
3. Is approved equipment used?
4. Has every participant received medical approval?
5. Is competent supervision always provided?
6. Are the participants properly trained and sufficiently skilled?
7. Is parental approval required for participation in vigorous athletic events?
8. Is parental approval required if students are to be transported for athletic contests?
9. Are adequate first aid and medical services available?

Going to and from school

1. Are studies made of hazards children may encounter going to or from school?
2. Are specific routes outlined for students?
3. Are the routes direct, requiring a minimal use of roadways and busy intersections?
4. Are stop and go signals, stop signs, school signs, police supervision, and one-way streets used to the greatest advantage?
5. Are ice, glass, and other hazardous obstructions removed from walks?
6. Do children stay on the walks and in crosswalk lanes, and do they obey rules, signs, and traffic directors?
7. If school traffic patrols are organized, are the patrols under proper adult supervision?
8. Is maximal use made of traffic enforcement officers and facilities?
9. Are bus riders given instruction on entering and leaving the bus as well as conduct in the bus?
10. Are bicycle riders given special instruction and supervision?
11. Are student motor vehicle drivers given special instruction and supervision?
12. Are the parents enlisted in the safety program to and from home?

indicates something of the health problems of young people and also indicates the types of services that school health personnel should be prepared to take care of.

In one small (240 students) midwestern elementary school (K through 6), all visits were carefully documented. Reasons for visiting the nurse's office ranged from minor excuses to avoid an unpopular class to major illness and injury that parents knew about and still sent the sick child to school to get "free" medical advice from the school nurse or aide. (NOTE: Students with wounds [trauma] should not visit the nurse. Rather, the nurse or first responder should visit the injured student at the scene of the accident. In many cases, an injured child should not be moved.) The data gathered in this school indicate that the way young people, even elementary school students, use health services (in this case the nurse's office) is very like the way adults use their health services (clinics and private physicians). More girls than boys come to the nurse's office in the course of a day. Occasionally the condition prompting care could have been attended to earlier and simply represented parental neglect. Accidents are the most common cause of a visit. And young people, like adults, frequently use sickness or at least sick role behavior to avoid doing things they do not enjoy.

The percentage distribution of complaints that students presented when they reported to the nurse's office is shown in Table 9-5. It is interesting to note that the incidence of headache was most frequent during the winter months when children had little opportunity to play and exercise out of doors during the school day. In the second year the rate of headaches declined. This decline was associated with a conscious effort to provide activities and exercise and recreation during the school day, including going out of doors for recreation unless the weather was especially bad.

This implies that student health, at least as reflected by visits to the nurse's office, is affected by such things as physical hazards and accidents but also by administrative organizational patterns.

In this school it was also noticed that students who used the nurse's office more frequently were not the same students who were absent most frequently. Respiratory complaints accounted for the largest number of health-illness-related absences (20.4%), followed by gastrointestinal problems (11.1%), fever (10.2%), and skin problems (10.2%). Interest-

TABLE 9-5. Elementary students' reasons for visiting school nurse's office[*]

Boys				Girls		
	Year 1	Year 2			Year 1	Year 2
Wounds (trauma)	39.5	51.5		Wounds (trauma)	30.5	43
Headache	19.5	8.5		Headache	19	11
Gastrointestinal	14.5	12.5		Gastrointestinal	17	12
Skin	8	9.5		Skin	10	14
Mouth	5.5	2.5		Mouth	9.5	6
Eye	5	4		General malaise	6	3.5
General malaise	3.5	3.5		Respiratory	4	5.5
Respiratory	3	4.5		Ear	2.5	2.5
Ear	2.5	3.5		Eye	2	2.5

[*]All figures are given as percentages.

ingly, respiratory complaints were neither prominent among the causes of sick room use nor was fever. The skin problems seen by the nurse or health aide (sunburn and exposure to cold) were very different from those causing absence. Gastrointestinal complaints were the only category of complaints where visits to the nurse's office and absenteeism appeared to be related. This relationship is probably a direct result of the nature of the illness with early symptoms occurring at school and convalescence taking place at home.

A total of 7.3% of all school absences were attributed to visits to the physician or dentist. Only 5% of the reported absences were on a physician's recommendation. Nonmedical reasons ranging from helping with harvest to baby-sitting and accompanying parents on vacation accounted for 25% of the absences.

Facilities and procedures for emergency care

Effective emergency care begins with adequate facilities and well-established procedures. These include:

1. Nurse's office or health room with at least two cots, adequate blankets, pillows, washbasin, soap, towels, and chair (A contingency plan should exist that identifies space and supplies for more than two children in case of a major emergency.)
2. Established procedures in case of an emergency and the clear posting of emergency phone numbers for police, fire department, physicians, ambulance, and hospital
3. Student files listing location and phone numbers (home and work) for all children's parents
4. Established protocols concerning the role of the principal, nurse, aide, secretaries, and teachers in case of emergencies
5. Adequate first aid supplies

With an organized plan of action the school is well prepared to meet its responsibility during emergencies. If the school emergency program is part of the community emergency response program, the school should rehearse its procedures as part of the community rehearsal. Otherwise, on its own initiative the school should go through simulated emergencies.

PLAN OF ACTION WHEN ACCIDENTS OCCUR

Most people do not recognize that accidents are an expected part of daily living. Therefore, when an accident occurs, these same people are taken by surprise. Because of this, all too often victims lose the critical and timely benefit of the necessary and appropriate care. Many school systems because of requirement have written guidelines for handling emergencies, but that is generally the extent of their action response to accidents. Whether these plans are realistic and up to date with regard to current practices in emergency medical care is always in question. Because society still views the saving of lives as an activity reserved for physicians inside hospitals, the important actions that need to take place when an emergency occurs in the school often go unnoticed. Emergency medical services (EMS) is a relatively new area of health care and the critical role that lay bystanders (e.g., general public, teachers) play in saving lives has not been totally realized. A person can die or suffer permanent disability when care is not rendered during the first critical moments. On the other hand, untrained bystanders relying on "common sense" can cause real harm and need to be controlled. The critical role of the trained bystander is to first recognize that an emergency situation exists and effectively summon help and maintain life function until EMS arrives. Without this lives can't be saved. Sadly, an uninformed public often assumes that accidental death is an inevitable consequence of accident, when in many cases it can be the failure of an untrained bystander. It is caused by lack of or inappropriate emergency care in the first few minutes. When an emergency occurs, the right things often do not happen. Not only are personnel not trained, but also plans are unrealistic, inappropriate, or based on outdated regulations and *not practiced*.

THE MODEL FOR SAVING LIVES: The Community Emergency Medical Services (EMS) System

Local governments save lives in the streets of your community with an organized EMS system. An EMS system is a coordinated means of providing care to victims of injury and sudden illness. It involves many of your community's human and physical resources linked together and trained to provide specialized emergency care. It involves police, fire, ambulance, and hospital personnel all joined together by strict and well thought-out planning to provide specialized care within precise times that relate to the physiologic life-death function of the victim. EMS systems have had tremendous "save" rates when victims are readily accessible and appropriate care can be rendered quickly. For example, when a victim is located on the street or in a home, access to care can be virtually unimpeded. But lives are lost quite often when care is delayed because the victim becomes a victim of the facility where the accident occurs. When an accident occurs in a facility such as a school, shopping mall, or stadium, access to care and adequately trained personnel often do not exist. Or, as in some cases as in the schools, barriers to care are present. Unrealistic procedures such as delaying necessary care in order to contact parents during a life-threatening emergency costs lives. Relying on untrained personnel or on school staff assumed to be trained in first aid can lead to negative consequences.

The school system should be an integrated submodel of the community's EMS system when an emergency occurs. When an emergency situation occurs, everyone inside the school environment should know what to do. This includes teachers, bystander students, and all other school personnel. For certain emergencies, the care that is provided immediately and continued to the hospital can be definitely consequential with regard to whether the child will live or suffer disability. Personnel must not only be trained, but also practiced in what to do.

TRAINING OF SCHOOL PERSONNEL

It may be advantageous but cost prohibitive to have all school personnel trained in advanced techniques of emergency care. Advanced training for all personnel may not be necessary. To have effective management of most medical emergencies, there must be at least two levels of personnel training present at the school.

1. All personnel on the school staff should have basic training in the management of emergency situations and the basic ABCs of first aid (Airway, Breathing, Circulation–heartbeat and bleeding; Fig. 9-3). This training does not necessarily contain extensive first aid procedures but teaches the teacher how to recognize an emergency situation, check that

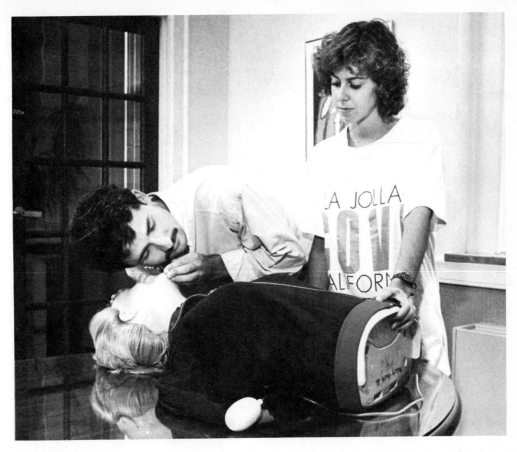

FIG. 9-3. Teachers practicing the ABCs of emergency care: *Airway, Breathing, Circulation*—heartbeat and bleeding.

conditions are safe for the injured and bystanders, efficiently and correctly notify the school and community's EMS systems, protect the victim from other inappropriate acts, and provide basic care until the school's first responder and community's EMS system arrives. This basic care includes managing problems that could lead to death during the first few minutes while the next level of care is being summoned or is responding. This care would include keeping the victim's airway open to breath, rescue breathing, cardiopulmonary resuscitation (CPR), and control of severe bleeding. Training that goes beyond the ABCs and being able to call for help and scene control are not necessary if the school has the next critical provider immediately available. Basic first-level training is sometimes difficult to find. Be careful to tell the training organization what you need to learn. Many training programs overtrain and teach unnecessary skills for this level of training such as splinting available from the American Red Cross. This type of training can confuse the lay audience through overtraining and does not foster helping behavior by the provider when the emergency occurs.

2. Within each school building and grounds, there should be one person trained to the first responder level. *First responder* is the first level of professional training designed to

respond and augment lay activities while the ambulance and other EMS system components are responding. This person has sufficient training in scene management and basic life support to sustain life until the EMS system arrives. There should be one trained first responder within each building or located where he or she can be contacted and respond to the emergency scene within 3 to 5 minutes. A lay person can be taught these skills. The school nurse may or may not be the best candidate for this training depending on such factors as his or her availability to the school and physical condition to be able to effectively respond to an accident scene in a short time. Notice that first aid training, especially the recommended first responder training, is not typically part of the training of a physician or nurse. So do not assume that your school nurse or doctor is trained and certified in emergency care. This type of training is available if you contact your community's local EMS office.

Adequately trained personnel along with well conceived and practiced EMS planning will prepare the school to deal effectively with typical emergency situations and offer a good defense in the event of litigation.

FIRST AID SUPPLIES

Every school building should have at least one fully stocked, conveniently located first aid cabinet. The cabinet should be placed in the nurse's office if there is one. Otherwise the emergency rest room or principal's office is an acceptable place to store these items. (See next page.)

SUMMARY

Accidental injury is the leading cause of death for age groups 1 to 44 years. Accidents result from uncontrolled behavior or uncontrolled environmental factors. However, the school environment is a relatively controlled environment and the activities in which the student participates are usually prescribed and controlled. Consequently, teachers and school officials have a greater responsibility for anticipating situations that could cause injury to students.

An injury control model that includes the student, the tool or equipment, and the environment is proposed. The external factors of the model include the tool and the environment. Examples of external control includes rules, regulations, and laws such as speed limits. Internal controls are designed to modify the person's behavior so that safe practices on the part of the student are promoted. The emphasis of safety education is strengthening internal controls.

Legal concepts of what constitutes prudent behavior on the part of the teacher or school administration is the basis for determining whether a person is negligent in carrying out his or her duties. If one's acts of commission or omission fail to meet a standard of acceptability, he or she may be held legally liable for injuries suffered by the student. All schools should have a written plan of the procedures along with facilities needed in the event of an emergency. The purpose of such a plan is to enable the school to respond appropriately in the first critical moments of an emergency. This includes maintaining life if necessary until the community's emergency medical care service arrives. In this regard, it is especially important that the school's emergency care program be planned as an integral part of the community's emergency medical care service. This implies that the school has appropriately trained personnel who would be able to maintain life until medical help arrives. Such a first responder should be able to manage the emergency scene, be on the scene in 3 to 5 minutes, and be able to administer the ABCs of first aid, which are *airway*, *breathing*, *circulation*—heartbeat and bleeding.

Inventory for First Aid Cabinet

Suggested Supplies	Purpose
Glass jars (2)	For applicators and blades
Blades, wood (500)	Splints, depressors
Wooden applicators (1000)	Swabs, remove particles
Toothpicks (750)	Remove particles
Tincture of green soap	Wash injured parts
Absorbent cotton roll	Large pads or dressings
Sterile gauze, 4 in roll	Dressings
Sterile gauze, 3 × 3 inch (7.5 × 7.5 cm) squares (100)	Protect injuries
Sterile gauze, 2 × 2 inch (5 × 5 cm) squares (100)	Protect injuries
Compress on adhesive band, 1 inch (2.5 cm) (100)	Protect injuries
Roller bandage, 1 inch (2.5 cm) (12 rolls)	Dressings
Roller bandage, 2 inches (5 cm) (12 rolls)	Dressings
Roller bandage, 4 inches (10 cm) (12 rolls)	Dressings
Triangular bandage (4)	Sling, area coverings
Safety pins (24)	For triangular bandage
Adhesive tape, roll (widths ½ to 2 inches [1.25 to 5 cm])	Fasten splints and dressings
Scissors (blunt or bandage)	Cut dressings
Forceps (3 inches [7.5 cm], pincer or tweezer type)	Grasp small objects
Tourniquet (3-foot ¼-inch rubber tube)	Check excessive bleeding
Splints (metal or yucca) (10)	Support
Quick cold packs	Relief of swelling
Hot-water bottle (with cover) (2)	Local relief of pain
Mineral oil or petroleum jelly (nonmedicated)	Relieve irritation
Paper cups (100)	Receptacle
Thermometer	Temperature checking
Elastic bandage	Sprains and strains
Inflatable splints	Fractures
Ample supply of ice	Bone and joint injuries
Pocket resuscitation mask	For protection of first responder from disease during rescue breathing

Inventory for First Aid Kit

Suggested Supplies	
Compress on adhesive band, 1 inch (2.5 cm) (20)	Adhesive tape, roll ½ and 1 inch (1.25 and 2.5 cm)
Sterile gauze, 2 × 2 inch (5 × 5 cm) squares (10)	Scissors
Roller bandage, 1 inch (2.5 cm) (1 roll)	Forceps
Roller bandage, 2 inches (5 cm) (1 roll)	Paper cups (10)

STUDY QUESTIONS

1. Should a school board and the faculty of a school district be held legally responsible for preventing risks of injury to students?
2. What are the elements of an "injury control" model?
3. In reference to your model of "injury control" above, where should the emphasis be placed to reduce the threat of injury to children and youth?
4. What is the minimum level of training required of all school staff to be able to respond to serious injury?
5. What constitutes a community emergency medical service (EMS) and how does a school relate to such services?
6. What is meant by the expression "teachers may be held legally liable for acts of commission and omission in situations of accidental injury to students?"
7. What do we mean by the ABCs of first aid?
8. For schools to respond effectively and efficiently to a medical emergency there should be two levels of training for school personnel. What are they?
9. Why do authorities on school health advise against giving medications to students?
10. Assume that you are the director of safety education in a school district. Where in the curriculum would you place emphasis on safety education and what faculty should receive training in safety education?

REFERENCES

American Red Cross: Adult CPR, Washington, D.C., 1987.

American Red Cross: Infant and Child CPR, Washington, D.C., 1988.

American Red Cross: Standard first aid, Washington, D.C., 1988.

Bergeron, D.: First responder, ed. 2, Bowie, Md., 1986, Robert J. Brady Co.

Committee on Trauma Research, Commission on Life Sciences, National Research Council, and the Institute of Medicine: Injury in America, a continuing public health problem, Washington, D.C., 1985, National Academy Press.

Florio, A., Alles, W., and Stafford, G.: Safety education, ed. 4, New York, 1979, McGraw-Hill Book Co.

Green, L., Kreuter, M., Deeds, S., and Partridge, K.: Health education planning, a diagnostic approach, Palo Alto, Calif., 1980, Mayfield Publishing Co.

Hafen, B.: First aid for health emergencies, St. Paul, Minn., 1985, West Publishing Co.

National Safety Council: Accident facts 1987, Chicago, 1987, the Council.

Reinberg, S., and Pendagast, E.: The first minutes, what to do until the ambulance arrives, Westport, Conn., 1984, Emergency Training.

Waller, J.: Injury control, a guide to the causes and prevention of trauma, Lexington, Mass., 1985, Lexington Books.

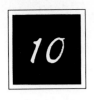

Tertiary Prevention and Special Populations

OVERVIEW   *Schools exist to educate students, but at times the school must go beyond education to actually facilitate education. Although schools teach about cigarette smoking and its accompanying risks, it is not the primary responsibility of the schools to "treat" students who smoke by providing clinics to help them quit smoking. On the other hand, schools do have a responsibility to help students with specific handicaps to receive the best education possible. This may mean providing services to deal directly with the handicapping conditions in order to facilitate the education process for these students.*

Because education is in part a social process, schools have a responsibility to educate all students, including students with special handicapping conditions, in a similar environment and in the company of others. So important is this principle that the U.S. Congress in 1977 passed PL 94-142, the Education for All Handicapped Children Act, to ensure that all students, regardless of their special needs, receive the best possible education in the least restrictive environment, carried out as often as possible in the normal school setting.

This chapter outlines the responsibilities of the school and especially the school health personnel in meeting the needs of special students. In this chapter special students include those with physically handicapping conditions, chronic health problems, handicaps brought on by family financial situations, and also students with unusual learning abilities.

OBJECTIVES   **After reading this chapter, the student should be able to:**

1. Describe how the goals of tertiary prevention complement the goals of education
2. Identify the major clauses specified in PL 94-142 (Education for All Handicapped Children Act), and explain the implications of each for the school health worker
3. State the meaning and significance of the terms *mainstreaming* and *least restrictive environment*
4. Explain the principal handicapping conditions found among the school-aged population and briefly discuss implications of each condition for school personnel
5. Outline the major steps in the medical and psychosocial assessments of handicapped students
6. Describe various specific actions school personnel can take to ensure the least restrictive environment for all students
7. Illustrate the role and functions of related services in the education of a handicapped student
8. Identify the elements of an individualized educational program
9. Justify the need for and nature of a school policy addressing the giving of medication to students during school hours
10. Outline how the Early Periodic Screening Diagnosis and Treatment Program of the Social Security Act can contribute to a school's health service program

Primary prevention involves efforts to prevent a health problem before it occurs. Secondary prevention involves the early detection and treatment of a health problem to limit its effects. Tertiary prevention addresses the need to carry treatment forward into full rehabilitation and ensure complete recovery or adaptation to any long-term disabilities. Ensuring that treatment continues through full rehabilitation decreases the chances of recurrence or the development of a secondary condition. This chapter describes the school's involvement in tertiary prevention.

At any given time a significant number of students will be experiencing handicapping conditions. However, for a large number of these students the conditions will be transitory in nature, including such things as common colds, asthma, allergies, mild emotional disturbances, gastrointestinal upsets, and minor injuries. In most cases these minor handicapping conditions will have little effect on the educational process. However, there are many students who experience handicapping conditions in the more traditional sense.

The term *handicap* usually refers to severe musculoskeletal disorders, neural disorders, cardiac disorders, disorders of vision and hearing, and intellectual and emotional disorders. For the school's purposes handicapping conditions identify students with special needs who require changes in one or more elements of the regular school program. Changes may be required in classroom facilities, classroom activities, teaching equipment, transportation, or the nature of auxiliary school personnel.

The extent and distribution of handicapping conditions are described in Table 10-1. The most frequent are speech impairments, mental retardation, learning disabilities, and emotional disturbances. Even the smaller school district will include students with these problems.

TABLE 10-1.   Handicapped children receiving special education and related services

Type of handicap	Total	Population (%)*	Handicapped population (%)
Mentally retarded	881,739	1.80	21.8
Hard of hearing	41,383	0.08	1.0
Deaf	41,489	0.08	1.0
Speech impaired	1,188,973	2.43	29.4
Visually handicapped	32,676	0.06	0.8
Emotionally disturbed	330,999	0.67	8.2
Orthopedically impaired	66,243	0.13	1.6
Other health impaired	106,287	0.21	2.6
Learning disabled	1,281,395	2.62	31.7
Deaf-blind	2578	0.00	0.0
Multihandicapped	61,923	0.12	1.5
TOTAL	4,035,685	8.25	100.0

Data from Office of the U.S. Secretary of Education, Assistant Secretary for Special Education and Rehabilitative Services, as reprinted in the American Academy of Pediatrics: School Health: a guide for health professionals, Evanston, Ill., 1981.
*Percentages of school-aged population 5 through 17 years in the nation. The last column indicates what percentage the number in each handicapping condition is of the total number reported as handicapped.

EDUCATION FOR ALL HANDICAPPED CHILDREN

Today there are approximately 40 million schoolchildren enrolled in 87,000 schools across the country. These students are served by an estimated 30,000 school health nurses and an unknown number of school health aides. Within this population some 4 million students have specific handicaps. For these 4 million people Congress passed PL 94-142, the Education for All Handicapped Children Act, in November 1975 and implemented nationwide in 1977. The principal intent of this legislation includes the following:

1. Guarantee free, appropriate public education at no cost to the parents of all handicapped children 3 to 21 years of age
2. Identify, locate, and evaluate all handicapped children regardless of the severity of their disabilities
3. Evaluate yearly each handicapped student and develop an individualized education plan
4. Provide educational services in the *least restrictive environment*, a process that often has been referred to as *mainstreaming*
5. Ensure for parents a clear role as a participant in the identification, evaluation, and placement of students
6. Ensure that students who are placed in private schools or special schools receive special educational services at no cost to parents; also that these students receive the same rights and programs as children enrolled in public education institutions
7. Provide in-service training for all teachers and support staff
8. Develop and implement public awareness programs to ensure greater sensitivity to and understanding of handicapped students

This legislation describes supportive services, including speech pathology, audiology, psychologic services, physical and occupational therapy, recreation, counseling services, and medical diagnosis and evaluation. This list, of course, could go on to include art therapy, music therapy, social work services, and other services that could be recommended for students with special needs. The intent of the legislation is to guarantee for handicapped children the removal of all obstacles denying access, excellence, and equity in education (Fig. 10-1).

An important consideration in working with students and parents of students who qualify for services under PL 94-142 is to remind them that the provision of services does not promise the complete remedy of all the student's problems. Students, parents, medical personnel, and all involved in developing each student's educational plan need to come to a realistic understanding of expectations. Unrealistically high expectations can be just as destructive as unrealistically low expectations. However, educational research does indicate that if we do err it would be better to err on the high side.

PRINCIPAL HANDICAPPING CONDITIONS
Mental retardation

Mental retardation is a major category of developmental disabilities, which also includes learning disabilities, cerebral palsy, and several other conditions such as autism, epilepsy, congenital rubella, and fetal alcohol syndrome. Mental retardation, the third most prevalent

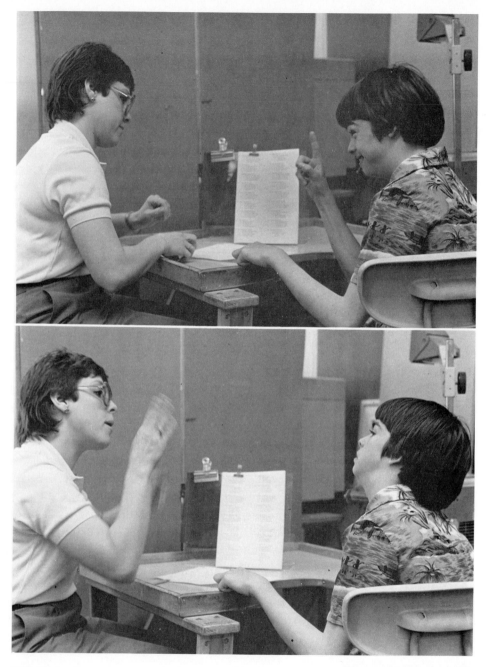

FIG. 10-1. Programs in special education enable children to achieve their optimum growth and development potential.

(Copyright 1983 by David Riecks.)

handicapping condition of school-aged children, follows speech impairments and learning disabilities. Functional mental retardation simply identifies a state of impairment recognized in the person's behavior. Severe retardation is frequently the result of overt brain damage; approximately 11% of children described as mentally retarded fall into this category. Mild retardation frequently results from cultural or familial conditions, and these children can benefit significantly from special education programs and early efforts at developmental stimulation.

Generally two types of programs address varying degrees of mental retardation. The first type is directed at infants and children with clearly recognized early developmental delays usually diagnosed by physicians. Carefully structured educational programs, designed to maximize the developmental potential of these children, can prevent secondary contributions to retardation that develop from within the student's social environment as a result of the handicapping condition. The other type of educational program focuses principally on students whose retardation has a cultural or familial base. Project Head Start is a program aimed at the developmentally deprived young person. The goal of programs such as this is to prevent borderline mental retardation from resulting in school failures and subsequent social, emotional, and cognitive difficulties. This type of program aims to give children maximal stimulation and reward frequently missing in their own social environments and to provide a structure in which they can function at maximal potential. Frequently these programs involve parents in an attempt to overcome the lack of stimulation or support that may exist in the family or social community.

Learning disabilities

Students with attentional deficit disorders, described on p. 113, are categorized as learning disabled. So are students with multiple forms of dysfunction, initially quite severe but that can be improved by special education. Again special education techniques are designed to strengthen the student's existing abilities and to discourage inappropriate behavior in the school or social setting.

The development of educational programs for mentally retarded and learning disabled students is frequently produced by interdisciplinary effort. Individualized educational programs for these students may involve close collaboration of the child's family physician, teachers, therapists in the areas of various deficits, and school counselors. Developing individualized educational programs is not easy, but when children's difficulties are clearly identified, objectives aimed at overcoming these difficulties and educational programs and activities designed to achieve these objectives can be developed. In this way PL 94-142 strives to provide for handicapped students educational programs designed specifically for their needs but that can be carried out, in the main, in the traditional educational setting. Although the intent of mainstreaming has always been part of the educational system, frequently in the past schools have not had to meet the challenge of students with these special educational needs. Consequently school health workers and school health educators may have to lead the way within the existing school structure and with existing school staff to meet the special needs of these students.

Hearing difficulties and deafness

Approximately 2% of handicapped students have significant hearing deficits. Because speech patterns clearly depend on hearing ability, it is critical that hearing loss be identified before school age.

Many students with hearing difficulties can be accommodated in the traditional classroom, if teachers are sensitive to such things as seating arrangements, supplemental speech and lip-reading instruction, the acceptance of hearing aids by fellow students, and occasionally the seeking of support services through community organizations. It is not the school's responsibility to treat these conditions, but one of the school's objectives is to facilitate education, and thus it is often in the interest of education for school personnel to stimulate family, community, or agency action to ensure that students have appropriate assistance. Frequently school personnel have been effective in getting necessary services for students with hearing and vision difficulties simply by making contact with appropriate community agencies and initiating action that ultimately leads to the improvement of the student's education.

Vision difficulties

Less than 1% of the handicapped population have severe vision difficulties, and unless the impairment to vision is severe (beyond 20/70 on the Snellen chart), students can usually be accommodated in the traditional classroom. Students who are partially sighted (20/70 to 20/200) cannot function in traditional classrooms without special aids, and although these children are not specifically defined as blind, special provision must be made to facilitate their education.

Because of difficulty in determining the exact status of vision in very young children, quite frequently children in kindergarten and the early grades manifest vision difficulties that have not been recognized by parents. Screening and observation of children therefore become especially important. There are several relatively simple steps the school can take to accommodate children with impaired vision. These range from making available large-type books printed on low-glare paper to using special dark pencils or felt pens, large-faced typewriters, and special seating arrangements in the classroom.

Orthopedic handicaps

Problems for orthopedically handicapped children are not so much problems of learning as those of ambulation and transportation. Accordingly the schools are faced with the problems of removing architectural barriers and providing special transportation. In addition, special facilities may be necessary (1) for orthopedically handicapped students to participate in adaptive physical education programs and to receive physical and occupational therapy and (2) to provide special assistance for students who may be catheterized.

Emotional disturbances

As many as 5 million, or 10%, of schoolchildren in the United States are described as having emotional problems, but as few as 14% of these receive specific care. Although some of these students will need therapeutic treatment outside the school's competency, significant numbers can benefit from school organization. The addition of special classroom activities, specially trained teachers, and supporting counselors and psychologists can present a low-cost alternative to the possible intensive care that may be required later in life if these conditions are overlooked.

Gifted students

Students with special talents and with ability for especially high performance should also be the subject of special concern from the school. As many as 5% of the school-aged population fall into this category and have been generally ignored, especially at the elementary school level. Consequently a large number of gifted students become frustrated and bored with the educational process. Although gifted students do not present any special health problems for the school to deal with, failure to provide adequate stimulation for these students is no less detrimental than the failure of the school to accommodate the able-minded student with a major orthopedic handicap.

MEDICAL ASSESSMENT

The medical examination of the student with a handicap differs only in terms of detail and focus from the medical examination of an apparently healthy child. Because of the detailed nature of the examination, it will likely be carried out by a team of specialists who will confer after the results of all tests are received and will plan a specific course of action. The intent of the examination, any resulting prescriptions, and the development of a prognosis will clearly identify the student's strengths and establish objectives to develop these strengths. Limitations and specific pathologic conditions will, of course, be explored, but from the school's view guidance concerning positive developments is just as important, if not more important, than statements of specific limitations and problems.

The health examination begins with a specific and detailed history that explores family history to identify possible hereditary trends and seeks data on the mother's health during the pregnancy. Detailed information from prenatal records often helps in understanding handicapping conditions. A detailed neurologic examination is completed; growth and development records are examined; and vision and hearing are carefully tested. In addition, a careful examination of the skin is carried out. Often the skin provides useful information concerning neurologic disorders. Anatomic defects are assessed to identify the extent of limitations and activity restrictions, and ways to maximize movement potentials are identified.

Like most examinations, medical examinations provide an opportunity to gain new knowledge and increase understanding. In the course of the examination, physicians will seek to better understand the parents' knowledge of the handicapping conditions and identify any misconceptions that may exist. They will show parents how they can better assist their child's growth and development.

PSYCHOSOCIAL ASSESSMENT

The most critical point in the psychosocial assessment of students is the final designation of handicapped. PL 94-142 calls for the identification of all handicapped students; it also clearly specifies that assessment must be nondiscriminatory. Because of the tendency for many tests to exhibit a degree of bias and also for factors of ethnicity, poverty, and culture to affect test outcomes, considerable caution is needed to avoid the unfortunate outcomes of labeling. To reduce the risks associated with assessments several points are important (Johnson, 1980).

1. Because so many handicapping conditions are health related, a comprehensive medical assessment should be completed before any psychosocial assessment.
2. Parents should be involved in all phases of the screening and assessment program to ensure that they understand what is being done and why. Fully informed parents will give greater cooperation and support when and if special programs need to be established.
3. Assessment should focus on the present level of educational functioning and what can realistically be achieved, rather than identifying what cannot be achieved. Such information should include but is not limited to the following:
   a. Academic level in the essential subjects
   b. Communication and language skills
   c. Motor and perceptual skills
   d. Social and emotional skills
   e. Prevocational and vocational skills

A comprehensive assessment of a student cannot be carried out without careful attention to the environment in which the student learns: the school. In the past, students have frequently been assessed in isolation from their environment. Handicapping conditions and their resulting psychosocial behaviors are influenced by the environment, and therefore the environment must be assessed. Among other things that affect the psychosocial development of the student and should be examined are the following:

1. Organizational climate of the classroom
2. Management style of the principal
3. Behavior of the teachers

Deviant social behavior indicative of emotional or physical problems can be the result of real handicapping conditions or reactions to specific environmental cues. Psychosocial assessment is therefore carried out with a recognition that the person being assessed is not a lone individual but is actually part of a social system, and the system must also be examined to understand the individual. Recognition of the social system's interconnecting nature decreases the likelihood of incorrect assessment results and the potentially damaging effect of inappropriate labeling.

Assessment is a team process and therein lies a significant safeguard. However, for a team approach to work, all members must have complementary ways of viewing the task. Recognizing the interaction of person and environment makes the assessment more difficult but increases the likelihood of a quality process and results leading to an effective individual education program.

IMPLICATIONS FOR SCHOOL HEALTH PERSONNEL

Most handicapping conditions are related to health problems; therefore school health personnel, nurses, health teachers, physicians, and aides are likely to be the first to notice them. Once noticed, and even when treatment is initiated, there is frequently a need for an advocate within the school to ensure that specific needs are met. Again health service and health education personnel are the most likely advocates to ensure that architectural barriers are modified, special classes or learning opportunities are provided, special services are available, and arrangements for medication, special meals, and transportation are made.

Architectural barriers

Architectural barriers deny equal access but can be dealt with in several ways. Barriers can be removed or modified to reduce their obstructiveness. Often a less costly alternative is to organize available spaces so that students who have difficulty can avoid architectural barriers and still participate fully in their educational program. This may not always be possible. School health personnel should carefully survey the school for barriers that exceed the limits of any student and then work actively with the school authorities to modify problem areas. On occasion a compromise between the student's needs and the economy of making changes must be found. The critical point is the provision of the "least restrictive environment," not an unrestricted environment. In this process, however, handicapped students will need an advocate within the school. Again school health personnel, health teachers, school nurses, physicians, and aides constitute the most obvious advocate group.

Adaptive physical education

The law assumes that handicapped students are essentially healthy and therefore should be provided access to a full curriculum. Physical education is the only area actually mentioned in the law's description of special education. Regulations specify motor development, body mechanics, and physical and motor fitness, all central to the objectives of any physical education program but especially to adaptive physical education. Adaptive physical education is defined as "the science of analyzing movement, identifying deficiencies within the psychomotor domain and developing instructional strategies to remediate identified deficiencies" (Sherrill, 1976).

Adaptive physical education, like regular physical education, contributes to the goals of education through physical activity. As such, the teachers concern goes beyond the qualitative and quantitative issues of biomechanics to include such concerns as posture, weight control, diet, stress management skills, relaxation, and mental health.

Depending on the extent of the handicapping conditions, the skill of the teacher, and the planned activities of the curriculum, handicapped students can be integrated into regular classes or they can participate in an exclusive class designed to meet their needs. Exclusive classes are not prohibited by the law but must be justified as the most appropriate for the particular student.

As with all curricular areas individual educational plans need to be developed, with the identification of the current level of psychomotor functioning, specific goals for psychomotor achievement, specific instructional objectives, suggestions for placement in classes, and evaluation plans and a specific time line.

Related services

Two essential services are outlined in the standards of PL 94-142. These are the provision of special education and related services. Special education is described as "specifically designed instruction at no cost to the parent to meet the unique needs of a handicapped child inclusive of home or hospital or classroom instruction as well as physical education" (*Education of Handicapped Children*, 1977). Related services include "professional services provided with the major goal to assist the handicapped child to benefit from special education" (*Education of Handicapped Children*, 1977). Steenson and Sullivan (1980) in identifying the relationship of related services to education suggest that "related services" could be called "student support services" and further suggest the following:

- Art therapy
- Audiologic services
- Corrective therapy
- Social work services
- School health services
- Occupational therapy
- Counseling services
- Drama therapy
- Physical therapy
- Psychologic services
- Speech therapy
- Transportation
- Orientation and mobility instruction
- Visual training therapy
- Recreation therapy
- Music therapy

The law did not intend for every student to receive every service but meant that services like these should be considered in the development of individualized educational plans.

Steenson and Sullivan (1980) further clarify the instructional goals for handicapped youth by collapsing various educational elements into eight areas: ambulation, self-care, emotion and behavior, vision, communications, hearing, health problems, and academic achievement. These areas of concern illustrates the role of school health service personnel, teachers, nurses, physicians, and aides in the planning of individualized educational programs.

Ensuring education for all in the least restrictive environment also breaks down the traditional separation of care providers (nurses and physicians) and educators (teachers). Now there is a need for partnership between health and medical personnel and educators to ensure the best possible program for all students. However, the goal of the program is not the medical goal of curing but is closer to the nursing-teaching goal of providing support services and immediate care while developing skills to enhance the ability to cope and survive.

In this way the objectives of prevention are served by enhancing a person's ability to achieve his or her full potential and reducing the chances of additional complications. Tertiary prevention, exhibited through full rehabilitation, essentially recycles a person back to the domain of primary prevention where the task is to reduce the likelihood that further regression occurs or that other health problems develop.

MEDICATIONS

In the majority of states, school nurses are responsible for administering medications during school hours. Medications may include those prescribed by physicians as part of ongoing treatment or maintenance therapy, as is frequently the case with handicapped students, but they can also include over-the-counter medications (OTCs) purchased without prescriptions by parents. Regular medication administration can become problematic for school personnel because of assignment of persons to the task and also because of the added responsibility for treatment and maintenance services rather than preventive and educational services, the school's traditional responsibilities. Schools with full-time nurses or aides can usually perform the task of providing medications, but schools that must rely on office personnel to carry out this function have greater difficulty.

Education of parents and communications with physicians are important in establishing a school medication policy.

For example, most medications that are prescribed three times a day do not need to be given during school hours. Administration before school, immediately after school, and before going to bed in the evening meets the instructions. Medications taken with meals, however, will need to be taken at school. Parents need to understand the difference so that they do not ask school personnel to carry out an unnecessary chore. Physicians sometimes overlook this option to avoid school-time administration when explaining a prescription to parents, and so it is frequently necessary for the nurse or principal to have parents question their physician about this option. Time-release medication may also be a possibility, reducing the needed number of daily doses. Again, a simple inquiry from parents to physicians may simplify the regimen and avoid an extra task for the school.

Dorsett (1982) has noted a series of points that should be included in a school's medication policy and has suggested that such a policy should have two major concerns: (1) safety—the assurance that the correct medication is given correctly to the right person, and (2) efficiency—minimizing the time needed for administration and minimizing the time taken from the teaching-learning process.

The following are points for school medication administration:

1. The principal of each school should ensure that a medication policy exists and is followed.
2. The principal must designate certain persons to administer medications according to specific guidelines.
3. The policy should clearly state that whenever possible medications should be given outside school hours and that only essential medications will be given by school personnel.
4. A form should be filled out by the prescribing physician for all medications to be administered during school hours, specifying the name of the medication, how often it should be given, the expected duration of the treatment, and whether a reaction is likely and if so, what type of reaction. The medication form should be signed by the parent or guardian authorizing the school personnel to administer the medication.
5. The school personnel should not be responsible for administering the first dose of any medication in case of an allergic reaction.
6. Medications properly labeled and accompanied by an authorization form should be hand carried to the school by the parent. Medications in containers other than the original one provided by the pharmacy should not be accepted.
7. Medication should be kept in a separate, locked facility or refrigerator accessible only to authorized persons.
8. A record should be completed for all medications administered. If for some reason a dosage of medication is not administered, a specific reason should be stated and parents notified.
9. A copy of the daily medication schedule should be kept by the principal or the school nurse.

EARLY PERIODIC SCREENING, DIAGNOSIS, AND TREATMENT

A growing concern of educators and physicians alike are children who come to school from homes where the parents either cannot afford or do not accept responsibility for the needed health and medical care of their children. Another complication is the lack of medical services available to the disadvantaged and to children in lower socioeconomic levels. This problem is particularly acute in many of the major cities in the United States today. Special federal legislation has been enacted, such as the amendments to the Social Security Act and Titles V and XIX (popularly known as Medicaid), which are designed to provide comprehensive health services for children and youth. This legislation intends to provide medical care for all those who are unable to pay for it. Although providing direct health care for children is not the school's responsibility, school personnel should not overlook students' health care needs. School officials should know state and federal legislative provisions for child health services. Indeed, school administrators, teachers, and school nurses, as advocates for the health of school-aged children and youths, must communicate health needs to families and to appropriate community health officials.

Although not focusing on a tertiary prevention issue, the Early Periodic Screening, Diagnosis, and Treatment Program does address an important need for children of low-income families who meet the standard to receive Medicaid or Aid to Dependent Children as authorized by Title XIX of the Social Security Act. This extension to Title XIX of the Medicaid program is commonly known as Early Periodic Screening, Diagnosis, and Treatment (EPSDT). The details of the way this program is administered may differ slightly from state to state. In Illinois, for example, children who receive Aid to Dependent Children or medical assistance are eligible for services under this program for the period from birth to 20 years of age. In Illinois the program is administered jointly by the Department of Public Aid and the Department of Public Health. In Nebraska it is administered by the Department of Social Services.

The extended services provided under the Medicaid (Title XIX) program include:

1. Periodic health appraisals including health history and physical examination, with emphasis on growth, development, and nutritional status (The schedule includes four medical checkups during the first year, annual checkups to age 6 years, and then at ages 10, 14, 17, and 20 years.)
2. A comprehensive immunization program and updating of previous immunization, including measles, poliomyelitis, diphtheria, pertussis, and tetanus
3. The periodic screening for urine sugar and protein, hemoglobin, or hematocrit determinations and tuberculosis testing (Vision and hearing screenings are provided annually from ages 3 to 8 years and thereafter at ages 10, 12, 14, and 16 years.)
4. Screening when indicated to detect specific conditions including lead poisoning, sickle-cell abnormality, and venereal disease
5. Dental examinations as provided on an annual basis from age 3 through 20 years

Emphasis is given to follow-up care and treatment of the health problems discovered through screening activities.

School officials and health educators should be informed about these federal and state services available to the children of their respective communities. With the development of new programs of health services, school health education should accept the responsibility for informing children and parents about these important community services and resources.

SUMMARY

Children with disabilities are no different from children without disabilities in their need for basic health care and educational services. The concept of mainstreaming emphasizes this principle.

Public Law 94-142, The Education for All Handicapped Children Act of 1975, defines handicapped children as those mentally retarded, hard of hearing, deaf, speech impaired, visually handicapped, seriously emotionally disturbed, orthopedically impaired, or suffering from other forms of health impairment such as limited strength or vitality, rheumatic fever, asthma, epilepsy, sickle-cell anemia, blood poisoning, diabetes, and other conditions that would affect educational performance.

For school personnel the challenge is to incorporate these children fully into the life of the school. School staff have the responsibility for planning and managing individual educational plans that involve a full range of human service professionals and helping other children learn from participating in activities with handicapped students.

All people in the school learn about human health, adaptability, the meaning of normal, and the difference between primary, secondary, and tertiary prevention when they work and learn together with handicapped students and modify the educational environment and activities to accommodate their special needs.

STUDY QUESTIONS

1. How can a physical defect adversely affect mental health?
2. What can be the relationships between a physical defect and academic performance?
3. Lack of family financial means should but increase the determination of the school to obtain the necessary medical services for the child needing correction of a defect. Explain the implications of this statement.
4. What can be done for children with noncorrective orthopedic defects to help them be normal members of their class and to give them the type of self-gratification from accomplishment that all normal youngsters want and need?
5. In any rehabilitation why is it important that one person have primary responsibility, even though the services of many persons may be utilized?
6. When a teacher recognizes that a child has a physical disorder, why should the teacher relate this to the school nurse and then to the school principal before anything is done on behalf of the child?
7. In a program to help a student adjust to a physical defect, why is it important to have the student develop a strong insight in terms of his or her status, needs, and progress?
8. How would you get a child to wear prescribed glasses when he or she does not want to wear them?
9. What can a small school system do to provide a modified program for the handicapped pupil?

10. How does the medical assessment for a healthy student differ from that for a handicapped student?
11. What does the term *handicapped* mean?
12. Why should a medical assessment always precede a psychosocial assessment?
13. Define tertiary prevention, and explain how it is different from primary and secondary prevention.
14. How does the concept of mainstreaming differ from the concept of education in a minimally restrictive environment?
15. Differentiate between acute and chronic handicapping conditions.
16. Explain the significance of PL 94-142 to (a) the health teacher, (b) the school nurse, and (c) the school principal.
17. List the major handicapping conditions found in the school-aged population.
18. Describe the major aspects of a school's environment and program that should be reviewed to ensure the school is best serving its handicapped students.
19. Should school personnel be expected to give medications to students during school hours? If so, why and under what conditions?
20. What is Title XIX of the Social Security Act, and why is it important to educators?

REFERENCES

American Academy of Pediatrics: School health: a guide for health professionals, Elk Grove Village, Ill., 1987, the Academy.

Accardo, P., and Capute, A.: The pediatrician and the developmentally delayed child, Baltimore, 1979, University Park Press.

Bleck, E.: Integrating the physically handicapped child, J. Sch. Health **49**:141, 1979.

Bogle, M.: Relationship between deviant behavior and reading disability: a retrospective study of the role of the nurse, J. Sch. Health **43**:312, 1973.

Bryan, E.: Administrative concerns and schools' relationship with private practicing physicians, J. Sch. Health **49**:157, 1979.

Dorsett, T.: Administration of medications during school hours, J. Sch. Health **52**:444, 1982.

Education of handicapped children: implementation of part B of the education of the handicapped act, Fed. Reg., Aug. 23, 1977.

Gleidman, J., and Roth, W.: The unexpected minority: handicapped children in America, New York, 1980, Harcourt Brace Jovanovich, Inc.

Johnson, J.: Psychosocial assessment of the handicapped, J. Sch. Health **50**:252, 1980.

Jones, E.: PL 94-142 and the role of the school nurse in caring for handicapped children, J. Sch. Health **49**:147, 1979.

Levenson, P.M., and Cooper, M.A.: School health education for the chronically impaired individual, J. Sch. Health **54**:446, 1984.

Martin, J.: Attitudes toward epileptic students in city high school system, J. Sch. Health **44**:144, 1974.

McCubbin, J., Combs, C.S., Jansma, P., et al.: Personal health training and the severly handicapped: a curriculum based research investigation, Health Educ. Q. **15**(2):217-223, 1988.

Menolascino, F., and Egger, M.: Medical dimensions of mental retardation, Lincoln, Neb., 1978, University of Nebraska Press.

Reed, H.: Biologic defects and special education — an issue of personnel preparation, J. Special Educ. **13**:9, 1979.

Rose, T.: The education of all handicapped children act (PL 94-142): new responsibilities or opportunities for the school nurse, J. Sch. Health **50**:30, 1980.

Shaffer, A., and Avery, M.: Diseases of the newborn, Philadelphia, 1977, W.B. Saunders Co.

Sherrill, C.: Adapted physical education and recreation, Dubuque, Iowa, 1976, Wm. C. Brown Group.

Steenson, C., and Sullivan, A.: Support services in the school setting: the nursing model, J. Sch. Health **50**:246, 1980.

Swisher, J.: Developmental restaging: meeting the mental health needs of handicapped students in the schools, J. Sch. Health **48**:548, 1978.

Vlasak, J.: Mainstreaming handicapped children: the underlying legal concept, J. Sch. Health **50**:5, 1980.

Zeitlin, S.: Assessing coping behavior, Am. J. Orthopsych. **50**:139, 1980.

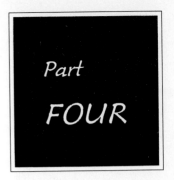

Part

FOUR

HEALTH INSTRUCTION

A Theoretical Foundation for Health Instruction

OVERVIEW   *This chapter begins with an examination of several widely published statements on health education including definitions and purposes. These statements are discussed in the light of changing conditions and needs in order to determine the most appropriate role for health education. The differing perspectives of education and public health are noted: the field of education emphasizing cognitive outcomes and public health placing greater emphasis on the health behavior outcomes. A code of ethics for health education is presented with the reminder that health educators have a special responsibility to serve the public in accordance with the highest standards of professional and ethical conduct. Since much of today's illness and disability is attributed to life-style factors and poor health habits, health education has taken on additional importance as a means of improving health. With this new recognition has come increased criticism of health education. The field is often criticized because of its lack of a sound theoretical basis to give direction to program activities as well as to research. In an effort to establish a theoretical basis two major theories of learning are discussed: (1) the connectionist, or behaviorist, position and (2) the cognitive position. Several of the theories and models now being applied to the field of health education are analyzed in terms of these two major theories of learning in order to gain a better understanding of both the theory and the methods being advocated. Among the health education applications discussed are (1) the health belief model, (2) social learning theory, (3) Fishbein's behavioral intention model, and (4) persuasive communication theory. The chapter concludes with suggested guidelines for planning effective health instruction programs.*

OBJECTIVES   **After reading this chapter, the student should be able to:**

1. Relate various statements of definition, purposes, and goals of health education

2. Demonstrate familiarity with major purposes and goals of health education that have been adopted by professional and government agencies

3. Explain why a code of ethics is of special importance to health educators

4. Explain why theories are important to the profession of health education

5. Identify the connectionist and cognitive theories of learning and explain some of the characteristic differences between these two major orientations

6. Show how learning theory is related to several different health education models and instructional programs

7. Identify several determinants of health behavior

8. Identify several models of behavior change that have been offered to the field of health education

9. Determine how one would use the persuasive communication matrix model in developing a health teaching plan

10. List several guidelines for developing a health instruction program

Health educators and other health professionals have long called for a national commitment to good health as a way of life. Health education should be one of the most dynamic components of the entire school curriculum, a program to achieve the goals of both education and public health.

Research has demonstrated that certain aspects of individual behavior are related to major causes of death in American society. In particular, long-term patterns of behavior or life-style factors have been determined to be risk factors for such major health problems as accidents, cardiovascular diseases, and cancer (Hamburg et al., 1982). Public health officials have long contended that there is a strong scientific basis for believing that habits and patterns of living and their associated diseases have their origins early in life (Epstein, 1980). This places a challenge before the school health education program to intervene early in the life of a person to prevent disease. Health education can make its greatest impact during the formative years of the school child to develop positive health-promoting behavior relating to habits of diet, exercise, use of health products and services, avoidance of cigarette smoking, excessive consumption of alcoholic beverages, and reckless driving.

It has become increasingly evident to medical researchers and the general public alike that many of today's health problems are caused by factors that are not responsive to medical solutions. For example, at this time there is no vaccine to prevent heart disease and no cure for the problem of alcoholism. Short of a dramatic breakthrough, such as the development of a cure for cancer, it is becoming apparent that further expansion in the nation's health care system will produce only marginal improvements in the health status of Americans. Although it is obvious that providing the best health care for all citizens is of great importance, it is also apparent that, in the long run, the greatest benefits to the health of the public are most likely to come from efforts to improve the life-style and the environment in which they live and work (U.S. Department of Health, Education and Welfare, 1975).

As a result of this thinking, a new emphasis is being placed on the behavioral aspects of health. Richmond (Nightingale et al., 1978), on taking the oath of office as the nation's highest ranking health officer, stated that the importance of behavioral research must be recognized so that we can:

> . . . discover how to enlist people into preventing disease and in promoting their own health. This means that health education encompasses not only the transmission of knowledge but also the full range of activities designed to provide the skills, the interest and the motivation to help make people's lives more fulfilling and free from disease and disability.

PURPOSE AND ETHICS OF HEALTH EDUCATION

Over the years members of the field of health education have attempted to develop a philosophy or point of view and have articulated a set of goals or a statement of purpose. These definitions not only reveal the intent of the particular time but also illustrate the growth and change in purpose that have occurred.

In 1934 the Joint Committee (NEA-AMA) on Health Problems in Education proposed the following definition: "Health education is the sum of all experiences which favorably influence habits, attitudes, and knowledge relating to individual, community, and racial health." This statement recognized that all of life's experiences, both in and out of school, contribute to the individual's attitudes toward health as well as patterns of living. Any formal health education planned by the school must recognize those forces outside the school that shape the health behaviors of children and youth.

The 1948 Joint Committee (NEA-AMA) statement emphasized that "health education is the process of providing learning experiences for the purpose of influencing knowledge, attitudes, or conduct relating to individual, community, and world health." This definition stresses the role of the school in providing learning experiences through a formal and planned program of health instruction. The statement also provides guidance as to the purpose of the curriculum. For classroom learning to have a positive effect on what students think, feel, and do about health in the community and the world at large, it must deal with contemporary problems of society.

The inclusion of world health in this definition reflects awareness of the World Health Organization (WHO), which had been created during this period. WHO issued its widely quoted definition on health as a state of complete physical, mental, and social well-being and not merely the absence of disease and disability. In 1954 WHO (Expert Committee on Health Education of the Public, 1954) addressed the subject of health education with the following statement:

> The aim of health education is to help people achieve health by their own actions and efforts. Health education begins, therefore, with the interests of people in improving their condition of living. . . in developing a sense of responsibility for their own health betterment and for. . . the health of their families and governments.

This statement has proved especially useful to health educators working in countries other than the United States, enabling them to relate more effectively to people of different cultures and ethnic groups. It has served as a reminder to public health and school officials that health education is not something to be done for or to be given to people. Rather, if it is to be truly educational, it is a process that causes change within the person through changes in knowledge and attitudes. In turn, health education is reflected in what a person does for himself or herself and for others in order to promote well-being and prevent illness and injury.

With the upsurge of public interest in health education in the 1970's, more statements have been issued. Like the earlier statements, these served to clarify the evolving and emerging role of health education. The statement of the President's Committee on Health Education (1973), issued in 1972, is illustrative:

> Health education is a process that bridges the gap between health information and health practices. Health education motivates the person to take information and do something with it, to keep himself/ herself healthier by avoiding actions that are harmful and by forming habits that are beneficial.

Here again, the emphasis on process is apparent, speaking to the relationship between health information and health education. Only after health information is translated into health knowledge, understanding, and action does it become health education. In the schools the process of health instruction translates health information into health outcomes.

After the President's Committee statement, the Joint Committee on Health Education Terminology (1972–1973) issued a revised definition of health education as:

> ...a process with intellectual, psychological, and social dimensions relating to activities which increase the abilities of people to make informed decisions affecting their personal, family, and community well-being. This process, based on scientific principles, facilitates learning and behavioral change in both health personnel and consumers including children and youth.

This statement also emphasizes the idea of process, but it recognizes that education is more than an intellectual experience. Emotional and social factors also shape health understandings and behaviors. But perhaps the part of the definition that is of most importance in the development of a philosophy of health education is the expression "the abilities of people to make informed decisions." This suggests that enabling the individual to make an informed decision about health is the central purpose of health education. Moreover, it implies that decision making is the prerogative of the individual. Although it is the teacher's responsibility to create the opportunities for decision making through the health instruction program, students must be given freedom to make decisions. If children and youth are to grow to full maturity and are to become health-educated citizens of tomorrow, they must be allowed to make decisions, choices, and even mistakes in the realm of health. The challenge of the health teacher and of parents in matters affecting health is to know when to lead, when to guide or control, and when to let the young person make the choice.

Sullivan (U.S. Department of Health, Education, and Welfare, 1977), in writting for health planning agencies, has suggested that a program of health education should meet the following criteria:

1. It should be consistent with current knowledge about how people learn.
2. It should be consistent with the rights of individuals to make their own decisions about health practices as long as these practices do not infringe on the rights of others.
3. The definition should be readily understood not only by the health educator specialist but also by the public at large.

The fact that these criteria apply primarily to programs geared to the health needs of the adult population indicates the need for an additional criterion. It should emphasize that adults must accept responsibility for the health and safety of the young and immature. For example, it is one thing for college students to make decisions and choices about their diets or about their physical exercise program, but it is quite another matter for primary grade children to make a choice about crossing the street. Health-related decisions and actions are highly specific to the individual and to the social and environmental setting. It must also be emphasized that in defining any program in health education, the information presented must be consistent with the scientifically established knowledge.

CODE OF ETHICS

Health educators, in addition to establishing criteria for health education, have attempted to clarify the relationship between the health educator and the student or client. The Society for Public Health Education, Inc., has adopted the code of ethics given below to guide health educators in their efforts to promote the health of all people through education.

Code of Ethics

Health educators, in utilizing educational processes to influence human well-being and to change health behavior, take on profound and grave responsibilities. Although ethical beliefs are a matter of personal choice, the values we have selected for ourselves must be constantly reexamined and modified. The nature, importance, and magnitude of health education are such that there is a potential for ethical abuse. To reduce the chances of abuse in health education and to guide professional behaviors of health educators toward the highest standards, the following code of ethics is adopted by and for the profession.

Principles

1. Health educators do not discriminate because of race, color, religion, age, sex, national ancestry, or socioeconomic status in rendering service, hiring, promotion, or training.
2. Health educators observe the principle of informed consent with respect to individuals and groups served.
3. Health educators value privacy, dignity, and worth of the individual, and use skills consistent with these values.
4. Health educators maintain their competence at the highest levels through continuing study, training, and research.
5. Health educators foster an educational environment which nurtures individual growth and development.
6. Health educators support change by choice, not by coercion.
7. Health educators as researchers or practitioners report activities and findings honestly and without distortion.
8. Health educators accurately represent their competence, education, training, and experience and act within the boundaries of their professional competence.
9. Health educators are aware of unprofessional practices, and are accountable for taking appropriate action to eliminate these practices.

Courtesy Society for Public Health Education: Code of ethics, San Francisco, Oct. 15, 1976, Society for Public Health Education, Inc.

CONTRIBUTION OF HEALTH EDUCATION TO HEALTH

The American Public Health Association, at its annual meeting in 1977, formally acknowledged the essential relationship of health education to the achievement of the association's goal of optimal health for the nation's population. Today, more than ever, methods of improving the public's health status focus on health education. The conviction is growing among health professionals that major advances in health status will come from changes in the life-styles of individuals and from the control of health hazards in the environment. It is through the process of education that citizens in a democratic society are alerted to the personal and societal obstacles to good health. Health education offers a channel for achieving the needed changes.

Because of the complexity of factors that interact to affect health, including the environment, social conditions, and institutional and economic politics (Fig. 11-1), the solving of health problems often requires coordinated action on the part of informed citizens. From

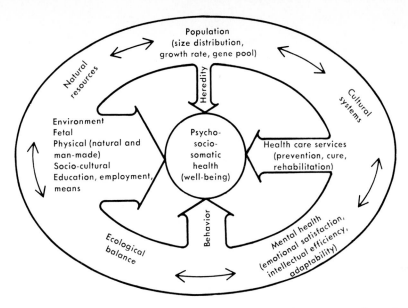

FIG. 11-1. Blum's inputs to health. The relative widths of the arrows indicate the relative importance attached to the various inputs. By inference, health education (behavior) is seen to make a major contribution to health.
(From Blum, H.L.: Planning for health: development and application of social change theory, New York, 1974, Human Sciences Press.)

the public health perspective, then, the goal of health education is the health-educated consumer-citizen who adopts a health-promoting life-style and wisely selects and uses health care resources, products, and services. Ideally, this citizen will actively participate in the formulation of public policy and planning on health care issues and in the larger environmental matters that affect health (American Public Health Association, 1977).

One of the most useful of statements issued thus far on the goals of consumer health is that of the Task Force Report on Consumer Health Education (Preventive Medicine USA, 1976). This report, one of eight provided by the American College of Preventive Medicine and the Fogarty International Center for Advanced Study in the Health Sciences, has served as the basis for the Department of Health, Education and Welfare *Forward Plan for Health*, FY 1977-1981. According to the task force, the term *consumer health education* subsumes a set of activities that serve the following purposes:

1. Inform people about health, illness, disability, and ways in which they can improve and protect their own health, including more efficient use of the delivery system
2. Motivate people to want to change to more healthful practices
3. Help them to learn the necessary skills to adopt and maintain healthful practices and life-styles
4. Foster teaching and communications skills in all those engaged in educating consumers about health
5. Advocate changes in the environment that facilitate healthful conditions and healthful behavior

6. Add to knowledge via research and evaluation concerning the most effective ways of achieving the above objectives

The task force continues as follows:

> In brief, consumer health education is a process that informs, motivates, and helps people to adopt and maintain healthy practices and life-styles, advocates environmental changes as needed to facilitate this goal, and conducts professional training and research to the same end.

If the American Public Health Association statement provides the broad general goal for health education, the task force statement spells out the details and activities that characterize an effective action program. The specificity of these activities makes it clear that health education includes informing, motivating, and helping people to acquire the skills needed to protect and promote health and to recover from illness. The program pertains to people of all ages and levels of health — the young, the aged, the handicapped, and the healthy. It covers more than academic, scientifically derived knowledge, including actions and practical skills ranging from the principles of diet selection to the life-saving skills of cardiopulmonary resuscitation (CPR) (Fig. 11-2). For the professional health educator, this statement carries a special message: to function effectively, teaching and communication

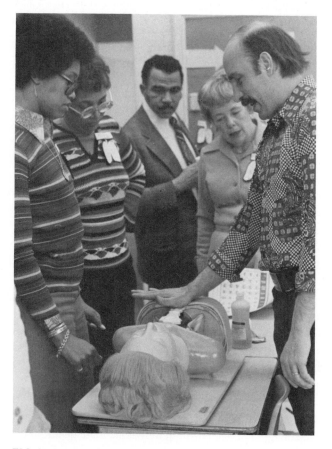

FIG. 11-2. Health educator explaining cardiopulmonary resuscitation (CPR) technique to a group of fellow teachers.

skills are essential. Moreover, like any other successful program activity, health education must rest on a scientific basis of on-going research and evaluation.

A THEORETICAL BASIS FOR HEALTH EDUCATION

A theoretical statement involves terms that cannot be observed directly but that are inferred from a great deal of data. According to Snow (Travers, 1978), what first may be considered a theoretical term later may be found to refer to real objects or events. An abstract idea or theory may become fact. This relationship between theoretical statements and factual reality is well illustrated by Darwin's early ideas about evolution. Two theoretical statements, the theory of "natural selection" and the "survival of the fittest," served to guide his observations and collection of data. Darwin observed that many more individual organisms were born than could survive. Among those that survived, Darwin noted that some were born stronger, swifter, with more protective coating, or with less conspicuous marking, blending more readily into their natural surroundings. Those born stronger, swifter, and more suited to their environments were more likely to survive, thus perpetuating those organisms having the more favorable variations (Moore and Editors of Life, 1964). Hence through evolution the surviving species or organism becomes ever more attuned to the environment.

A *theory* is a set of interacting, interlocking, or independent principles designed to account for a wide range of observations or facts (Bugelski, 1971). Travers (1978) contends that the behavioral sciences have been much less successful than the physical sciences in developing theories that eventually can be proved in the real world. In fact, many of the behavioral science theories have remained just that—theoretical abstractions, with little or no progress toward predicting real events. This discouraging fact does not diminish the importance of theories in science, for no science or any consequence has yet been built without employing theoretical terms. Therefore it becomes necessary to develop a productive theory of health behavior change on which to base health education programs.

What purpose does theory serve and how does it serve the field of health education? In the broadest sense, a theory is a way of interpreting knowledge. The interest in theories reflects a desire for unity and simplicity (Hill, 1963). Theories provide a person with useful ways of conceptualizing his or her world. For the health educator, theories can provide an orientation, a systematic interpretation of the field, as well as a rational approach to the practice of health education.

Researchers are rarely content merely to collect more and more facts about learning. To satisfy the individual's desire for understanding, knowledge must be organized. Broad, general laws or principles from which specific principles may be deduced help to organize facts and knowledge. Unlike research in physical science, which uses general acceptance and understanding of concepts such as mass, space, and time, research in education offers no comparable agreements or general understandings on which to base a theory of learning. It is necessary to examine terms such as health and education in order to establish a common ground.

Theories of learning

A theory of learning is concerned with describing how learning takes place. As defined by Hilgard and associates (1971), learning is a relatively permanent change in behavior that occurs as the result of practice. Establishing the desired changes and bringing them about constitute the role of schools and education. It follows then that schools are interested in both theories of learning and theories of teaching or instruction. A theory of learning describes what happens when learning occurs, whereas a theory of instruction is concerned with the teaching methods and the instructional material required for something to be learned.

According to Hill (1963), most of the different theories of learning, no matter how diverse, derive from two general sources, the connectionist and the cognitive theorists. The connectionists, or associationists, as they are sometimes called, view learning as a matter of making connections between stimuli and responses. This theory assumes that all responses are caused by stimuli. Other terms used to describe these connections are habits, stimulus-response bonds, and conditional response. Research is conducted on the responses that occur, on the stimuli that elicit the response, and on the ways in which experience affects these relationships.

Those employing a cognitive theory of learning are concerned with the perceptions or attitudes and beliefs that a person has about his or her environment and the ways these cognitions affect behavior. Attention is directed to these cognitions to define and describe them and to determine how they are modified by experience.

Of course, there is no "either-or" approach to learning. Both kinds of interpretations are used. The connectionist's interpretation of learning can often be identified by comments such as "I have developed a bad habit" or "His long hours of practice produced a flawless performance." Statements such as "He has a very positive attitude about school" reveal a cognitive interpretation of learning.

Connectionist theory.   Preference for one theory over another may relate, in part, to the nature of the learning task. For example, the connectionist theories lend themselves to greater precision and are used when there is need to define learning in objective and quantifiable terms that can be measured. The applied psychologists or the educational psychologists are more likely to employ the cognitive interpretation. Learning, in this sense, refers to the concepts of beliefs and purpose. This interpretation holds that behavior change results from a change in what one knows or from a change in cognition. Such learning is more likely to deal with complex problems and behavior.

Whereas learning theorists may be strongly biased toward one or the other of the major learning theories, it is apparent that no one approach is followed when theories are applied in the field. A review of educational research shows how the different learning theories are reflected in educational developments. In the early 1930s, when the progressive education movement had identified "critical thinking" as an outcome of major importance for schools, Tyler (Travers, 1978) led the way in writing behavioral objectives that were detailed, objective, and explicit. His purpose was to clarify the goals of education that had been, until then, so vague that it was virtually impossible to determine whether schools were accomplishing their intended purpose. Tyler's objectives were written in behaviors that could be observed, measured, and evaluated. On this basis Skinner developed operant psychology and insisted on definitions of behavior that met the standards of objectivity and accuracy necessary for laboratory research. This trend characterized the period of the 1960s and 1970s, when great emphasis was placed on the precision of objectives as illustrated in Mager's behavioral objectives (1961).

Concepts such as readiness, motivation, and stimulus are central features of the connectionist approach, as is the importance of practice (Fig. 11-3). Thorndike, in his "laws of exercise" (Hill, 1963) stated that one learns by practicing the correct response or skill. Through repetition and practice the behavior to be learned is strengthened or is "stamped in" to the individual's neurologic processes. A key concept in the learning theory is recognition of the importance of rewarding the learner's correct or desired responses. This principle is expressed in such terms as reinforcement, operant conditioning, and feedback, which are derived from cybernetics and from the study of control mechanisms, as in engineering. Reinforcement, or positive feedback, used in today's classrooms, rewards the students for giving the correct response to a classroom learning activity, such as answering a question, solving a problem, or demonstrating the appropriate behavior, as in performing a skill in using the computer. Providing students with immediate and positive feedback has proved very effective in influencing student learning (Fig. 11-4). Examples of positive feedback would include the teacher's written comments on students' papers, class work assignments, and comments on examinations. The value or benefits of negative reinforcement, where the stimulus to an undesired response is removed, are less clear. However, negative feedback, as displayed in the learning of a skill when the individual observes his or her error of performance and is able to make the necessary adjustments to achieve correct performance, is also widely accepted in educational practice.

Much in the connectionist theories, as revealed in the works of Thorndike, Watson, and Skinner (Zais, 1976) has influenced present-day curriculum planning. For example, principles derived from these theories advocated the subdividing of curriculum content and learning activities into their most elemental components. Once separated into the basic parts, content and activities then can be restructured or arranged into an optimal sequence

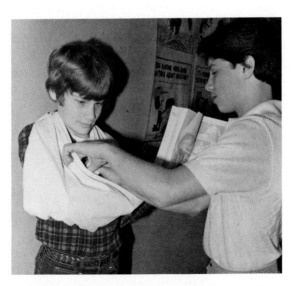

FIG. 11-3. Following directions. Gaining valuable learning experience in trying to figure out how to make a sling for a broken arm by reading directions from a first aid manual and learning an important skill through practice.
(Courtesy Corvallis Public Schools, Corvallis, Ore.)

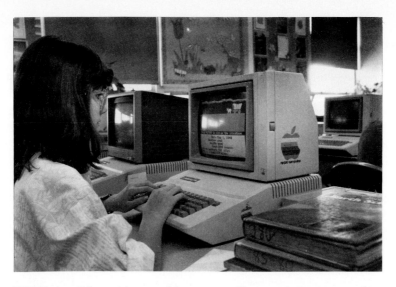

FIG. 11-4.   Girl practicing use of the computer illustrates the importance of repetition and feedback in learning a skill.
(Courtesy Champaign Public Schools, Champaign, Ill.).

for learning. According to this approach, the student learns by being taught first the simplest learning task and then the more difficult. By building on prior learning, complex learning is attained.

In addition, the process of bringing the curriculum together with the learner illustrates the classic stimulus-response principle of the connectionist theory.

Although this development helped to overcome the vagueness of earlier educational thinking and goals, it did not produce the hoped-for advances in education. A chief criticism of the connectionist approach to learning is that it is too mechanistic and simplistic. According to Travers (1978) the problem with this approach is the fact that it never succeeded in providing an adequate description of human intellectual performance. Although it is useful in rote learning tasks, it does not contribute to the higher levels of intellectual learning and to general understanding.

Cognitive theory.   The cognitive learning approach, as represented by those who accept the gestalt and field theories, holds that learning is determined by one's perceptions. One perceives in terms of a pattern or in dynamic, structured wholes. For example, according to this theory, the listener is not aware of all the separate tones when listening to a musical performance but rather perceives the whole, or the melody. Nor does one perceive each separate skill of all the many related skills in an athletic performance. Instead, one perceives the total configuration of integrated skills in a gymnastic stunt.

Lewin (Hill, 1963), a leader among the field theorists, argues that a clear picture of learning cannot be attained unless the entire complex, psychologic world that he calls the "life space" of an individual is considered. According to Lewin, the life space includes all the forces within which the individual operates. These include both internal forces, such as the basic psychologic drives for food, water, and sex, and external forces such as the interaction with people met, objects encountered and used, and geographic places within which the individual moves. It must be stressed that life space means those forces recognized by the individual's psychologic perceptions. If an individual does not perceive an object in the environment, then it simply does not exist insofar as that individual's life space is concerned.

Lewin contends that there are four different kinds of changes that compose the process of learning. These include changes in (1) cognitive structure, (2) motivation, (3) group membership, and (4) voluntary muscle control, as in skills and motor performances (Fig. 11-5). Of central importance to Lewin's field theory are perception and motivation. He argues that the connectionist theory of learning is inadequate to explain the different types of learning. For example, he contends that the learning of a skill is not the same as learning to like a person or learning to live without alcohol.

Applying Lewin's principles to teaching and curriculum planning would involve giving increased attention to the relationships of the individual and studying the individual's motivation and behavior in the school. Small classes would be important in order for the individuals to know each other and to emphasize those classroom activities that would place greater stress on interpersonal class activities. This approach recognizes the importance of motivation in learning and makes a distinction between the goals of the curriculum and the individual's psychologic goals (Fig. 11-6).

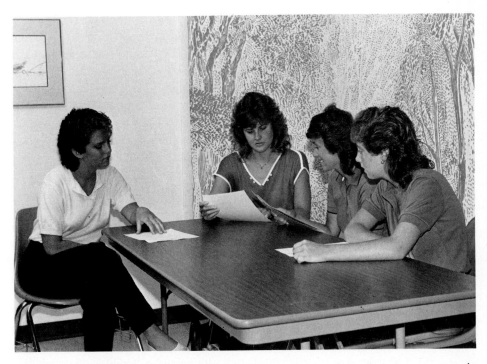

FIG. 11-5. Communication and mental health. Without talking, students are trying to put a puzzle together to illustrate nonverbal communication and interaction.
(Copyright 1983 by David Riecks.)

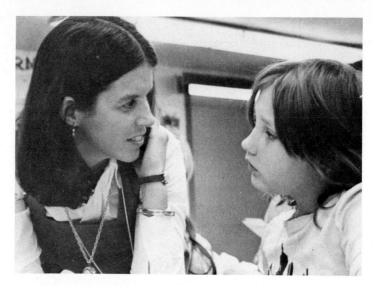

FIG. 11-6.   Cognitive theory of learning emphasizes motivation and the importance of interpersonal relationships.

HEALTH EDUCATION APPLICATION: THEORIES AND MODELS

Every health education program has as its major, long-range objective the outcome of health behavior change: the development of a life-style that will lead to good health. Traditionally, these objectives have been defined in terms of health knowledge, health attitudes, and health practices. However, health educators have long been aware of the troublesome gap that often exists between health knowledge, health attitudes, and health practices or between what the individual knows about health and what he or she does about it. The physician who fails to care for his or her own health is an often-cited example, as is the obese nutritionist, the physical educator who fails to exercise, and the health educator who smokes.

Despite this evidence, the pressure of the public's growing interest in health education as a method for preventing disease, eliminating social problems, and achieving better health often causes schools to adopt unrealistic and unattainable objectives for their health education program. As Kreuter and Green (1978) have warned, it is naïve to expect health education to produce health behavior changes that result in significant improvements in health. Instead, school health education can make its most important contribution in the development of specific knowledge and skills. The school's health instruction program, since it is directed to healthy children and youth, is designed to intervene in or to prevent illness and disease before signs or symptoms are apparent.

Health behavior change is not a favorable goal or objective for schools because of the very complex nature of health behavior. Even in a situation offering optimal control, as in an experimental study, it is very difficult to determine which influences of many affecting children are causally related to health behavior. Although children do spend a considerable portion of their lives in school, its influence is relatively weak compared to pressure exerted by their homes, their neighborhoods and communities, and particularly their peer group.

Under optimal conditions, such as an ideal school health instruction program, the time available for formal health instruction is relatively limited.

Therefore it becomes apparent that the major role of health instruction is to develop health knowledge and positive health attitudes (Fig. 11-7). Additionally, certain health behavior skills are taught, such as those related to hygienic measures, personal and interpersonal skills, selecting nutritious diets, selecting health care, participating in fitness and exercise activities, and acquiring the skills necessary to apply first aid and emergency care procedures. It is assumed that this approach will provide the developing students with the basis for making wise decisions and appropriate choices about healthful life-styles and behavior patterns that will contribute to their health and well-being.

Clarification of health behavior goals

With the development of health education and its expansion into a variety of settings outside the schools, such as public health, health care, rehabilitation, and occupational centers, it becomes important to recognize that objectives and approaches will differ. Professionals in health care settings have called attention to the need for making distinctions in the health behavior outcome in order to clarify the program objectives and related activity. This behavior can be classified as (1) health behavior — that which is related to the prevention of illness and disease, (2) sick role behavior — that which occurs after the appearance of symptoms of illness, and (3) illness behavior — that which occurs after the diagnosis of disease (Society for Public Health Education, 1976).

In light of these distinctions, the school's health instruction program will, to a large extent, focus on health behavior. Schools must also give some attention to sick role behavior,

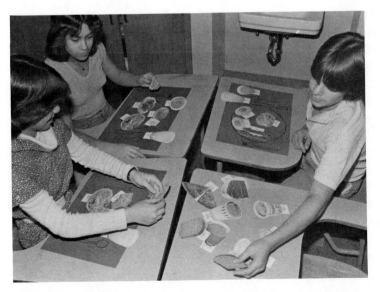

FIG. 11-7.   Nutrition. Designing menus for breakfast, lunch, and dinner using models from the National Dairy Council.
(Courtesy Corvallis Public Schools, Corvallis, Ore.)

helping persons to understand their own feelings and to know how to care for themselves when symptoms appear. Also, learning how to use health services and how to relate to health service personnel is an important aspect of health instruction. Illness behavior, though it may be beyond the scope of the school, is within the realm of health education. It has long been recognized that a sick person is much easier to motivate to adopt a recommended health practice or to accept medical advice than is a well person. A task force of the American College of Preventive Medicine (Preventive Medicine USA, 1976) concluded that the most effective health education programs have involved persons who already had strong motivation, such as chronic illness or disability, an acute crisis such as surgery, or a job-threatening condition such as alcoholism. It is out of this experience of working with the ill that the logic of health education seems most appealing. If the person understands his or her disease, recognizes how to control the disease, and understands why the medication should be taken or why the treatment should be followed, than he or she is more likely to comply with the physician's recommendations (Podell, 1976).

Although health education is involved with the total spectrum of the population, the three general arenas where it takes place may include only a portion of the whole. School health education deals with young people in a generally healthy state. Therefore the instructional emphasis is on primary prevention, and the curriculum covers a wide range of topics. The objectives of school health education would emphasize specific knowledge and attitudes, with health behavior change receiving much less emphasis. This is not because the health outcome is less important, but because, practically speaking, the opportunity to practice the health outcome is not always present.

Community health education covers the widest range of subjects, since it includes the total community: old, young, sick, and well. The instructional objectives for community health, however, are quite specific, focusing on programs such as glaucoma screening or measles immunization campaigns. There is greater emphasis on health behavior change, with specific actions being required to carry out the program.

Health care education deals with a narrow spectrum of subjects—sick people. The instructional objectives are very specific, concerning patient education on a particular disease, diet, or medical therapy. There is great emphasis on health behavior change, involving actions required by specific treatment, diet, or follow-up procedure.

Health belief model

How have the connectionist and cognitive theories affected the field of health education? The health belief model represents the most extensive work done thus far in an effort to develop a theory and a science of health behavior change. This model was influenced by the theories of Lewin and his phenomenologic orientation, which holds that it is the individual's perception or psychologic environment that determines what his or her action will be (Rosenstock, 1974). This complex of psychologic forces, which Lewin calls the "life space of the individual," explains how learning takes place. The life space includes regions of positive and negative valence that exert forces causing the individual to move away from negative and toward positive forces. Lewin considers motivation to be very important to learning, explaining that learning involves changes in both cognition (knowledge) structure and motivation (Zais, 1976).

Fig. 11-8 illustrates the health belief model and the three distinct phases leading up to

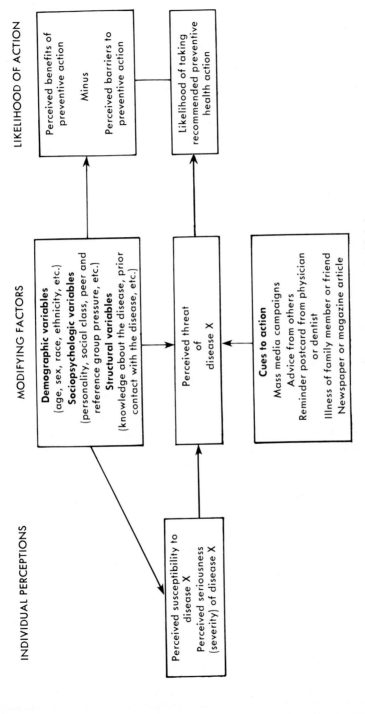

FIG. 11-8. The health belief model as predictor of preventive health behavior.
(From Becker, M.H., editor: The health belief model and personal health behavior, Thorofare, N.J., 1974, Charles B. Slack, Inc.)

a health action. The three phases are individual perception, modifying factors, and likelihood of action.

Individual perceptions.   Individual perceptions include the individual's subjective risk of contracting the disease. For example, consider the issue of teenage smoking. The disease in question is a smoking-related disease such as lung cancer, emphysema, or heart disease. According to the principle of this model, the teenager's smoking behavior will be influenced away from smoking to a reduced or nonsmoking state or will continue in a nonsmoking state if the teenager perceives the effects of smoking as presenting a serious threat to health and perceives that conditions such as lung cancer, emphysema, and heart disease are very serious diseases. In addition, cigarette smoking must be perceived as behavior that greatly increases the likelihood of developing one of these diseases. Thus the two perceptions, personal susceptibility to the disease and the severity or seriousness of disease as a personal threat, are interacting perceptions that are the necessary conditions for modifying the smoking behavior or maintaining the nonsmoking behavior.

Modifying factors.   Assuming that the foregoing perceptions or conditions are present, the ultimate decision of the individual to change or maintain his or her smoking behavior depends, to a great extent, on the modifying factors present in the teenager's situation. For example, if the individual comes from a home where smoking has not been part of the family culture and if his or her peers are nonsmokers, the prospects of changing smoking behavior to nonsmoking or for continuing as a nonsmoker are greatly enhanced. If, also, this young person has just gained knowledge from the high school health science course that further demonstrates the hazardous effects of smoking on health, the change in the student's cognitive structure (knowledge) adds an important factor to behavior change. The combined influence of the home, peer group pressure, and health knowledge gained at school acts either to modify the teenager's smoking behavior or to reinforce the continuation of nonsmoking.

The calls to action issued by the mass media and other sources are interpreted in the context of these perceptions. If the cues encourage smoking, the individual is more likely to reject them because they are inconsistent with the major predisposing forces identified in this situation. Nonsmoking media presentations and similar advice from friends and respected adults are interpreted as consistent with the many other factors that support the nonsmoking position.

Likelihood of action.   According to the health belief model, individual action is determined by the balance or imbalance between the individual's perceived positive and negative forces affecting his or her health behavior. In the foregoing example, the action of stopping smoking or continuing nonsmoking wins approval for the individual from family and friends. This action also assures consistency with the knowledge (cognitive structure) that the individual has acquired in the school health education course.

•　　•　　•

Admittedly, this example illustrates a situation in which all of what Lewin describes as the complex of psychologic forces favor nonsmoking. In terms of the health belief model, the modifying factors and the perceived benefits favor nonsmoking. Another example might show the major forces in the student's life space as encouraging the continuation of smoking or encouraging its initiation. A more true-to-life example would show both negative and positive valences (values), some favoring and some opposing smoking, that combine to pose a genuine dilemma for the teenager. In this situation the student's health education experiences can play a major role in decision making. Obviously, the quality of this instruction, the preparation of the teacher, and the teacher's sensitivities to the student's dilemma are of critical importance.

Social learning theory

According to social learning theory there is a continuous, reciprocal interaction among the individual's behavior, other personal factors (thoughts, emotional reactions, and expectations), and the environmental consequences of behavior. Bandura calls this reciprocal determinism, a process in which all factors are interlocking determinants of each other.

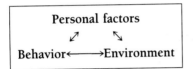

The distinction between social learning theory and the extreme behaviorist (connectionist) position is the importance attached to inner causes of behavior. The behaviorists deny that cognitive functions have any effect on behavior. In fact, behaviorists reject the concept of cognitive functions on the grounds that cognitions are unassessable or fictitious constructs that do not exist in reality. After extensive analysis of stimulus conditions, many behavioral psychologists have reached the conclusion that environmental forces control behavior.

Although proponents of social learning theory recognize the importance of environment, they believe that interaction among the three components (i.e., behavior, personal factors, and the environmental consequences) ultimately determines human behavior.

According to the social learning theory, the most important factor affecting behavior is the continuous, reciprocal interaction or feedback that occurs. The relative influence exerted by these factors may vary in accordance with the changing environment, with the particular behavior, and with the variations of personal factors. For instance, there may be situations in which the environment is the all-powerful constraining force on behavior; correspondingly, there may be instances when personal factors such as emotional reactions may become the overriding control of behavior.

The feedback from behavior and the consequent effect on future behavior might be illustrated by the example of the person who attempts to engage a fellow worker in conversation by extending a friendly greeting. However, when such efforts are repeatedly rebuffed, it is highly probable that this person will cease efforts to initiate conversations. On the other hand, if the greetings are met with a friendly response, future conversations between the two persons are more likely to develop.

The social learning theory proponents also differ with the stimulus-response psychologists, who have assumed that the individual learns by directly *performing* responses and from directly *experiencing* their effects. However, according to the social learning view, nearly all learning occurs vicariously, by observing other people's behavior and its consequences. This capacity to learn through observation enables a person to acquire more rapidly large, integrated patterns of behavior without having to learn everything through the long and tedious process of trial and error. This capacity to learn through observation enables a person to accelerate the process of learning. In fact, history offers many instances wherein individual survival has been determined by the ability to learn from the experience of others.

Bandura and others argue that there is much research that demonstrates that cognitions can be activated by instruction and that cognitive effects can be assessed indirectly. Bandura points to studies that have demonstrated that people learn and retain behavior much better by using instructional techniques and other cognitive aids than by the use of repeated practice.

In addition to learning from the experience of others, Bandura points out that a person learns from observation, from reading, from listening, and through the capacity to use symbols. Perhaps one of the most useful concepts of social learning theory is that a person has the capacity to determine many of the consequences of his or her actions (i.e., to establish a standard of behavior). Having adopted a standard of behavior or a level of expectation, the individual is now able to provide his or her own rewards and punishments, depending on whether the personal standard of behavior has been achieved.

The social learning theory, that is, that personal standards of behavior can be acquired in many different ways, is of great practical significance to the health educator. Some of the ways in which this learning of a new behavior is attained are as follows:

1. *Learning by direct experience.* A person learns from the consequences of his or her own behavior. A student seeking advice from a teacher about a personal problem such as drug abuse will respond in terms of behavior, in accordance with the way he or she is treated by the teacher. If the student is treated with respectful attentiveness, he or she is more likely to continue to seek the counsel of the teacher (Fig. 11-9). If the consequences of the session with the teacher are perceived as threatening and unsympathetic, the student will behave negatively. In each instance, the behavior is modified, but it is the direction of change that is of critical importance from the health education perspective.

2. *Learning by observing.* Other students may learn quickly from observing the behavior of their classmates and the consequences of their actions. If students observe that their teacher is open, friendly, and supportive and that other students react favorably to interaction with the teacher, the future behavior of the observing student concerning contacting the teacher for advice will be positively reinforced.

3. *Learning by listening and reading.* Here again, the student learns about how a specific behavior (seeking advice from the teacher) and the consequences of such action are related. The "acceptance of the student by the teacher" and the "giving of valued counsel" are likely to be determining factors in the student's future behavior.

4. *Learning discriminating and generalizing.* The student develops a more sophisticated level of both understanding and consequences by analyzing human behavior. As Zimbardo and associates (1977) have explained, people learn "if-this" relationships.

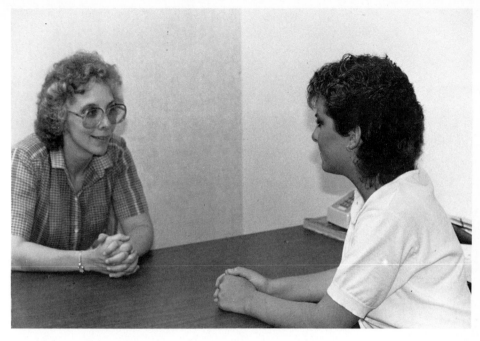

FIG. 11-9. Positive interpersonal relationships between students and school counselors are important resources for enabling students to develop health-promoting behaviors.
(Copyright 1983 by David Riecks.)

They learn by adopting tentative hypotheses about the relationships between observed events, phenomena, or variables. They also learn under which conditions these relationships are true.

Behavior modification

The behavior modification approach is a direct application of the connectionist theory of learning and emphasizes relating observable activity or responses to antecedents and subsequent events or stimuli. The stimulus-response association and the reinforcement of the desired activity or behavior compose essential elements.

One concept that has emerged from the behavior modification approach is *contingency management,* which is based on the experimental observations that the consequences of behavior, the reinforcing stimuli, determine the pattern of behavior. The reinforcer is a consequence that has the effect of making the behavior that preceded it more likely to be repeated. For example, if praise (reinforcement) is given to a boy for washing his hands before eating, he is more likely to repeat this act in the future.

The second important concept of behavior modification is *stimulus control.* This involves an analysis of how a stimulus provides the context for ongoing behavior. Stimulus control analysis is used in many behavior applications to determine exactly how the environment controls a particular problem behavior. Such an analysis usually begins with the keeping of a detailed record of the times when the behavior occurs, the physical location, the current mood, and the social context of the behavior. For example, the characteristics of each occurrence of an unwanted behavior such as overeating or cigarette smoking would be carefully defined.

Bandura (1969) has developed a five-part process for applying a behavior modification approach that includes the following:

1. Analyzing existing relevant behavior and developing behavioral objectives
2. Modeling of the new behavior by the instructor
3. Providing guided practice of the new behavior by the learners
4. Providing for reinforcement of the new behavior
5. Being able to maintain the new behavior without further assistance from the instructor

Of these five parts, reinforcement devices for new behavior are particularly important. Changes in diet, smoking, and exercise, for example, might develop such reinforcements as encouragement from the instructor, support from family members, and approval from friends and peers.

A recent development that has made behavior modification more acceptable to the health educator is self-control behavioral strategems. As expressed in the code of ethics statement for health education, self-control is in keeping with the principle of fostering an educational environment that nurtures individual growth and development. It is also consistent with the idea of helping people to make behavior changes by conscious choices rather than by coercion.

In behavior modification, changes are often brought about by environmental manipulations that force the person with the problem to modify or change behavior. Examples of such manipulation include putting a substance in the cigarette to create an unpleasant taste to the smoker, thus causing the smoker to consider stopping smoking, or, in an effort to get the automobile driver to wear safety belts, installing a device that creates a loud, unpleasant noise when the key is inserted into the starter switch and the seat belt is not fastened. Such environmental manipulation is designed to force compliance rather than to help the person make a conscious choice of health actions.

Under a self-managed approach, the person with the problem behavior becomes an active participant in changing or modifying his or her own behavior.

Although educators find the self-control strategem a more acceptable method than environmental manipulation, it often proves unsuccessful because of vague or poorly defined instructions. Also, as Bandura (1969) contends, such instructions may have no immediate implications. In addition, persons using this approach have often failed to provide the necessary support that comes from reinforcement. To assure the success of self-managed behavioral change, research has demonstrated the importance of the following steps:

1. Both immediate and long-range goals require carefully defined objectives. In keeping with the self-control approach, the person involved should choose the objectives or goals.
2. Adopting contractual agreements is an important means of increasing a person's commitment to goal achievement. For example, an agreement recommended for smoking behavior change would call for gradually restricting cigarette smoking by reducing the number of times and places where smoking is permitted. To succeed,

persons must personally set the objectives and then voluntarily commit themselves to attaining these immediate objectives on a day-to-day basis.

3. Negative self-evaluations that result from deviation from a person's contractual agreement are an important element in helping counteract the undesired behavior.

4. The satisfaction resulting from an agreement and receiving a favorable social reaction from family and friends for adopting the new health behavior represents an important source of reinforcement.

5. Keeping a detailed record of behavior changes is an additional source of reinforcement, since it provides a tangible and objective measure of the progress. Experience has shown that those who record their daily activities continue to work toward achieving objectives until they have exceeded preceding performances, thus ensuring continued improvement.

The altering of stimulus conditions under which the maladaptive or undesired behavior occurs is an effective technique in changing or modifying behavior. For example, research has shown that the problem of overeating often arises in situations where appetizing foods are prominently displayed. In order to counteract this influence, altering the stimulus condition by storing foods out of sight and in less accessible places is effective. Another way of helping control the overeating problem involves limiting the circumstances under which a person eats. Special efforts are made to avoid eating in nondining settings (e.g., while watching television, reading, or listening to the radio).

It must be recognized that many of the undesired behaviors, such as smoking, overeating, and drinking, provide immediate gratification or reinforcement to a person. Because these behaviors occur in many and diverse situations and times, it is necessary for a person to narrow this stimulus control over his or her behavior.

The need for developing self-reinforcing techniques must also be recognized in self-control behavior modification. To do this, persons are taught to arrange for contingencies that serve as reinforcements. This is done by selection of a variety of activities that they find rewarding. For example, after refraining from smoking for a certain period of time, persons then reward themselves by engaging in an enjoyable activity, such as taking a recreational break or watching a favorite television program.

The Stanford Heart Disease Prevention Program

The Stanford Heart Disease Prevention Program experiment is an example of behavior modification, using three California towns employing two different experimental conditions while the third town served as the control. The study sought to produce changes in people's cognitive structure, motivational structure, and behavior skills in order to reduce their risks of heart disease. The specific program objectives were to produce both knowledge and behavior changes relating to diet, exercise, and smoking. The study compared the effectiveness of mass media used alone and used with personal instruction, including a self-control behavior modification approach. It is interesting in the context of learning theory, since both cognitive learning strategies and connectionist learning theory were employed in the personalized behavior modification phase of the study.

Results from the study showed that the mass media approach produced almost as much information gain as did the personalized instruction and also was effective in changing simple behaviors. However, to achieve complex behavior change, it was necessary to have the reinforcement or social support that was supplied by the personal instruction or self-control behavior modification approach (McAlister and Berger, 1979). The implications to be drawn from this study are that in order to achieve significant long-range health behavior outcomes the schools must play a major role in complementing mass media instructional programs. Schools can provide personalized instruction about health hazards and can help children develop the necessary knowledge and the self-help, self-management behavior skills needed to sustain health action that will lessen the risk of future chronic diseases.

Fishbein's behavioral intention theory

Although it is helpful to simplify the analysis of learning theories by grouping them into one of two broad categories—cognitive and connectionist, or associationist, learning theory— further attempts have been made to combine the advantages of these two theories. Many researchers have been attracted by the connectionist's objectivity in identifying behavior and precision in measuring behavior, but others have been dissatisfied with a stimulus-response analysis of behavior. These researchers have argued that in addition to this effect the person's behavior is also a result of his or her beliefs, attitudes, and desires to achieve a goal. The Fishbein conceptual framework is one example of the attempt to combine cognitive and connectionist approaches to learning.

According to Fishbein's theory (Fishbein and Ajzen, 1975) beliefs are the fundamental building blocks. The individual, through direct observation or by other methods such as receiving information from an outside source, as in health instruction, learns or forms some beliefs about a particular object. The individual also develops beliefs about the various attributes of the object. Through this process, beliefs about health, illness, cigarettes, food, physicians, hospitals, health behavior, and many other things in life are acquired. The totality of a person's beliefs serves as the information or knowledge base that ultimately determines the person's attitudes, intentions, and behavior. This approach views the individual as an entirely rational being, one who uses the information available to make judgments, to form evaluations, and to arrive at decisions. An adapted and simplified illustration of the behavioral intentions model is presented in Fig. 11-10.

Formally stated, the theory holds that an individual has many beliefs about a given object. Moreover, the object is seen as having various attributes or characteristics. For example, the object *cigarette* may be seen as having various attributes, such that cigarette smoke may represent odor, the cause of disease, and an offense to friends. If these beliefs about the attributes of cigarettes are associated with unfavorable attitudes, then, through the process of conditioning, the attitude of the individual toward cigarettes and smoking is likely to be negative. According to this theory, attitudes toward an object are conditioned by beliefs about the attributes of the object and by evaluation of those attributes. Also, according to this theory, a person's attitude toward an object is related to his or her intention to perform a variety of behaviors relating to the object, in this case, cigarettes. If a person's overall attitude toward cigarettes is negative, his or her intention to perform certain behaviors with respect to cigarettes may be something like the following:

1. To decide against smoking a cigarette

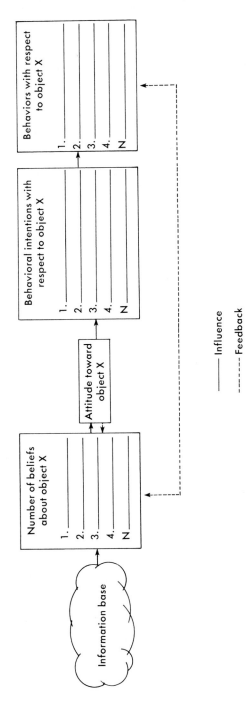

FIG. 11-10. Fishbein's conceptual framework. Adapted from Fishbein's conceptual framework relating beliefs, attitudes, intentions, and behaviors with respect to a given object.
(From Martin Fishbein and Icek Ajzen: Belief, Attitude, and Behavior, New York, © 1975, Random House, Inc. Reprinted with permission.)

2. To continue not smoking

3. To avoid areas where cigarettes are smoked

Fishbein points out that there may not be a direct and consistent relationship between beliefs, attitudes, and behavioral interactions. He contends that a person's intention to perform a particular behavior is a function of two basic determinants, one attitudinal and the other normative (Fig. 11-11). The attitudinal component refers to the person's attitude toward performing the behavior in question. The normative component (subject norm) is related to the individual's beliefs about people who are very important to him or her and what such people's expectations of him or her are. For example, if the individual sees all the attributes of cigarettes as being bad or negative (attitude) and believes parents and friends (subjective norm) do not want him or her to smoke, it is more likely that he or she will *intend not* to smoke.

In summary, a person's intentions (to smoke or not to smoke) are a function of two variables intervening between the stimulus conditions and the intention. These variables are (1) attitude toward the behavior and (2) the subjective norm. The individual's attitude is determined by the stimulus conditions, by beliefs about what others think he or she should do and by his or her own desire to comply with their standards of behavior. Fishbein's general framework for behavior change with its stimulus conditions, intervening variables, and behavioral intentions response is clearly in the connectionist tradition of learning and its well-known model of stimulus-response. However, many of the percepts from the cognitive theory of learning have also been included in Fishbein's model. For example, the intervening variables of knowledge, beliefs, attitudes, and the influence of others on the individual's decisions are closely related to cognitive theories and Lewin's concept of life space.

Persuasive communication theory

The effort to influence other people by arguing, presenting facts, drawing conclusions, and predicting the future consequences of a proposed behavior has become one of the most widely used influence techniques. The adult's attempt to influence the child, the father's

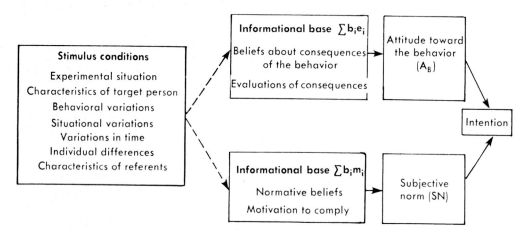

FIG. 11-11. Fishbein's behavioral intentions model.
(From Martin Fishbein and Icek Ajzen: Belief, Attitude, and Behavior, New York, © 1975, Random House, Inc. Reprinted with permission.)

efforts to mold the son, and the teacher's approach to educating the pupil represent varying degrees of sophistication in applying what has become known as *persuasive communication*.

The premise of persuasive communication theory holds that an individual's attitudes (the affective component) are influenced or changed by alteration of that individual's opinions or beliefs (the cognitive or knowledge component) (Zimbardo et al., 1977). For example, it should be possible for the heatlh educator to change people's attitudes toward proposed legislation to raise the qualifying age for a driver's license by changing their beliefs about the advantages, the disadvantages, and the potential impact on traffic accidents of such a law. Persuasive communication theory holds that previously unknown information will affect beliefs.

An examination of school health education curriculums and teaching plans provides evidence that this assumption, though rarely made explicit, is the premise for most of today's health teaching. As Wallack (1980) has observed, common sense tells us that a change of attitude will ultimately lead to a change in behavior. Attractive as this theory may be, it is not the reality of behavioral science research. Although a positive relationship between knowledge and attitude often exists, it is painfully small; studies of the relationship between attitude and behavior have found the connection to be disappointingly small or insignificant (McGuire, 1981).

However, these apparent inconsistencies in the studies of attitude and behavior change stimulated the interest of several behavioral scientists. Their efforts to clarify the relationship between feelings and actions has led to a delineation of the persuasive communication theory. This research has identified four processes that determine the extent to which a person will be persuaded by a communication. As applied to health education, the processes are as follows:

1. *Attention.* Obviously, the attention of students must be gained before the communication can have the effect. Regardless of how appealing, logical, or well organized the argument may be, it will not change anyone's attitude until the message has been received.

2. *Comprehension.* Even if the student is attentive to the message, it must be understood. People must first understand the argument if they are to change their attitudes or comprehend which behavior is being advocated.

3. *Acceptance.* Once the message has been comprehended, the important question is the extent to which the student agrees with or accepts the argument. Ultimately this will be determined by what the student perceives the rewards of the message to be.

4. *Retention.* How effective has the communication been? This will be determined by its retention and application at some future time.

Although these processes are all important to successful communication, they constitute only half of the communication equation. The outcome depends on the effectiveness of the inputs or the message and its transmission. Whether a message is accepted and effects a behavior change depends on several factors. Often "who said what to whom" is the critical factor in determining whether a communication is persuasive. Accordingly, researchers have identified several factors that affect the acceptance of a communication. Some of the most important factors include the following:

1. *The source.* The source of the communication often has an important effect on the attitude of the recipient. For example, if the person communicating the message is seen as one who is credible and trustworthy, that person's ability to persuade others is greatly enhanced. Other important perceived characteristics of the speaker include intelligence, experience, sincerity, likability, and attractiveness of the manner of speaking. Another favorable characteristic of the communicator as perceived by the listener is the appearance of familiarity—someone with whom the audience can identify.

2. *Communication.* The characteristics of the message can enhance or reduce its effectiveness. Such things as good organization and clear order of presentation (one sided or two sided) improve the presentation. The use of logic and emotions, fear techniques, the extent of the analysis, and documentation are all part of the effectiveness of the message.

3. *Audience.* The characteristics of the audience, their predispositions and attitudes,

TABLE 11-1. Adaptation of McGuire's persuasive communication matrix for antismoking education

Output variables	Input variables	
	Source of the message	Characteristics of the message
	Viewed as credible, likable, trustworthy; attractiveness; teaching style: knowledgeable, authoritative, powerful	Effectively organized; salient information organized appeals to student's autonomy to make own decisions
Exposure to the communication: health education program designed to provide maximal exposure to message presenting arguments against smoking	Teacher designed 5-day module on hazards of smoking	
Attention: teaching methods are interesting; hold students' attention to hear message advocating nonsmoking	Introduces unit with color film on teenaged smoking	Reviews trends depicting teenaged smoking
Comprehension: communication well organized; numerous examples and illustrations enable student to understand message	Teacher conducts frequent reviews to assess students' understanding	Formal testing of students' knowledge on smoking
Acceptance: arguments and conclusions of message abstaining from smoking are accepted; appeal to student to use information in decision making; possible models for nonsmoking	Teacher discusses epidemiologic evidence linking smoking to disease	Students conduct discussions on more effective labeling of cigarettes
Retention and application: reinforcement is provided; recalls information for future use; applies information to decision making; learns; wants to resist pressure to smoke; maintains nonsmoking status	Appeals made to student to use information on smoking in decision making	Analyzes data on health benefits realized from quitting

their knowledge of the subject, their previous experience, their level of intelligence, and their self-esteem all enter into the final acceptance or rejection of the communication.

4. *Audience reaction.* Reaction to communication influences its acceptance. If the message presents an opportunity for a response or counterargument, it may be more effective than a "hard sell" approach, which may put people on the defensive, causing them to become suspicious and fearful of being manipulated. Overemphasis on a fear approach can cause people to reject, avoid, or fail to hear the argument.

Finally, McGuire has developed the social-influences communications matrix. It is a process by which a person (the source) communicates with another person (the receiver) about some object for the purpose of changing the person's (receiver's) attitude or behavior about the object. The *input* component of the social influence process is the communication, and the *output* is the persuasive communication effect. Table 11-1 gives an adaptation of McGuire's communications matrix applied to school health education.

Input variables		
Characteristics of the students	**Channel or method of delivery**	**Target objective of the communication**
Age; grade level; background experience; intelligence; attitude of acceptance; committed willingness to listen	Appropriate uses of visual and auditory stimuli; example of model behavior; effective use of teaching-learning activities Bulletin board advertising appeals to smoking	Specific attitude or behavior change objective (e.g., favorable attitude toward nonsmoking; avoids experimental smoking)
Conducts class experiment on composition of tar acid smoke (i.e., tar)	Collects and analyzes (e.g., smoking ads in popular magazines)	Students display attentiveness to class activities
Students practice assertive methods to resist pressure to smoke	Class discussion of nonsmokers' rights	
Students do volunteer, peer-led counseling with younger students on antismoking theme		

SUMMARY

The purpose or goals of health education are to help people prevent disease and promote health through their own efforts. From the perspective of the practicing health educator persuading people to change their health behavior involves an important moral and ethical problem. Changing one's health behavior implies that such decisions are made freely without coercion.

With respect to health education's contribution to the health of the nation, health and medical authorities now recognize that major advances in health improvement will come from changes in people's life-style and from the controlling of environmental hazards. At the same time a national task force has called for a broader health education responsibility — to serve as an advocate for changes in the environment in order to facilitate healthful conditions as well as healthful behaviors.

To develop effective strategies for health education and health behaviors changes requires an understanding of the theories of learning. Most theories derive from two sources (1) the connectionist and the (2) cognitive learning theory. Learning according to the connectionist is recognition of the importance of rewards or reinforcing the learner's correct or desired responses as expressed in Skinner's operant conditioning and feedback. Cognitive learning, on the other hand, refers to concepts of belief. Learning is determined by one's perceptions. Advocates of the cognitive theory argue that connectionist theory is too limited and fails to explain the different types of learning. Learning a skill is not the same as learning to like someone.

Several models of behavior change are illustrated to show different applications of learning theory. The health belief model holds that a person's perception of psychologic environment determines the action a person will take.

Social learning theory proponents recognize the importance of the environmental forces on behavior. They believe the interaction among behavior, personal factors, and the environment determine human behavior. Behavior modification, which is widely used in the health field, is a direct application of connectionist theory. The essential elements in this process includes stimulus-response and reinforcement of the desired action.

The Stanford Heart Disease Prevention Program is cited as a project that has made use of both cognitive and connectionist learning theory. In Fishbein's model, the totality of a person's beliefs or knowledge base determine that person's attitude. However, the connectionist theory is reflected in the model that shows how one's beliefs become a process of conditioning the attitude one holds toward an object.

McGuire's persuasive communication theory provides a final example of the processes of changing behavior. The premise of this theory holds that one's attitudes are influenced or changed when his or her opinions and beliefs are changed. A change in attitude will ultimately lead to a behavior change. The apparent inconsistencies of this model has led to the identification of four processes: (1) attention, (2) comprehension, (3) acceptance, and (4) retention. In addition, a second set of factors that determine whether a message is accepted were identified. This includes the source of the message, the way a message is communicated, the characteristics of the audience, and the reaction of the audience to the message.

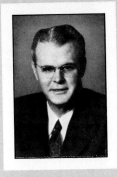

Delbert Oberteuffer

BORN 1902
DIED March 26, 1981, Hyannis, Massachusetts
EDUCATION B.A., University of Oregon, 1923; M.A. and Ph.D., Columbia University, 1930

Dr. Delbert "Obie" Oberteuffer was one of the few professionals recognized as an authority in both physical education and health education. An articulate spokesperson for the philosophy and essential interrelatedness of the two fields, Oberteuffer contributed significantly to the development of curriculum, having authored significant texts in both fields. He was the only person to receive both the William A. Howe Award, the highest honor of the American School Health Association, and the Luther H. Gulick Award, the most distinguished honor of the American Association for Health, Physical Education, Recreation, and Dance.

Before his long and distinguished career at Ohio State University, Oberteuffer taught at the University of Oregon for 5 years. He then served as the state of Ohio's supervisor of physical education and health education, where his leadership was nationally recognized for the development of outstanding programs in health education and physical education in the public schools of Ohio. Oberteuffer was a member of the Ohio State University faculty from 1932 to 1966, serving as head of the Physical Education Department for 25 years. Many of today's leaders in health education were students of Dr. Oberteuffer during his tenure at Ohio State University.

Oberteuffer was a prolific writer and one of the profession's most stirring speakers. He contributed over 100 articles to the literature and wrote two basic textbooks, *Physical Education* and *School Health Education*, which are still in use. He served as president of the American School Health Association in 1958 and was, for the next 14 years, the editor-in-chief of the association's journal. In commemoration of his speaking skills and contributions to the field, the Ohio State University School of Health, Physical Education, and Recreation has established a lecture series in his name.

STUDY QUESTIONS

1. Discuss the program implications of the following definitions of health education: (a) a process that enables the individual to make an informal decision and (b) a process whose aim is to help people achieve health by their own actions.

2. With respect to a code of ethics what does the following statement imply for the health educator, "Health education supports change by choice, not by coercion."

3. In his model of health, Blum illustrates several inputs to health including the gene pool, health services, and health behavior. What would you consider to be the *outputs*, or the effects, of these inputs?

4. Assume that a connectionist or behaviorist is conducting an intervention program designed to improve students' nutritional status. Which measures would he or she use? How might a cognitive theorist approach this measurement problem differently?

5. How would a health education program based on social learning theory differ from an approach based on behavior modification?

6. Explain the key elements of the health belief model.

7. Discuss the problem of unrealistic expectations for school health education.

8. What do you consider to be the major determinants of health behavior?

9. Of the theories and models discussed in this chapter, which of these do you think will be of most value to your health education efforts? Explain.

10. Assume that you have responsibility for planning a health instruction program. Which guideline does your text have to offer?

REFERENCES

American Public Health Association: Toward a policy on health education and public health. Position paper adopted by the governing council of the American Public Health Association, Washington, D.C., Nov. 2, 1977.

Bandura, A.: Social learning theory, Englewood Cliffs, N.J., 1977, Prentice-Hall, Inc.

Bugelski, B.R.: The psychology of learning applied to teaching, Indianapolis, 1971, The Bobbs-Merrill Co., Inc.

Davidson, P.O., and Davidson, S.M.: Behavioral medicine: changing health lifestyles, New York, 1980, Brunner/Mazel, Inc.

Elder, J., Hovell, M., Lasater, T., et al.: Applications of behavior modification to community health education: the case of heart disease prevention, Health Educ. Q. 12:151, 1985.

Epstein, F.: Forward. In Berenson, G.S., et al.: Cardiovascular risk factors in children: the early natural history of atherosclerosis and essential hypertension, New York, 1980, Oxford University Press.

Expert Committee on Health Education of the Public: First report. World Health Organization Technical Report Series no. 89, Geneva, 1954, World Health Organization.

Fishbein, M., and Ajzen, I.: Belief, attitude, intention, and behavior: an introduction to theory and research, Menlo Park, Calif., 1975, Addison-Wesley Publishing Co., Inc.

Flay, B.R., Ryan, K.B., Best, J.A., et al: Are social psychological smoking prevention programs effective? The Waterloo Study, J. Behav. Med. 8:37, 1985.

Givner, A., and Grantard, P.S.: A handbook of behavior modification for the classroom, New York, 1974, Holt, Rinehart & Winston.

Golaszewski, T.J.: Influencing behavior through instruction: methodology in health education, Washington, D.C., Feb. 1979, ERIC Clearinghouse on Teacher Education.

Hamburg, D.A., et al., editors: Health behavior: frontiers of research in the biobehavioral sciences, Washington, D.C., 1982, National Academy Press, Institute of Medicine.

Hansen, W.B., and Malotte, C.K.: Perceived personal immunity: the development of beliefs about susceptibility to the consequences of smoking, Prev. Med. 15:363, 1986.

Hilgard, E.R., Atkinson, R.C., and Atkinson, R.L.: Introduction to psychology, ed. 5, New York, 1971, Harcourt, Brace, Jovanovich, Inc.

Hill, W.F.: Learning: a survey of psychological interpretations, Scranton, Pa., 1963, Chandler Publishing Co.

Kreuter, M.W., and Green, L.W.: Evaluation of school health education: identifying purposes, keeping perspective, J. Sch. Health 48(4):228, 1978.

Leventhal, H., Glynn, K., and Flemming, R.: Is the smoking decision an 'informed choice'? JAMA 257(24):3373, 1987.

Mager, R.F.: Preparing objectives for programmed instruction, Belmont, Calif., 1961, Fearon Publishers.

Matthew, A., and Creswell, W.H., Jr.: The relationship among attitudes, behaviors, and biomedical measures of adolescents "at risk" for cardiovascular disease, J. Sch. Health 57:326, 1987.

McGuire, W.J.: Attitude theory and management. In Food and nutrition research: proceedings of a symposium, University Park, Pa., 1980, The Pennsylvania State University Press.

McGuire, W.J.: Behavioral medicine, public health and communication theories, Health Educ., p. 8, May-June 1981.

Moore, R., and the Editors of Life: Evolution, New York, 1964, Life Nature Library, Time, Inc.

Nightingale, E.O., et al.: Perspective on health promotion and disease prevention in the United States, Washington, D.C., 1978, Institute of Medicine, National Academy of Sciences.

Parcel, G.S.: Theoretical models for application in school health education research, J. Sch. Health **54**:39, 1984.

Petrosa, R.: Enhancing the health competence of school-age children through behavioral self-management skills, J. Sch. Health **56**:211, 1986.

Podell, R.N.: Appendix V: physician's guide to compliance in hypertension. In Preventive medicine USA: health promotion and consumer health education, New York, 1976, Prodist, Division of Neale Watson Academic Publications, Inc.

President's Committee on Health Education: The report of the President's Committee on Health Education, New York, 1973, the Committee.

Preventive medicine USA: Theory, practice and application of prevention in personal health services: quality control and evaluation of preventive health services. Task force reports sponsored by the John E. Fogarty International Center for Advanced Study in the Health Sciences, National Institutes of Health, and the American College of Preventive Medicine, New York, 1975, Prodist, Division of Neale Watson Academic Publications, Inc.

Report of the 1972-1973 Joint Committee on Health Education Terminology, prepared by representatives of the American Academy of Pediatrics, American Association for Health, Physical Education and Recreation, American School Health Association, American Public Health Association, and Society for Public Health Education, Washington, D.C.

Rosenstock, I.M.: Historical origins of the health belief model. In Becker, M.H., editor: The health belief model and personal health educator, Thorofare, N.J., 1974, Charles B. Slack, Inc.

Rosenstock, I.M., Strecher, V.J., and Becker, M.H.: Social learning theory and the health belief model, Health Educ. Q. **15**(2):175, 1988.

St. Pierre, R., and Lawrence, P.S.: Reducing smoking using positive self-management, J. Sch. Health **45**(1):7, 1975.

Society for Public Health Education: Code of ethics, San Francisco, Oct. 15, 1976, the Society.

Travers, R.M.W.: An introduction to educational research, ed. 4, New York, 1978, Macmillan Publishing Co., Inc.

U.S. Department of Health, Education and Welfare: Forward plan for health, FY 1977-1981, Washington, D.C., June 1975, U.S. Government Printing Office.

U.S. Department of Health, Education and Welfare: Educating the public about health: a planning guide, Washington, D.C., 1977, Public Health Service, Health Resources Administration.

U.S. Department of Health, Education and Welfare: The school health curriculum project. Public Health Service Center for Disease Control Bureau of Health Education, Atlanta, Dec. 1977, U.S. Government Printing Office.

Wallack, L.M.: Assessing effects of mass media campaigns: an alternative perspective, Alcohol Health Res. World, p. 18, Fall 1980.

Weight management: a summary of current theory and practice, Rosemont, Ill., 1985, National Dairy Council.

Werch, C.E., McNab, W.L., et al.: Motivations and strategies for quitting and preventing tobacco and alcohol use, J. Sch. Health **58**(4):156, 1988.

Zais, R.S.: Curriculum principles and foundations, New York, 1976, Thomas Y. Crowell Co.

Zimbardo, P.G., Ebbesen, E.B., and Maslath, C.: Influencing attitudes and changing behavior, Menlo Park, Calif., 1977, Addison-Wesley Publishing Co., Inc.

12

Planning the Health Education Curriculum

OVERVIEW　　*It is generally accepted that health education as an academic discipline originated with the 1918 report on the cardinal principles of secondary education. Health was identified as one of the seven major goals of education. The school's curriculum and the curriculum development processes are presented as background for the planning of the health education curriculum. Differing views over the goals of health education are examined from the perspectives of education and public health. Educators have stressed knowledge as a major goal, whereas public health officials have emphasized the goal of changing health behavior to promote health and to prevent disease.*

　　The issue of what to teach is discussed in the context of the controversy over the comparative effectiveness of the comprehensive or the categorical health problems curriculum.

　　Forces affecting the school health curriculum are identified, beginning with the early temperance movement and continuing through to the present influences of the surgeon general's report on health goals for the nation, which stressed the importance of health promotion and disease prevention. The influence of these developments on schools is most evident in the health education risk reduction programs sponsored by the U.S. Public Health Service. The personal health risk behaviors of smoking, inadequate diets, alcohol and drug use, lack of exercise, stress, and accidents are receiving increasing attention.

　　Examples of curriculum organized according to a comprehensive conceptual scheme and a categorical problems approach are discussed. The identification of health risk factors has given rise to health curriculum focused on correcting unhealthy behaviors of diet, drinking, smoking, lack of exercise, and stress-producing behaviors. The strengths and weaknesses of these curriculums are reviewed. Finally, the chapter outlines a series of steps (to guide school officials) in planning an effective health instruction unit.

OBJECTIVES　　**After reading this chapter, the student should be able to:**

1. Identify historical events that help explain why health education has become part of the public school curriculum

2. List several steps in the curriculum development process

3. Explain why public health authorities have stressed the importance of life-style factors and health behavior in preventing disease

4. Identify and explain three different levels of decision making that determine the nature of the health curriculum

5. Identify past developments that have helped to determine the health topics or content of health education

6. Discuss the arguments favoring either a categorical health problem or a comprehensive health education approach to curriculum planning

7. Explain the increased interest on the part of schools in the health-education risk-reduction programs

8. Explain how Goodlad's conceptual framework would help in planning a comprehensive health education curriculum

9. Identify the elements of the teaching unit

10. Explain the necessary steps involved in developing the health teaching unit

HEALTH EDUCATION IN SCHOOLS

Although the adult's concern for the schooling of the young has existed throughout civilized history, the origin of health education in today's schools in America is most frequently identified as 1918, an important starting point for curriculum studies in the United States. On this date one of the most influential statements affecting the curriculum of American schools was issued, the report of the Commission on the Reorganization of Secondary Education, entitled "The Cardinal Principles of Education."

These principles were intended to serve as the general goals of all secondary schools and are frequently cited as the basis for the establishment of health education in the school. The following areas were included:

1. Health
2. Command of fundamental processes
3. Worthy home membership
4. Vocation
5. Citizenship
6. Worthy use of leisure
7. Ethical character

This statement has been of singular importance to education because of its widespread influence on and recognition by educational leaders. Recognizing its historical significance, the National Education Association appointed a special commission to reexamine the seven cardinal principles. The results were issued as a part of the nation's bicentennial celebration in 1976. The commission members were among the nation's most prominent leaders, representing such fields as business, industry, and labor, as well as professional and scientific fields. The commission reaffirmed the validity of the cardinal principles and their value as goals for all secondary schools. However, the principles were restated and reinterpreted in order to make them more relevant in terms of the needs of today's society. For example, the commission's interpretation of the goal of health was as follows, "The scope and importance of health as an educational objective has become even more important than it was in 1918." Accordingly, greater emphasis should be placed on "the need for healthy interpersonal and intellectual attitudes. . . ." The importance of a world view of health and the worldwide challenge that that entails were emphasized. Support was given to a broad concept of health, including total mental, physical, and emotional health for each person. Support of the efforts to improve drug education and support for frank discussions of family living were included. This aspect of education, the commission stated, is necessary if the youth of today are to be guided toward acceptance of responsible citizenship as tomorrow's leaders.

As previously stated, the events and concerns of the day often have a pronounced effect on the schools. Because the institution of education is close to the average citizen, the curriculum is frequently determined by the immediate concerns of the people. For example, Kliebard (1982) has identified four different interest groups that at the turn of the century also exerted a major influence on what the schools taught. These groups were the (1) humanists, (2) social efficiency reformers, (3) child study movement, and (4) social meliorists. The child study group and the social meliorists were instrumental in obtaining the inclusion of health among the seven cardinal principles.

The rise and fall of public interest create a continuous change in the school's curriculum. Because health has been identified as a priority of education at one time does not ensure that it will always continue to be so.

The growing influence of political action groups in shaping public programs means that the position of health education in the schools could change very quickly. Unless the health education curriculum maintains an ongoing review and evaluation of its program, it could become irrelevant to the needs of both the individual and society.

THE SCHOOL CURRICULUM

Any discussion of the health education curriculum requires the establishment of a common definition for the term *curriculum*. It is most often identified as the plan for schooling, which is the content that curriculum planners expect the teachers to teach and that the students are expected to learn. Curriculum development entails the selection and organization of a set of intended learning outcomes (Posner and Rudnitsky, 1978).

The term *curriculum,* in addition to its use as a definition of an education plan for the learner, also refers to a field of study. It is helpful to consider some general principles that have derived from work done in the field of curriculum study and the application of such knowledge to a plan for action, or a plan that guides instruction, when the curriculum for health education is being considered (Zais, 1976).

Curriculum foundations

Most curriculum specialists agree that the determinants of a curriculum should reflect some, if not all, of the following considerations:

1. *Philosophy and the nature of knowledge.* Basic assumptions about the nature of knowledge and the philosophy that guides beliefs about knowledge have particular relevance to the formulation of the curriculum.
2. *Society and culture.* The school is the institution invented by society to transmit the cultural heritage and to ensure its survival. Societal values, assumptions, and concepts of good and bad are translated into the curriculum objectives and learning activities.
3. *The individual.* The nature of humankind and its biologic and psychologic characteristics, needs, and capacities to learn have placed certain limits on the curriculum,

such as the content included, the organization of the curriculum, and the types of learning activities to be selected.

4. *Theory of learning.* Some elements of learning theory enjoy wide acceptance (e.g., the social learning theory), whereas other theories (e.g., behavior modification) are more controversial. The particular theory of learning embraced by the curriculum developer will exert a pronounced influence on the design. For example, Dewey's theory that the school curriculum should serve as a preparation for living has been applied directly to certain types of learning activity, including use of the project method. The theory of learning and the importance that environment places on learning have significant implications for the contemporary curriculum developer.

Curriculum development

Tyler (1975) stresses the importance of conducting a careful preliminary analysis of a society to determine clearly the needs that the curriculum should serve. Such an analysis may call for extensive work with the local community, parents, peer groups, teachers, and school officials. If the curriculum to be developed is to be accepted and used by the teachers, special efforts must be made to seek their active involvement and to give careful consideration to their needs as well.

The process.   In this extensive work in curriculum development, Tyler (1975) has developed a series of steps to be followed:

1. *Selecting and defining the objectives.* Curriculum developers must resist the temptation to write their own objectives and must, instead, involve many different groups in the selection process, seeking group deliberation and judgment. Involvement of teachers is essential to their ultimate commitment to the curriculum. Subject matter specialists, curriculum specialists, psychologists, sociologists, and specialists in human development all offer judgments in this area. The level of generality for objectives must be considered; objectives that are too general are nonfunctional, and overly specific objectives are burdensome.
2. *Developing a philosophy.* The theory of learning that is adopted influences the philosophy or point of view of the curriculum developer.
3. *Selecting and creating learning experiences.* The purpose of the learning experience is to meet the curriculum objectives (i.e., to perform and to practice the behavior called for in the objective). Appropriate learning activities should invite the attention and interest of the learner and provide satisfaction. Activities should be balanced between those that can be carried out alone and those involving peer group cooperation.
4. *Organizing learning experiences.* The learning activities should provide maximal impact on the learner. They should be sequenced to build relationships, so that the student's learning builds from one activity to the next.
5. *Curriculum evaluation.* Evaluation of the curriculum involves determining (a) the effectiveness of the curriculum approach in its developmental stage; (b) whether teachers can, in fact, use the curriculum at the point of implementation; (c) the

effectiveness of the curriculum in its operational stage; and (d) the extent to which students have achieved the objectives selected for the curriculum.

Posner and Rudnitsky (1978) have provided a model of the curriculum development process including the various activities and sequence of steps or events that characterize the curriculum development enterprise (Fig. 12-1).

Making decisions about the curriculum

Goodlad (1979) has identified three levels of decision making that are involved in the curriculum development process. These include (1) the *societal level,* which includes the community and the local board of education; (2) the *institutional level,* which involves the superintendent and the central office or district staff; and (3) the *instructional level,* which involves schools and teachers. According to this scheme the societal decisions are performed by the board of education through powers it has been delegated by the state board of education or state legislating authority. For instance, the State Board of Education in Illinois (1983) has redefined schooling for public school students in Illinois to include the following areas: (1) mathematics, (2) language arts, (3) science, (4) social science, (5) fine arts, and (6) physical development and health. Moreover, the board has requested that for each of these suggestions schools must specify what students are to know and what they will be able to do as a consequence of having received this instruction.

The health instruction framework for California public schools is another example of decision making at the societal level. This document, which was issued by the California

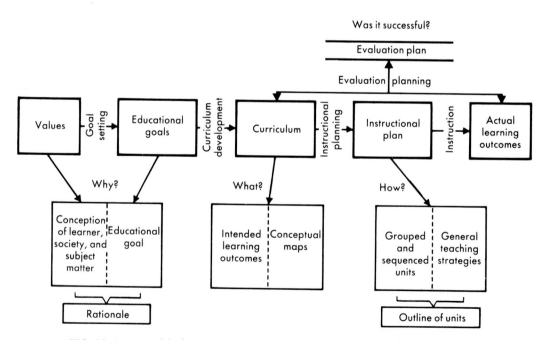

FIG. 12-1. A model of the components and processes of curriculum development sources. *(From George J. Posner and Alan N. Rudnitsky: Course design: a guide to curriculum development for teachers, ed. 2, New York, © 1978 and 1982 by Longman, Inc. Reprinted with permission.)*

State Department of Education (Curriculum Framework Criteria Committee on Health, 1978), was developed by a committee composed of health educators and curriculum specialists for the state department of education. The framework defines the scope and sequence of the health education curriculum for California schools. As such it is a very useful tool for local school district personnel in helping them decide on the specific objectives and specific classroom teaching plans and student learning experiences. The health instruction framework encompasses 10 topic areas:

1. Personal health
2. Family health
3. Nutrition
4. Mental-emotional health
5. Use and abuse of substances
6. Diseases and disorders
7. Consumer health
8. Accident prevention and emergency health services
9. Community health
10. Environment

The board's responsibilities are critical to the whole curriculum development process. Typically, such decisions are made at the beginning of the process and involve actions concerning matters of board policy and questions with budgetary implications. Also, the board must adopt or establish the central goals and functions that are to be served by the schools.

Decisions at the *institutional level,* made by the superintendent and his or her administrative staff, are more likely to be concerned with curricular questions pertaining to the whole school system. These decisions include questions about the subjects to be taught and the curricular framework to which each subject area of the district curriculum is to be related. Decisions at the institutional level are concerned with the coordination and articulation of the district's instructional program to ensure that the various elements of the program are related to the educational goals adopted by the board of education.

At the *instructional level,* decisions are made about the working elements of the curriculum. Ideally this should be a teamwork process among principals, teachers, students, and parents. More typically, the classroom teacher makes the decision about the specific teaching-learning activities that will ultimately be used in the classroom. Here the general societal goals of the curriculum are translated into instructional objectives and learning outcomes.

The California state curriculum provides a good illustration of how the different levels of decision making can function effectively in providing a quality program of instruction at the classroom level. The state department uses its resources to enlist the assistance of experts in determining the state's general goals and curriculum framework. However, because it is a framework, or an outline, the school district administration may benefit from the guidance of the framework in planning its district-wide program of instruction, while at the same time one local school is given a maximal degree of flexibility in selecting specific teaching materials and learning experiences to be employed in the classroom. Such flexibility enables the teacher to make the decisions necessary to meet the specific health education needs of the children in the local schools.

THE HEALTH EDUCATION CURRICULUM: DECIDING WHAT TO TEACH

The term *health* connotes a wholeness of mind and body, a condition free from disease and disability. The term *hygiene* is the forerunner of the term *health education*. Although hygiene has become archaic in today's usage, except in its limited application to industrial hygiene, the meaning (i.e., the science of preserving the health of both the individual and the community), is entirely appropriate. The teaching of hygiene was often narrowly focused because of the implied limited knowledge base of health and disease. Tracing the development of health education over the last century reveals a gradual expansion of knowledge concerning health and disease.

During the early nineteenth century the teaching of physiology and hygiene moved away from the teaching of facts about the structure or anatomy of the body to presenting information on the function or dynamic qualities of living.

Understanding the timing and events of history gives the student a greater appreciation for the growth of human knowledge and the effect of these events on the understanding of health. For example, the first law requiring the teaching of physiology and hygiene was passed in 1850, predating Pasteur's work and the development of the germ theory. With the enactment of laws requiring compulsory school attendance there also came outbreaks of epidemic diseases in the schools. These developments and the new knowledge about infectious diseases led to the teaching of information about communicable diseases and to a further expansion of the concept of health and disease. As a consequence, awareness of preventive measures, including the importance of environmental sanitation in controlling disease, increased.

Other developments during the first decades of the 1900s that influenced the teaching of health and the health education curriculum included the scientific temperance movement, the child study movement, and World War I. These events initiated teaching in such areas as alcohol, tobacco, narcotics, physical growth, exercise, and fresh air and ventilation. Unfortunately, not all developments had a completely positive impact on health teaching in the schools. The first breakthrough of new scientific knowledge was often incomplete, and partial truths often led to errors and the spreading of misconceptions as well as new facts. For example, early programs that were designed to prevent and control the spread of tuberculosis may not always have had a positive effect on the health of children. The emphasis on fresh air and ventilation may have led to an overexposure of children to the elements, thereby lowering their resistance to upper respiratory tract infections.

The scientific temperance movement provides yet another example of how a group in its zeal to stamp out the use of alcohol and tobacco can have a negative effect on education. Although the program advocated teaching scientifically verified facts (i.e., the effects of these substances on human health), often the teaching and instructional materials contained a mixture of misconceptions, myths, and facts. Moreover, the laws requiring the teaching of these subjects were often poorly conceived and educationally unworkable.

In the early decades of this century, acute infectious diseases represented one of the most serious health problems. As scientific knowledge progressed, these diseases were controlled, and chronic diseases became the focus of research.

Determining the goals and objectives of health education

The 1973 report of the President's Committee on Health Education revealed a general confusion and lack of agreement over the goals of health education. The public hearings conducted by the committee revealed the fact that two different approaches were being advocated for health education. One approach held that the goal of health education was to facilitate the achievement of the highest optimal level of health by the individual—a concept of health similar to that embraced by the World Health Organization. The other approach maintained that the goal of health education was disease prevention, emphasizing the prevention or management of specific conditions. The legislation that created the Office of Disease Prevention and Health Promotion, as well as recent publications of the Public Health Service issued under a similar title, indicate that the federal government is attempting to circumvent this controversy by including both the concept of positive health and that of disease prevention in its statement of the goal of health education.

The fact that health education originated in two fields, health and education, may explain this difference in orientation. The field of health has long been dominated by the influence of medicine, with its focus on the treatment and control of disease. Education's major influence on the field focuses on the nurturing of the individual's growth and development, or health promotion.

How are the goals of health education to be selected or defined? School programs, responsible for many different curriculums and program specialties, should maintain an ongoing process of selecting or defining goals. To ensure that a particular school program's goals are consistent with those of the larger mission or purpose of the educational enterprise, a careful survey of the educational literature pertaining to the fundamental purpose of schooling should be conducted. Sources that may be consulted when writing or selecting program goals include the following:

1. State and federal legislation (especially that which is mandatory)
2. Literature pertaining to local and national concerns
3. Goals of other programs, especially those considered to be exemplary
4. Parental concerns and requests and special study reports on program needs

In general terms the purposes or goals of education focus on the development of cognitive abilities and positive habits of the individual. In American society, schools play a major role in helping to establish an ideal democratic society where respect, justice, and fair play should provide firsthand experiences with ethical values. Thus a general goal of education is to provide students with an opportunity to learn the responsibilities of adulthood and citizenship (Tyler, 1975). Although these general goals of education may not be specifically identified as health goals, nevertheless, it is evident that health education can play a key role in the achievement of such aims.

Other goals of education stress personal, intellectual, creative, social, moral, emotional, and physical development. Here, the relationship to health education is more obvious. Such general concepts as personal development, including a social consciousness, hold important implications for health education (Taylor, 1975).

Traditionally health education has been characterized by its threefold objectives of health: knowledge, attitudes, and behavior. However, the degree to which these objectives are emphasized is determined largely by the point of view held regarding the purpose of health education and the theory of learning or theory of behavior change.

Two recent publications, the Surgeon General's report *Healthy People* and its companion publication, *Disease Prevention and Health Promotion: Objectives for the Nation,* have placed great emphasis on the role of education in developing health-promoting and disease-preventing behaviors. It is apparent that such expectations call for health education to play a key role in helping the nation to achieve its health goals. Perhaps this is best illustrated by the following statement from *Healthy People* (Office of the Assistant Secretary for Health and the Surgeon General, 1979):

> Personal habits play critical roles in the development of many serious diseases and in injuries from violence and automobile accidents.
>
> Many of today's most pressing health problems are related to excess — of smoking, drinking, faulty nutrition, overuse of medications, careless driving and the relentless pressure to achieve.
>
> In fact, of the ten leading causes of death in the United States, at least seven could be substantially reduced if persons at risk improved just five habits: diet, smoking, lack of exercise, alcohol abuse and use of antihypertensive medication.

Moreover, analysis of the various health problems posing serious threats to the different age groups in American society (infants, children, adolescents, and adults) unmistakably calls for changes in behavior or life-style. It is clear that health education programs committed to reducing many of these problems are attracting widespread support. The childhood accident problem is a case in point. With some 10,000 children below 14 years of age killed annually, the need for remediation of this problem can hardly be questioned. The accident problem, it is argued, is in large part the result of environmental and social factors; as such, it is not amenable to medical care or to methods of medical intervention.

This same point of view is expressed in former Governor Rockefeller's report on social problems and health and hospital services and costs (Governor's Steering Committee on Social Problems, 1971), "Prevention and sound maintenance are as much an individual responsibility as they are a medical responsibility."

In the field of health, education has established new concepts of disease prevention and health promotion, accepting a model of health (see Fig. 11-1) that recognizes the roles of (1) heredity, (2) environment (including physical, social, and psychologic factors), (3) health services, and (4) life-style factors and behavior in an expanding concept of health.

Deciding what to teach not only calls for an examination of the structure of knowledge about health but also a determination of the most effective approach to use from the standpoint of the teaching-learning process or curriculum design.

What should be the parameters of the health education curriculum? Can a comprehensive view of health be taught, as implied in Bruner's (1960) thesis that children can be taught to understand the essential intellectual concepts of *any* subject; or is a child-centered approach that focuses on the particular developmental stages of growth more appropriate? Regardless of the approach to be taken, Goodlad (1979) has called for the establishment of a comprehensive and coherent framework for curriculum design.

A FRAMEWORK FOR CURRICULUM DESIGN

According to Goodlad's conceptual scheme (1979), content and behavior are the organized elements of a curriculum design. Such a design may be depicted graphically in the form of a chart with the behavioral elements written along a *vertical* axis and the substantive elements (subject matter) presented along the *horizontal* axis (Table 12-1). This illustration provides an adaptation such as might be employed for the development of a health education curriculum. The specific learning objectives for students are determined by the points at which the columns of subject matter elements intersect the rows of the behavioral elements. Fig. 12-2 depicts three elements of the teaching-learning plan for each of four health topics that might be part of a larger comprehensive curriculum. There is a progression in both the level of behavioral outcomes and for each of the subject matter topics. The squares represent segments in the total design of a comprehensive curriculum.

In terms of the levels of decision making, the squares where the learning objectives are identified constitute the points at which the decision making of superintendent and school district staffs (institutional level) separates from the decisions that are now to be made at the instructional level. The responsibility for determining student learning outcomes, teaching methods, study materials, and the evaluation of student learning are decisions made at the school and classroom level. Again, according to Goodlad, the activities emanating from the learning objectives constitute the organizing centers. Traditionally these elements of the curriculum have been identified as teaching units or, in more contemporary terms, as teaching modules.

COMPREHENSIVE CURRICULUM VERSUS CATEGORICAL HEALTH PROBLEMS CURRICULUM

The scope of teaching about health and disease prevention has gradually evolved and expanded. This expansion results from the new knowledge gained from technologic advances, from society's accumulated experiences in learning to apply principles of disease prevention, and from the development of ways to promote health.

With this expanding knowledge, curriculum planners and learning theorists have generally advocated the adoption of a comprehensive approach to health education. Health

TABLE 12-1. Conceptual framework for health education curriculum

Behavior elements	Smoking, alcohol, and drugs	Diet and nutrition	Safety and first aid	Family life and sex education	Organizing elements (content + objectives)
Level III behavioral objectives	Differentiate between use and misuse of alcohol	Explain relationship between nutritional status and health	Analyze the relationship between accidents and emotions	Compare and contrast male and female reproductive systems	
Level II behavioral objectives	Explain the effect of alcohol on the body	Illustrate variety of food in a good diet	Illustrate relationships between accidents and human behavior	Explain body changes occurring in puberty	Learning objectives
Level I behavioral objectives	Identify uses of alcohol	Identify	Describe an accident and how to prevent it	List similarities and differences between boys and girls	

Adaptation from Goodlad, J.I., et al.: Curriculum inquiry: the study of curriculum practice, New York, 1979, McGraw-Hill Book Co.

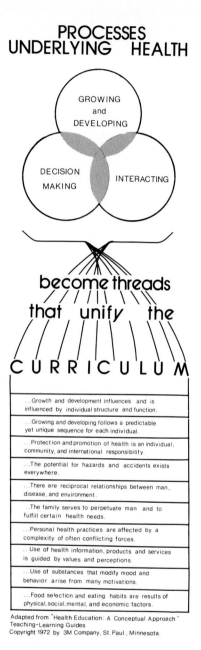

FIG. 12-2. SHES three key concepts.

(Modified from School Health Education Study, Inc.: Health education: a conceptual approach to curriculum design, Washington, D.C., © 1967, p. 20. Published by 3M Education Press, St. Paul, Minn., 1968; artwork by William H. Creswell III.)

education specialists and school policy-making groups also support this approach. For example, in a recent statement the Education Commission of the States (1981) recommends that "state education agencies should promote the development of *comprehensive* school health education programs."

In discussing the nature of such a curriculum the term *comprehensive* may be characterized in at least two ways. First, a comprehensive curriculum includes all grade levels from kindergarten to grade 12, and instruction should be provided for all students. Second, a comprehensive curriculum presents an all-inclusive treatment of health topics.

Essentially health educators do not differ as to whether a health education curriculum plan should be comprehensive and coherent. There are differences of opinion about *what* should be taught and *when* it should be taught to students. Some of these arguments stem from ideologic differences, whereas others are based on practical considerations and realistic expectations.

From the curriculum reform movement of the 1960s and 1970s, which supported a comprehensive treatment of subject matter, emerged the theory that the study of health can be organized into a conceptual structure, which in turn can be presented as a curriculum plan. This material can be taught in an articulated sequence of learning experiences, beginning in the elementary school and continuing through high school. The goal of this approach is the development of a health-educated citizenry.

As expressed in PL 95-561, the Health Education Act of 1978, the comprehensive school health program provides learning experiences based on the best available scientific information in an effort to promote the understanding, attitudes, behavioral skills, and practices of students (1) to prevent illness, disease, and injury and (2) to enhance the physical and mental health of the individual, family, and community.

The act identifies 21 different health topics, which are to be organized into a progressive sequence of learning activities taught through the elementary and secondary school years. California, Florida, Illinois, Michigan, and New York have adopted comprehensive health education program curriculum plans (Table 12-2).

Proponents of the comprehensive approach contend that health-promoting principles and theories of disease causation can be generalized and that such principles may be transferred and applied by the learner to all conditions to satisfy health needs. According to this view, health is a quality of life involving a dynamic interaction and interdependence among the different aspects of health. These include the physical, mental-emotional, social, as well as spiritual dimensions of health. Thus it is argued that if a person is to be truly healthy, health must be understood in its totality (School Health Education Study, 1968).

The advocates of a comprehensive health education curriculum criticize the categorical problem approach on the grounds that it often becomes the teaching of health education by crisis. Examples of a categorized problem approach would include teaching about a specific problem such as alcohol, drugs, smoking, sex education, or sexually transmitted disease. Such programs are usually launched with little planning and often without adequate resources or support. Typically, the program veers from one new development to another topical issue, vacillating from one crisis to the next, with health education forced to draw its support from whatever problem has temporarily captured the public's interest. For example, in the 1960s, it was the issue of the smoking problem, followed by the drug crisis of the

TABLE 12-2. A scope and sequence chart for a comprehensive health education curriculum

Suggested topics	Grade emphasis			
	K-3	4-6	Junior high	Senior high
Personal cleanliness and appearance	X	X	Omit	Omit
Physical activity, sleep, rest, and relaxation	X	X	X	Omit
Nutrition and growth	X	X	X	Omit
Dental health	X	X	X	Omit
Body structure and operation (including the senses and skin)	X	X	X	Omit *
Prevention and control of disease	X	X	X	Omit*
Safety and first aid	X	X	X	Omit
Mental health	X	X	X	X
Sex and family living education	X	X	X	X
Environmental and community health	X	X	X	X
Alcohol, drugs, and tobacco	Omit	X	X	X
Consumer health	Omit	X	X	X
World health	Omit	Omit	Omit	X
Health careers	Omit	Omit	X	X

From Willgoose, C.G.: J. Sch. Health **43**:189, 1973.
*Decisions regarding which topics will receive emphasis at a particular grade level are determined at the state and local school level. However, in view of the current AIDS epidemic, no doubt the topic of infectious disease would be emphasized at all educational levels.

1970s. The current problems are the unmarried parent, venereal disease (herpes), and increased drinking. This approach means a constant shifting of priorities as well as program activity. Programs lack the stability essential to long-range planning, as well as the systematic progress necessary for achievement of long-term goals.

It is argued that approaching health education from a categorical disease perspective is both limiting and artificial. Teaching about health by focusing on health problems is a negative orientation that falls far short of the goal of health education. The disease, or health problem, approach is inefficient, emphasizing the disease manifestation rather than the more positive and productive approaches of disease prevention and health promotion. There is not enough time in the curriculum for health education if every health problem is to be taught. Finally, a categorical disease approach is poor pedagogy. Teaching about specific diseases, apart from the general study of health and disease, is like teaching the concepts of multiplication apart from the context of mathematics.

On the other side of the argument, however, critics of the comprehensive program contend that it is too general and too vague to be meaningful or to be communicated effectively. Instead, they argue for a specific problem approach. Because this approach can be communicated to people, it takes advantage of their natural interest and motivation to solve problems. In support of this approach, they point to the many voluntary and governmental organizations that have successfully conducted programs to deal with categorical problems.

Further, it is argued that organizing health education around a problem approach need not fall into the trap of overemphasis on the disease entity to the exclusion of health concerns. Instead, this approach can also develop the students' understanding of general principles of disease prevention and health promotion that are applicable to all aspects of life. Also, directing the health education effort to the most important health problems for a particular age group offers the advantage of concentrating limited resources where the need is greatest and where the greatest benefits may be achieved.

Also critics of the comprehensive approach have argued that the failure of states to implement effective comprehensive school health education programs, even when such programs have carried the force of mandatory legislation, points up the weaknesses and impracticality of this approach. Such programs represent a major undertaking and commitment on the part of the school. In an era of limited budgets, state and local school systems lack the resources to implement a program of such magnitude.

Finally, in support of a categorical health problems curriculum several voluntary, commercial, and governmental agencies have developed several excellent curriculum modules around specific or categorical problems. Because there are high-quality materials already available, the school can implement specific health topic programs at relatively low cost. The fact that such programs are targeted for a specific problem often means that they are more likely to be undertaken by the school. Visibility of a categorical problem approach also may attract support from a community agency whose goals are closely related to those of the school. Instead of languishing on the shelf of the curriculum writer, these categorical programs have shown steady and consistent growth. In particular, those health education curriculums relating to cardiovascular disease, cancer, and personal risk behaviors such as smoking, diet, and alcohol are being implemented in a growing number of schools.

A major force that has moved schools toward a categorical health problems approach has been the availability of a small grants program entitled Health Education Risk Reduction Projects to schools through the state health department. The purpose is to develop and test school health education risk-reduction curriculums. Typically these programs include the health topics identified under the health promotion category of the report *Promoting Health and Preventing Disease: Objectives for the Nation* (Public Health Service, 1980). These health topics are included in the 15 priority areas identified in the U.S. Surgeon General's report *Healthy People* (1979) given in the box on p. 278. Schools have been strongly encouraged by the U.S. Public Health Service to develop health education programs around the five areas of health promotion.

School Health Education Study: comprehensive approach

Health Education: A Conceptual Design for Curriculum Development is an example of a comprehensive treatment of health or a conceptual structure of health as a subject. It also represents an effort to apply learning theory to curriculum planning in health education. Often such projects are eclectic, using several different principles of learning rather than following a particular approach. The School Health Education Study (SHES) is an example of this in some respects, drawing on principles derived from both the cognitive and the connectionist traditions. Whereas school practitioners have sometimes been criticized for failing to adopt a consistent overall theory to guide the instructional program, common sense may

Promoting health and preventing disease: objectives for the nation

Preventive health services

1. High blood pressure control
2. Family planning
3. Pregnancy and infant health
4. Immunization
5. Sexually transmitted diseases

Health protection

1. Toxic agent control
2. Occupational safety and health
3. Accident prevention and injury control
4. Fluoridation and dental health
5. Surveillance and control of infectious diseases

Health promotion

1. Smoking and health
2. Misuse of alcohol and drugs
3. Nutrition
4. Physical fitness and exercise
5. Control of stress and violent behavior

dictate the use of both kinds of interpretations in certain instances. As Hill (1963) has observed, some principles of learning appear to apply in all situations, whereas others are germane only in particular circumstances.

However, examination of the SHES conceptual model for curriculum design reveals that it is more characteristic of the field, or cognitive, theory of learning. The SHES model is based on the concept of health that serves as the focal point in formulating a structure of health and from which the framework for health education is derived (Table 12-1).

The term *health* implies a wholeness or, as modern-day philosophers and scholars have contended, a dynamic process in which the individual is functioning in harmony both with his or her total self and with the total environment. The next step undertaken is to determine what constitutes the principal ideas to be elaborated on if a structure is to be devised that is at once logical for curriculum development, meaningful to the learner, and a valid representation of ideas held to be true by the scientist and the philosopher.

Health is the comprehensive, unified concept at the apex of the hierarchy developed for the conceptual model for health and health education. It has three dimensions — physical, mental, and social. More specifically, physical health pertains to the structure and function of the biologic organism; mental health pertains to behavior and personality patterns; and social health includes the complex of interpersonal and societal forces. Health is a quality of life involving dynamic interaction and interdependence among the individual's physical well-being, his or her mental and emotional reactions, and the social complex in which he or she exists. Any one dimension may play a greater or lesser role than the other two at a given time, but the interdependence and interaction of the three dimensions still hold true (School Health Education Study, 1968).

This view of the individual and his or her health closely parallels Lewin's (Zais, 1976) contention that learning refers to a multitude of different phenomena. He argues that we cannot have a clear understanding of learning unless we take into account the entire complex psychologic world that he calls the life space of the individual.

The hierarchy of concepts portrays the unified concept of health at the apex or highest order in the model. Following immediately are the three key concepts of growing and developing, interacting, and decision making, which are considered to be the unifying threads of the curriculum (Fig. 12-2). These three features are peculiar to all human beings, and from the standpoint of health education they are essential to the understanding of the individual's health problems and the forces affecting health behavior. Thus they are considered to be the processes that underlie health.

These three concepts are consistent with the cognitive theory of motivation that may be regarded as a theory of preferential choice or of decision making. The decision to become involved is made on the basis of cognitive considerations (Hill, 1963). For example, consider the importance of the key concept of growth and development to the curriculum planner and health education teacher in the case of a 14-year-old boy whose pubescence is late in developing. Frequently such a boy suffers severe emotional disturbances because his associates of the same age are not only sexually more mature but are also bigger and stronger than he is. Consider the impact of his state of growth and development on his social interaction with boys and girls of his same age. What kind of effect will his physical development have on his choices and decisions about participating in sports and physical activity? Will it affect his decision about diet?

Next come the 10 concepts and subconcepts that represent the scope of the subject matter treated in health education. The 10 concepts and subconcepts together with the behavioral objectives, according to Goodlad's curriculum nomenclature (1963), are the "organizing elements" of the curriculum. According to this scheme, the concepts and subconcepts include 31 different health topics.

These broad content areas have been phrased in conceptual statements to give more meaning and direction to the teaching-learning process. For example, instead of using the term *accident prevention,* the following conceptual statement is given: "The potential for hazards and accidents exists, whatever the environment." This is considered to be more descriptive as well as prescriptive insofar as health education is concerned.

The long-range goals and behavioral objectives are derived from the conceptual structure representing that which is to be learned (Table 12-1). The goals and behavioral objectives represent the educational outcomes that are sought. These represent various health behaviors, including the way students think, feel, and act with regard to health. The goals are long-term, general outcomes, whereas the behavioral objectives are specific outcomes. Similarly, goals are the result of the total health education experience, whereas behavioral objectives are those designed for a particular educational level. Also in keeping with the instructional level of decision making, classroom teachers worked with the curriculum designers in developing the behavioral objectives for student instruction.

These characteristics of the SHES curriculum point to other similarities of the field, or cognitive theories, approach. For learning to occur, it is essential that the student pursue goals that the individual student considers to be his or her own. Adopting affective as well as cognitive goals with constant attention to the three unifying key concepts serves as a constant reminder to the curriculum planner to be ever aware of the individual student's needs.

In order to apply the SHES conceptual model to teaching, each concept was analyzed and translated into priority behavioral objectives at four different educational levels (as opposed to the three levels illustrated in Goodlad's framework) beginning with level I and progressing through level IV. Here the SHES model draws on the connectionist theory of learning, which calls for the writing of objectives in precise, observable, and measurable behaviors. Behaviors considered appropriate to the desired outcomes must be identified and carefully arranged in a progression of increasingly complex behaviors. This is similar to the approach used by the advocates of behavior modification, based on the principles developed by Thorndike, Guthrie, Watson, and Skinner. According to the behaviorist, establishing complex social behavior and modifying existing response patterns can be achieved most consistently through a gradual process in which the person participates in an orderly learning sequence that guides him or her stepwise toward more intricate or demanding performances (Bandura, 1969).

To illustrate how this progression is developed in the SHES model, behavioral objectives were developed from the concept *food selection and eating patterns are determined by physical, social, mental, economic, and cultural factors* (box below). Behavioral objectives from each of the four educational levels are illustrated to show the sequences and qrogressions of these behaviors. The similarity to Goodlad's conceptual scheme is readily apparent.

Behavior modification: categorical health problems approach

Golaszewski (1979) has developed an innovative composite behavior modification model for use in school health education programs. His proposal, similar to previous efforts to apply learning theory in schools, draws to some extent on both the connectionist and cognitive traditions of learning. This composite model provides a good example of behavior modification as the application of connectionist theory to school health education. As Golaszewski points out, in any attempt to develop an ideal program, the following points should be considered: (1) a multitude of environmental influences shape the child's behaviors; therefore the tendency to take an overly simplistic view of learning and behavior must be avoided; (2) many individual variations exist, resulting from ethnic and cultural differences; and (3)

Progression of behavioral objectives by education level

Concept 10: Food selection and eating patterns are determined by physical, social, mental, economic, and cultural factors

Level I   *Identifies* — many different kinds of foods
             ↓

Level II   *Illustrates* — that a variety of foods are necessary in maintaining a balanced diet
             ↓

Level III   *Describes* — the relationship between nutritional status and disease
             ↓

Level IV   *Applies*   — criteria for selecting foods and planning meals that provide for a balanced diet the constraints of school finances, school policies, and biases of the health educator affect curriculum decisions.

The three steps of the composite model include the following:

1. Providing for student participation through appropriate laboratory experiences. For example, in teaching a unit on heart disease, activities such as an exercise stress test, serum lipid evaluations, blood pressure measurements, and growth measurements might be included. Such measures can be related to results taken from actual student surveys of behavior, such as eating, exercise, and smoking habits. Data from this step can be used as the basis for developing goals for behavior change.

2. Providing students with the information necessary for them to build a knowledge base required for rational decision making. This procedure draws on the cognitive theory of learning for behavior change. Since the objectives of this unit are to reduce the risk of heart disease, information to be included should relate to the need to eat a nutritious diet low in fats, to avoid cigarette smoking, to exercise regularly, to control blood pressure, and to make appropriate use of health care services. A variety of teaching aids, including multimedia tapes, film reports, and guest appearances of experts, is needed to ensure the validity of the content material and to stimulate student interest.

3. Providing value clarification activities that delineate actual and ideal behavior patterns aimed at preventing disease and promoting health. A major purpose of this step is the use of student participation in the setting of personal goals. Each student is expected to formulate a written plan of action to meet this goal. The goal selected should be measurable, be related to a specific time period, and be realistic for the student. In keeping with the self-management or self-care approach, the student should provide a plan for monitoring progress and a system of rewarding or reinforcing the desired behavior.

To help ensure the success of a behavior modification approach in school health education, the following procedure for the teacher is recommended:

1. Review all student plans to determine their appropriateness as well as feasibility.

2. Follow a contract-grading procedure, where each step of progress is appropriately rewarded.

3. Organize the class into small groups of students having similar goals. Encourage students to make a group commitment and to share their progress as well as their problems.

4. Include the technique of mental imagery in student learning activities. This encourages the student to visualize goal achievement, such as losing 20 pounds (9 kg) of weight, being able to jog 3 miles, or stopping smoking. The student then imagines being rewarded for achieving the goal and receiving compliments on the results.

5. Provide opportunities for the students to give a public demonstration after goal achievement. For example, a diet group might give a "health meal" demonstration, an exercise group might sponsor a special road race, and an antismoking group might give a special class presentation to younger students in the school.

6. Arrange special booster sessions or programs that will provide reinforcement for student progress toward goal achievement, for example, giving awards to students for adopting a new behavior or recognizing students who lose weight.

School Health Curriculum Project

Originally, the School Health Curriculum Project (SHCP) represented a categorical health problems approach for health instruction at the elementary and middle or junior high school levels. However, since its inception the SHCP has been greatly expanded. It now includes an articulated curriculum plan beginning with the primary grades and continuing through high school. As such it can perhaps best be described as a middle-ground approach between that of a narrowly focused categoric health problems approach and that of a comprehensive curriculum. The curriculum began as an experimental project in California during the early 1960s and initially was taught to intermediate grade school children as an in-depth study of the heart and circulatory system. It was first known as the "Berkeley Project" but later was given the title of the School Health Curriculum Project (SHCP). Its general purpose is to help children learn how their bodies function in a normal, healthy state and the changes that occur when disease strikes. The effects of the environment and living habits on the body are stressed.

The goal of the SHCP is to help the child realize that the body is each person's greatest natural resource in life, is uniquely one's own, is exquisitely beautiful and complex in its structure and function, and is affected by the choices one makes throughout life (U.S. Department of Health, Education and Welfare, 1977). From a health perspective, children are taught about the importance of controlling events in their lives that might create a serious health problem, such as heart disease or cancer. In brief, the SHCP is (1) a curriculum, (2) a method of teaching, and (3) a training program for classroom teachers in health education. The curriculum focuses on the healthy body and ways of maintaining it. Acitivities are designed to involve and motivate a wide range of persons associated with the school, including students, teachers, school administrators, school health staff, community resource people, voluntary agencies' staffs, and parents.

The curriculum plan is designed for the elementary school, kindergarten through grade 7. The primary grades (K-3) unit studies the senses, whereas successive grade levels from four through seven develop study of a different organ system at each level, including units on digestion, the lungs, the heart, and the brain.

The curriculum employs a common organization (Fig. 12-3 and box on p. 284) for each of the units that includes the following:

- Introduction: curiosity arousal and motivation of students
- Phase one: overview of the body's system
- Phase two: appreciation of one of the body's systems and its unique function
- Phase three: structure and function of the body system
- Phase four: diseases and problems of the body system
- Phase five: care of the body and prevention of disease
- Culmination: synthesis, through group presentations of the previous phases

Developers of the curriculum contend that using the same teaching approach serves to reinforce the children's understanding of the concept that all body systems are related and that any single event affecting a part of the body affects the whole body and the total health of the person.

Audiovisual materials, including films, filmstrips, slides, tape recorders, and records, are used extensively to stimulate the children's interest. Models and dissection and analysis

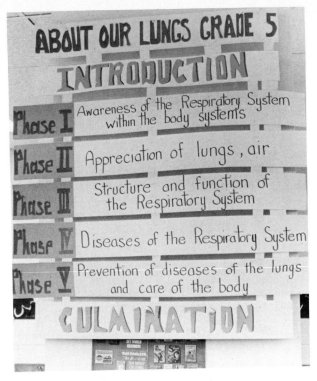

FIG. 12-3. Five phases of study about our lungs. This provides a logical sequence for understanding the progression of disease.
(From School Health Curriculum Project. Pub. No. [CDC] 78-8359, Atlanta, 1977, Public Health Service, Centers for Disease Control, U.S. Department of Health, Education and Welfare.)

of animal organs make the study of health more realistic. Such concrete experiences help the student to personalize the relationship between living habits and their effect on the body.

This curriculum involves the use of a learning center of five or six stations, enabling children to participate in several different learning activities simultaneously (Fig. 12-4). Children study in small groups, rotating through each of the stations in the learning center, actively involved in the learning process (Fig. 12-5). For example, a series of activities might be developed around the study of circulation, including tracing the locations of arteries and veins, examining red blood cells under the microscope, and learning to take blood pressure. Groups rotate every 30 minutes or at the end of each period, depending on the complexity of the task.

Schools wishing to initiate the curriculum are required to send a team of four or five members to a special training center. The team is composed of at least two classroom teachers who will teach the unit at a particular grade level. Other members of the team include the principal and two other persons such as a nurse, a health educator, or a curriculum specialist. These teams participate in a training session of 60 hours for each unit. During this intensive training workshop, teachers are introduced to each step of the unit exactly as it will be taught to their classes. After the teacher has successfully taught the

Unit 5 — About our lungs

Introduction: Curiosity arousal about air

The existence of air
The body's need for air
Life needs air
Artificial resuscitation demonstration
Your breath can save somebody's life

Phase one: Overview of the body's systems

Skeletal system	Excretory system
Muscular system	Endocrine system
Respiratory system	Reproductive system
Circulatory system	Nervous system
Digestive system	

Phase two: Appreciation of air and lungs

Essence of air
Properties of air
Functions of air
How the human body uses air
Pollution and its effects on the respiratory system

Phase three: Structure and function of the respiratory system

Nasal passages, trachea, bronchial tubes, bronchioles, alveoli, lungs, diaphragm, rib cage, cells
Inhalation, exhalation, oxygen–carbon dioxide exchange with blood, cleansing system

Phase four: Diseases and problems of the respiratory system

Communicable diseases: colds, flu, pneumonia, bronchitis, etc.
Noncommunicable diseases: allergy, asthma, emphysema, lung cancer, heart disease

Phase five: Care of body and prevention of respiratory diseases

Clean air/pollution
   Effects of tobacco smoke
   Good and harmful effects of drugs
   Nutrition
   Rest
   Exercise

Culmination: The respiratory system

Activities planned and executed by children, including skits, games, poster presentation, etc., presented to class or to the total school community, including parents

From The School Health Curriculum Project, Washington, D.C., DHEW Pub. No. (CDC) 78-8359, U.S. Department of Health, Education and Welfare, Public Health Service, Centers for Disease Control, Bureau of Health Education, Atlanta, 1977, HEW Publications.

program, he or she then must conduct a training session for other teachers in the school program, he or she then must conduct a training session for other teachers in the school district in order to ensure the dissemination of the model throughout the school system.

   Strengths of the SHCP approach include clear definition of each unit, which facilitates the classroom teacher's understanding and preparation. The variety of audiovisual aids, teaching materials, and learning activities makes the curriculum interesting to both students

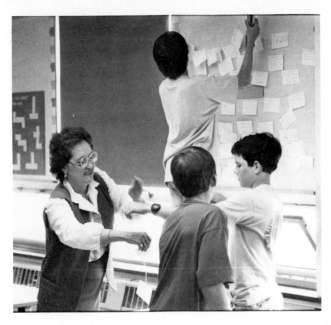

FIG. 12-4.   Teachers use a variety of classroom activities to stimulate student interest and motivation to learn.

and teachers. The active participation of the student in his or her learning, the involvement of community health agencies in providing resources for the curriculum, and the interest of parents in the health problem being studied not only facilitate learning but also provide a broad base of support and reinforcement to the student.

This curriculum has not been identified with a particular learning theory but is based on principles that have evolved from a distillation of empirically tested school practices. Widely accepted principles of instruction evident in the project include the following: (1) the active involvement of the learner, (2) the extensive use of concrete learning activities, (3) the use of cooperative group learning activities, and (4) the structured yet flexible program that allows for variation in student abilities. Several of the principles derived from the cognitive learning theory are employed in the emphasis on motivation and the recognition of structure and its interrelationship in the study of body systems. Perhaps the characteristic that would most closely relate this curriculum to connectionist theory is its recognition of individual differences and its use of a variety of individual learning activities.

THE HEALTH TEACHING UNIT

Once the goals and the general framework of the health education curriculum have been established, the planning organization, and instruction of the teaching unit can then proceed. Whether the unit is to be developed from its very inception or is to be adopted from a general teaching guide provided by the state or school district administration, the classroom teachers and personnel of the local school must play the central role in this final stage of curriculum construction. It is they, the teachers, who will make the decisions about the teaching strategies and learning activities that students will ultimately experience in the classroom.

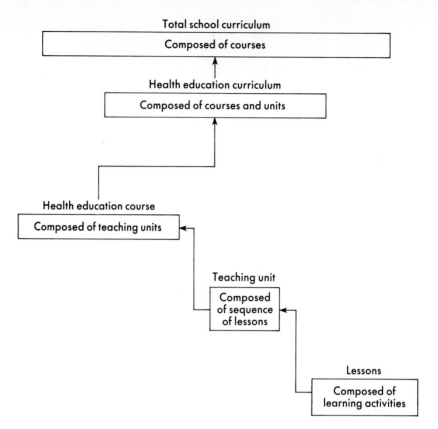

FIG. 12-5. A context for curriculum building.

The term *unit* implies a wholeness or unity of several elements. It has been defined as "an instructional sequence having distinct objectives and separate assessment" (Tyler, 1975). The unit is a manifestation of what Goodlad (1979) has called the "organizing centers of curriculum design" (see Table 12-1). Typically the unit includes (1) a title and an introduction or overview statement about the unit; (2) the goals, or long-range objectives; (3) the subject matter or health content to be learned by the student; (4) the methods or teaching strategies for presenting information or engaging the student in learning activities; (5) teaching aids to implement the effectiveness of classroom methods and learning activities; (6) the techniques for assessing the effects of the unit, in terms of the effectiveness of the teaching process and the degree to which students have achieved the intended learning outcomes; and (7) a compilation of resources for both the student and the teacher.

The unit of instruction is the basic building block of the total curriculum structure. It is the smallest complete teaching-learning segment of the curriculum (Fig. 12-5). How long should the unit be? Although no single time period meets all needs, there is general agreement that short units offer certain educational advantages. For example, a unit covering a shorter time frame provides early assessment and feedback to the student. This enables the teacher to assess the student's progress at an early point, when modification of the unit and student learning problems can be easily achieved. The demonstrated effectiveness of mastery teaching, with its relatively short teaching sequences and feedback to the student, has led to the recommendation that teaching units be planned for approximately 5 to 10 hours of instruction or 1 to 2 weeks in length.

Constructing the health unit

Title and overview. *The title and overview* of the unit often evolve from discussion and questions that are raised about a particular problem or health topic of interest. Discussions among teachers, students, school officials, parents, health officials, and other experts can be highly productive in identifying issues, concerns, and problems. Several sessions may be required to clarify questions and to determine the key ideas, focal points, or themes around which the unit can be developed. As Tyler (1975) has cautioned, teachers should resist the temptation to close this phase of planning too soon. There is much evidence to support the benefits to be derived from the appropriate involvement of such groups in planning for health instruction. Not the least of these benefits is the support for the health education program that is often engendered from such planning.

Depending on what the planning group and teaching faculty decide, the title selected for the unit may convey a particular theme. A catchy, provocative title or one that communicates simply and directly the health topic for the unit works best. For example, a title such as "The Psychology of Accidents" is intended to call attention to the importance of our emotions, attitudes, feelings, values, and interpersonal relationships as factors to be understood in the dynamics of accidents. Another example, "The Potential for Accidents Exists Whatever the Environment," serves both as a unit title and as one of the major ideas or conceptual statements making up the School Health Education Study Curriculum design. It is the organizing element for planning the teaching and learning activities that are designed to promote safety and prevent accidents.

The overview, or introduction to the unit, ideally provides a statement summarizing the characteristics, needs, and interests of the student group for whom the unit is designed. Additionally, the overview contains a statement about the subject (i.e., the health problem) and its importance to the student and to the larger community or societal concerns. For example, an overview statement for a senior high school teaching unit on safety and accident prevention might include reference to the motor vehicle accident death rate for teenagers. The fact that these accidents are often related to drinking and that the rates for this age group have recently shown an increase gives added meaning to the curriculum planning.

Curriculum goals. Traditionally, in health education such goals have been expressed as knowledge (cognitions), attitudes (affective domain), and health practices or applications. School curriculum goals have often been selected at the societal level (e.g., national or state goals). Examples of such goal statements are as follows:

- *Knowledge (cognitive domain)*: students will develop an understanding that accidents are related to human behavior, the physical environment, and the interaction of these factors (Fig. 12-6).
- *Attitude (affective domain)*: students will become sensitive to the dangerous aspects of a changing environment.
- *Practice (action or application)*: students will attempt to make the environment safe, and they will assist or cooperate with others in such efforts (School Health Education Study, 1968). (See Fig. 12-7.)

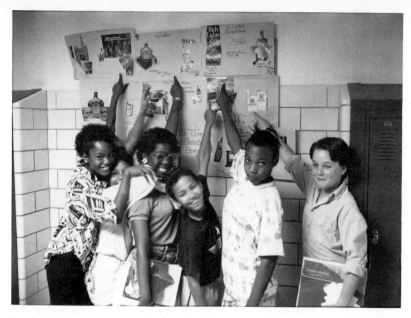

FIG. 12-6. Students identify harmful substances on a bulletin board they have constructed as a class activity.

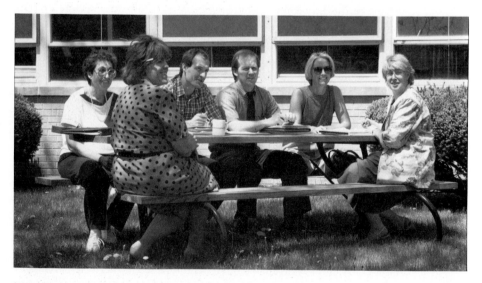

FIG. 12-7. Curriculum planning calls for the special knowledge and perspectives of teachers, counselors, parents, and community personnel.

Instructional or behavioral objectives. Instructional and behavioral objectives are derived from the goals as long-range objectives that have been adopted by the district for the health education curriculum. Although there may be differences of opinion as to the exact nature or degree of precision required of instructional objectives, there is agreement on the purposes they are to serve. They direct the teaching process and determine the learning outcomes that are intended for the student. Accomplishing such a purpose requires special care and skill on the part of the teacher. Moreover, the writing of these objectives becomes the primary responsibility of those teachers who will teach the unit. A well-stated objective must specify the observed behavior that a student will exhibit on achievement of the objective (Posner and Rudnitsky, 1978).

To continue with another example drawn from the area of safety and accident prevention, an instructional objective (cognitive domain) has been written for a unit on basic rescue and water safety procedures (American National Red Cross, 1983) taught to junior high school students: "Students will be able to explain the correct water safety assists to be used in attempting to rescue a potential drowning victim."

Specific behavior objectives shall also be written for the affective and practice or application domains.

Content outline.   This section of the teaching unit probably should take precedence over all other aspects. The importance of the content and its relevance to the instructional objectives are fundamental to the success of the whole teaching effort. There are several steps to be taken that will help the curriculum committee develop the content section. First, they should include or arrange to have the advice of a subject matter specialist. Because the health education curriculum includes such a wide array of health topics and technical subject matter, it becomes especially important to have the content reviewed and checked for both its timeliness and its accuracy. Although having the advice of a subject matter specialist or a discipline scholar will not assure a correct decision on matters of pedagogy, it will protect against error and misconceptions in subject matter.

In this regard, Pratt (1980) has offered a series of questions that are useful to the curriculum writer.

1. Is the content relevant?
2. Is the material comprehensive?
3. Is the material interesting and challenging?
4. Is the quality of the material consistent?
5. Is the content logically organized?
6. Is the material current or easily updated?

Second, a preliminary content outline should be prepared. Drawing on the ideas discussed earlier in relation to the goals, objectives, and overview statement will help to define and clarify the particular emphasis of the unit. Conducting a literature search, including the review of textbooks, periodic references, and other courses of study, is beneficial to the committee in helping them to become familiar with the subject matter. It is particularly important, at this juncture, that a well-developed and logically organized content outline be developed. Although the outline should have sufficient detail to reveal its structure, too much detail can be confusing.

Once a preliminary outline has been developed, it should be reviewed by a technical expert or subject matter specialist. This represents an important check on the curriculum committee's work—a content validation step to avoid the possibility of introducing errors into the curriculum. This step should be repeated periodically to ensure that the content is kept current and checked for scientific accuracy. The rapid growth of science and technology and its accompanying accelerated increase of information have caused psychologists and curriculum writers to seek new and more efficient ways to organize information in order to facilitate the teaching and learning process. The teacher and learner are confronted with a difficult problem in attempting to keep abreast of these new developments. This is the background that has given rise to a concept approach. This approach seeks out the basic principles, fundamental concepts, and methods that make up a large body of knowledge. Much of the interest in concepts learning stems from the belief that knowledge can be greatly simplified for teaching. Knowledge is not merely an accumulation of isolated bits of information but instead is composed of a network of ideas. Posner and Rudnitsky (1978) have described a method of "concept mapping" as a way of revealing the structure of a subject or discipline. Such a map provides a graphic representation of a conceptual structure and the various relationships completing the structure. Fig. 12-8 shows how a conceptual map on water safety might be developed.

As one of the curriculum writers for the School Health Education Study (1968), Means provided a much earlier example, given in the following paragraph, of how a conceptual approach could be used to organize a content outline for a senior high school unit on safety.

The conceptual statement is, "The potential for accidents exists regardless of the environment." Accordingly, one of the major subtopics or generalizations relating to this conceptual statement is presented with its supporting content materials.

WATER SAFETY RESCUE ASSISTS

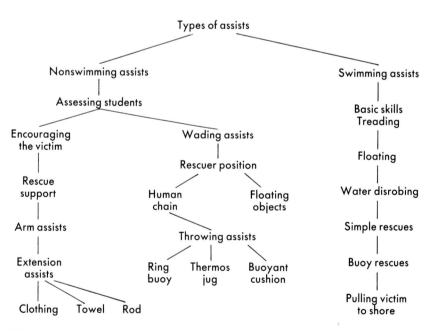

FIG. 12-8. Conceptual mapping for developing an instructional outline for teaching a unit on water safety.

Subtopic — interpretation of accident data reveals a variety of implications (e.g., physical, mental, social, and economic)

1. Consequences of accidents
   a. Temporary and permanent disability
   b. Mental anguish and human suffering
   c. Family and group disruption
   d. Economic costs
2. Individual factors relating to accidents
   a. Physical defects
   b. Risk factors vary with age and occupation
   c. Mental and emotional states
3. Social and environmental factors
   a. Group pressures
   b. Laws
   c. Weather conditions
   d. Defective equipment
4. Using accident data to prevent accidents
   a. Planning safer cities
   b. Improved laws and regulations
   c. Safe location of public facilities (parks; schools, airports, etc.)
   d. Educational programs

As each subtopic is written, it can be readily transformed into a student behavioral objective such as, "Students will be able to interpret accident data in terms of their various implications."

Teaching strategies.   Although there are no absolutes regarding the best method of teaching, there are several generalizations that can be made about teaching and that have been supported by experience and research. Certain teaching characteristics are known to have a positive effect on student achievement. For example, teachers who are effective tend to be warm, friendly, and outgoing; are enthusiastic about their teaching; are well organized in their presentations; are able to express themselves clearly; make effective use of gestures; and have a good sense of humor.

Pratt (1980) has offered a model composed of four key steps to guide the teacher and curriculum writer in selecting teaching strategies (Fig. 12-9).

Reviewing the instructional objectives should give a clear vision of what is intended as the learning outcomes for the student. This will also help the teacher decide on an effective teaching strategy. For example, the following instructional objective from the unit on water safety rescue indicates quite specifically the kind of teaching strategy to be used. "The student will be able to demonstrate how to rescue a victim using *nonswimming assists.*"

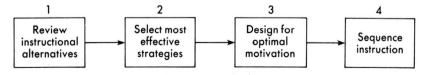

FIG. 12-9.   Main steps in selecting teaching strategies.
(From David Pratt: Curriculum: design and development, New York, © 1980, Harcourt Brace Jovanovich, Inc. Reprinted with permission of the publisher.)

Being able to maintain student interest is of such importance that the teacher may be justified in selecting some classroom activities primarily for their interest value. Once having caught the students' interest, the thoughtful teacher should be able to focus the students' attention on the desired learning objective. (See Fig. 12-5.)

Research on teaching reveals that most teachers tend to rely too much on a limited number of teaching activities, such as teacher talk or "telling the student," teacher questioning, and student recitation. Increasing the variety of teaching methods increases student interest and teacher effectiveness. Consequently, teachers are encouraged to make a concerted effort to expand their teaching repertoire by drawing on the vast resources that are available to them. Understandably, teachers will have their preferences as to teaching style. However, using different teaching methods also recognizes that students learn in different ways.

Student motivation is also greatly enhanced by student interest. Being able to match the instructional objective with the interests and needs of the student is one of the keys to motivation. A long-accepted axiom in education holds that "success breeds success, and failure breeds failure," which is further validation of the concept of positive reinforcement. In this regard the reward system is widely used in education. Although both external and internal rewards are used, students tend to lose interest in external rewards once the goal has been achieved.

An interrelationship appears to exist between the desire for success, as a motivator, and the fear of failure. If success is perceived as too easily achieved, the lesson or learning risk may lose its value as an incentive. Correspondingly, if the learning task is sufficiently difficult so that the probability of failure is about equal to that of success, the incentive value increases. Students tend to work hardest at tasks of intermediate difficulty. However, if the task is perceived as very difficult, with a high risk of failure, it is more likely to discourage the student from trying. Moreover, if the student tends to be too anxious, even a task of intermediate difficulty may lose its incentive value to the student (Atkinson, 1978).

Sequencing instruction has long been recognized as an important consideration in developing a teaching strategy. Furthermore, there is a consensus that learning should proceed from the simple to the complex, or from that which is familiar to that which is difficult and unknown. However, good reasons exist for varying the sequence of lessons. An unfamiliar, yet novel, learning activity may be effective in stimulating student interest. Introducing a unit by providing students with an overview or a general perspective of the problem before proceeding to the specifics may also increase student *interest* and *motivation* for learning.

Unit evaluation.   In unit evaluation the emphasis is on formative rather than summative evaluation. Because the unit typically represents only 5 to 10 hours of instruction, the teacher's concern at this point is to learn how much progress students have made (formative evaluation) toward achieving the objectives. Summative evaluation comes after instruction has been completed. It is designed to answer the question, "How much did students achieve?"

The emphasis on formative evaluation provides another effective teaching method. As such, this form of evaluation must provide immediate feedback to the students. It can be done with the usual classroom tests that check student work and by informal observation of the student in class. It is important that the test results be fed back immediately, so that students may learn of and correct any errors that they may have made. When tests are used as a learning activity, they should not be used for grading purposes. Again, the emphasis of formative evaluation is on assessing, feeding back, and reinforcing by providing further encouragement, in order for the student to reach the maximal level of achievement.

Materials.   There is an important distinction between the materials section of teaching and resource units. Teaching units include only those materials that have been selected by the teacher to serve a specific purpose, that is, to be used with a specific learning activity. The resource units, as the term implies, are a compilation of many materials from which the teacher may draw. Typically, the resource units are collected and kept in the curriculum library of the school district. Curriculum writing committees and classroom teachers use this resource in planning the teaching unit.

A major problem facing today's health education teaching is the challenge to keep up with all the new materials and teaching aids that are available. Fortunately, information systems such as bibliographies, indexes, abstracts, and periodicals are becoming available through computer-based information systems. Several information dissemination publications are available for health education. Two publications covering the general field of health education are the *Bibliographic Index of Health Education Periodicals* (BIHEP), published quarterly by Indiana University, and *Current Awareness in Health Education,* a publication of the Center for Health Promotion and Education in the Centers for Disease Control of the Public Health Service. The latter publication includes both abstracts of literature and program descriptions. In addition, there are several special subject indexes of topics such as smoking, drugs, and nutrition.

With the increasing availability of materials, more attention must be given to their evaluation. Teachers will need to develop their skills, using such criteria as appropriateness, coverage, and accuracy of the content. They will have to consider such questions as readability levels, suitability of the material for the school and the community, and cost of the material.

SUMMARY

This chapter provides a brief historical review of the school health education curriculum developments leading up to the present. Several events are examined including the Commission on Reorganizing Secondary Education and their Cardinal Principles of Education, which have had a major influence on the development of health education since the World War I. With respect to curriculum development the contributions of two leaders in the field role were discussed in some detail. Ralph Tyler, a national authority on theory and practice of curriculum development and John Goodlad's conceptual approach to curriculum have had a major influence on the teaching of health education. Events that have had an influence on contemporary health education curriculums were reviewed including the curriculum reform movement after Sputnik (1957), the President's Committee on Health Education in the 1970s, the Surgeon General's report *Healthy People* (1979), and the national health goals for 1990 (which appeared in the Surgeon General's report *Healthy People,* 1979).

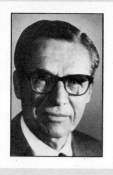

Howard S. Hoyman

BORN   January 21, 1902, Lancaster, Ohio

EDUCATION   B.S., Ohio State University, 1928; M.S., Columbia University, 1932; Ed.D., Columbia University, 1947

Howard "Mike" Hoyman is a premier educator whose major interest has always been curriculum. He has done pioneer work in developing curriculums for health education, particularly at the secondary school level.

After completing his undergraduate and master's level course work in the Midwest and the East, Hoyman moved to Oregon in 1932. There he began the work that later resulted in the publication *Developing Health Instruction in Oregon High Schools.* This was the first comprehensive series of functional health guide units covering all major areas of personal, family, and community health produced in the United States for use in high schools. Part I contained the first sex education unit distributed and used in the Oregon secondary schools. This was expanded to *Health Guide Units for Oregon Teachers,* which contained the so-called Oregon plan for including the sex education phase of family life education as an integral part of the high school health education curriculum for boys and girls in grades 7 to 12. It was the first statewide plan for providing such instruction in the United States. Subsequently other states issued courses of study in health education containing sex education topics and units. This plan of including sex education as an integral part of the health curriculum instead of as a separate unit, course, or lecture has been widely accepted.

The Four Cycle Curriculum for health instruction has also been widely adopted and is considered a major contribution to the theory and practice of health education. Hoyman has always had a strong interest in philosophy and has written widely on the subject of health and human ecology. His ecologic model of health has had a major influence on the thinking of health educators.

Hoyman was always a teacher — for 17 years at the University of Oregon and for 21 years at the University of Illinois. He was a member of the graduate faculty and also served as head of the Department of Health and Safety Education at the University of Illinois from its inception in 1957. He prepared the 4-year undergraduate health education curriculum at the University of Oregon and prepared both the undergraduate and graduate programs in health education at the University of Illinois. He has served on many professional committees and has belonged to many professional organizations, but his main interest has always been the training of teachers and the teaching of chidren.

Examples of comprehensive and categorical health curriculums are also discussed. The rationale for these different approaches and the events that have influenced their development are also presented. The chapter concludes with a detailed analysis of the teaching unit, the foundation upon which all curriculums are based.

STUDY QUESTIONS

1. Why is the 1918 report of the Commission on Reorganization of Secondary Education of importance to health education?
2. What are the foundations of today's school curriculum?
3. How might the curriculum planner's theory of learning affect the organization of the health education curriculum?
4. How might the report *Health Promotion and Disease Prevention: Objectives for the Nation* influence the decision making for the health education curriculum? What level of decision making is most likely to be affected?
5. Although many leaders in health education have advocated a comprehensive health education curriculum, why does the categorical health problems approach enjoy increased interest and emphasis?
6. What is the rationale for a conceptual approach to curriculum development?
7. What are the formulations of curriculum development?
8. What is the principal difference in point of view or theory between the School Health Curriculum Project and the School Health Education Study?
9. What is the difference between a goal of the health education curriculum and a health instruction objective?

REFERENCES

American National Red Cross: Life saving: rescue and water safety, Washington, D.C., 1982.

Atkinson, J.W.: An introduction to motivation, ed. 2, Princeton, N.J., 1978, Van Nostrand Reinhold Co., Inc.

Bandura, A.: Principles of behavior modification, New York, 1969, Holt, Rinehart & Winston, Inc.

Brink, S.G., Simons-Morton, D., et al.: Developing comprehensive smoking control programs in schools, J. Sch. Health **58:**177, 1988.

Bruner, J.S.: The process of education, Cambridge, Mass., 1963, Harvard University Press.

Commission on the Reorganization of Secondary Education: Cardinal principles of secondary education, Washington, D.C., 1918, U.S. Government Printing Office.

Cornacchia, H.J., Olsen, H.K., and Nickerson, C.J.: Health in elementary schools, ed. 6, St. Louis, 1984, The C.V. Mosby Co.

Curriculum Framework Criteria Committee on Health: Health instruction framework for California Public Schools, Sacramento, Calif., 1978, California State Department of Education.

Del Greco, L., and others: Four-year results of a youth smoking prevention program using assertiveness training, Adolescence **21:**631, 1986.

Downey, A.M., Virgilio, S.J., Serpas, D.C., Nicklas, T.A., Arbeit, M.L., and Berenson, G.S.: "Heart Smart"—a staff development model for a school-based cardiovascular health intervention, Health Educ. **19:**12, 1988.

Education Commission of the States: Recommendations for school health education: a handbook for state policymakers, report no. 130, Denver, 1981, Education Commission of the States.

Education Commission of the States: State policy support for school health education: a review and analysis, report no. 182, Denver, 1982, Education Commission of the States.

Eisner, E., and Valloner, E., editors: Conflicting conceptions of curriculum, Berkely, Calif., 1974, McCutchan Publishing Corp.

Fodor, J.T., and Dalis, G.T.: Health instruction: theory and application, ed. 3, Philadelphia, 1981, Lea & Febiger.

Garrard, J.: Health education and science education: changing roles, common goals? Studies in Science Education **13:**26, 1986.

Golaszewski, T.J.: Influencing behavior through instruction: methodology in health education, Washington, D.C., 1979, ERIC Clearinghouse on Teacher Education.

Goodlad, J.I.: Planning and organizing for teaching. Project on instruction, Washington, D.C., 1963, National Education Association.

Goodlad, J.I., et al.: Curriculum inquiry: the study of curriculum practice, New York, 1979, McGraw-Hill Book Co.

Goodlad, J.I.: A study of schooling: some findings and hypothesis, Phi Delta Kappan, p. 465, March 1983.

Governor's Steering Committee on Social Problems: Report from the Governor's Steering Committee on Social Problems in Health and Hospital Costs, New York, 1971, State of New York.

Gow, D.T., and Casey, T.W.: Selected learning activities. In Finwich, W.E., editor: Yearbook fundamental curriculum decisions, Alexandria, Va., 1983, Association for Supervision and Curriculum Development.

Green, L.W.: Three ways research influences policy and practice: the public's right to know and the scientist's responsibility to educate, Health Educ. **18:**44, 1987.

Hansen, W.B., Malotte, C.K., and Fielding, J.E.: Evaluation of a tobacco and alcohol abuse prevention curriculum for adolescents, Health Educ. Q. **15**:93, 1988.

Hill, W.F.: Learning: a survey of psychological interpretations, Scranton, Pa., 1963, Chandler Publishing Co.

Illinois State Board of Education: Phase I mandate studies final staff recommendations, Springfield, Ill., 1983, Illinois State Board of Education.

Killip, D.E., and others: Integrated school and community programs, J. Sch. Health **57**:437, 1987.

Kleibard, H.: Education at the turn of the century: a crucible for curriculum change, Ed. Res. **11**(1):16, 1982.

Lohmann, D.K., and DeJoy, D.M.: Utilizing the competency-based curriculum framework for curriculum revision: a case study, Health Educ. **18**:36, 1988.

Means, R.K.: Historical perspective on school health, Thorofare, N.J., 1975, Charles B. Slack, Inc.

Office of the Assistant Secretary for Health and the Surgeon General: Healthy people: the Surgeon General's report on health promotion and disease prevention. DHEW Pub. no. (PHS) 79-55071, Washington, D.C., 1979, U.S. Government Printing Office.

Pollock, M.B., and Oberteuffer, D.: Health science and the young child, New York, 1974, Harper & Row, Publishers, Inc.

Posner, G.J., and Rudnitsky, A.N.: Course design: a guide to curriculum development for teachers, New York, 1978, Longman, Inc.

Pratt, D.: Curriculum design and development, New York, 1980, Harcourt Bruce Jovanovich, Inc.

President's Committee on Health Education: The report of the President's Committee on Health Education, New York, 1973, the Committee.

Public Health Service: Promoting health, preventing diseases — objectives for the nation, Washington, D.C., 1980, U.S. Government Printing Office.

Redican, K.J., Olsen, L.K., and Stone, D.B.: Health education: a positive force in increasing the reading skills of low socio-economic elementary students, Urban Rev. **2**(4):215, 1979.

Rist, M.C.: Antismoking policies can work in schools, Educ. Dig. **52**:53, 1987.

Schlaadt, R.G.: School health education. In Brandt, R.S., editor: Yearbook content of the curriculum, Alexandria, Va., 1988, Association for Supervision and Curriculum Development.

School Health Education Study: Health education: a conceptual approach to curriculum design, St. Paul, 1968, 3M Education Press.

Simpson, M.: School-based and centrally directed curriculum development — the middle ground, Scott. Educ. Rev. **2**:16, 1986.

Tyler, R.W. In Schaffarzich, J., and Hampton, D.H., editors: Strategies for curriculum development, Berkeley, Calif., 1975, McCutchan Publishing Corp.

Tyler, R.W.: A place called school, Phi Delta Kappan, p. 462, March 1983.

U.S. Department of Health, Education and Welfare: The School Health Curriculum Project, Public Health Service, Center for Disease Control, Bureau of Health Education, Atlanta, 1977, U.S. Government Printing Office.

U.S. Department of Health, Education and Welfare, Office of Education, Health Education Program: Proposed regulations governing award of grants to state and local educational leagues. II, Fed. Reg. **44**(115):34024, June 13, 1979.

U.S. Department of Health and Human Services, Public Health Service: Promoting health and preventing disease: objectives for the nation, Washington, D.C., 1980, U.S. Government Printing Office.

Willgoose, C.E.: Health teaching in secondary schools, ed. 3, Philadelphia, 1982, W.B. Saunders Co.

Willgoose, C.E.: Saving the curriculum for health education, J. Sch. Health **43**:189, 1973.

Zais, R.: Curriculum principles and foundations, New York, 1976, Thomas Y. Crowell Co.

13

Elementary School Health Instruction

OVERVIEW   *Several curriculum and scheduling patterns for health instruction in elementary schools are discussed; these include integration, correlation, and direct teaching. Successful programs employ each of these approaches. There are many opportunities for the alert teacher to integrate and to correlate health-related activities and opportunities for health education in all areas of the curriculum as well as the regular school activities. However, for a program to be fully successful, the direct formal teaching of health is basic. Such a program has a planned set of learning activities, teaching materials, and a formally designated schedule for health instruction. The program is directed toward the accomplishing of clearly defined health education objectives. The role of the school health coordinator is discussed both at the school district and school building level. Emphasis is placed on the coordinating function in contrast to the administering or directing function. Coordination calls for cooperating and facilitating and in general providing support for the classroom teacher who is the central figure in the elementary school health instruction program. The health interest of primary and intermediate level students are identified together with ways of motivating students. Providing opportunities for students to achieve and to gain recognition for their improved health status is emphasized. Showing a person how he or she can accept responsibility for self-care and take pride in self is part of effective teaching.*

Criteria are offered for evaluating textbooks and other health education materials in order that materials of high quality may be selected. Several examples of available health education curriculums are presented to aid the teacher in his or her own curriculum planning. Health teaching units and sample teaching plans for several health topics such as sex education, or human relationships, environmental health, smoking, and dental health are included. Also included in an outline of the Primary Grades Health Curriculum Project (PGHCP). This guide for the primary grades is a companion curriculum to the School Health Curriculum Project, which is designed for the intermediate and junior high school grades (see Chapter 12).

OBJECTIVES   **After reading this chapter, the student should be able to:**

1. Explain several patterns for offering health instruction at the elementary school level

2. Name several health topics to be included in the health curriculum for an elementary school

3. Explain the role of a school health coordinator in the health instruction programs

4. Suggest criteria for evaluating textbooks as well as criteria for evaluating other forms of health education literature

5. Identify several topics that would be included in sex education at the primary and intermediate grade levels

6. Explain some of the typical concerns parents are likely to have about a sex education program

7. Explain the several different unit formats that are represented by the various curriculums now available

8. Explain the general organization of the Primary Grades Health Curriculum Project and show how it is related to the School Health Curriculum Project

The school is not the sole agency that contributes to the health education of a child. However, the core of health instruction must come for the school. Other health instruction should not be considered an embellishment of the program of the school but an intensification and extension of what the school is doing (Fig. 13-1). The school must proceed on the principle that it will provide the best possible health instruction for the pupils and that other sources of health instruction will add to it. This is altogether sound because some children have limited opportunities for health instruction outside of school.

In the elementary school, health instruction, like all other instructional areas, should be a meaningful experience of permanent value. In an effort to make health interesting and enjoyable, the means should not become so important that it obscures the real purpose of the

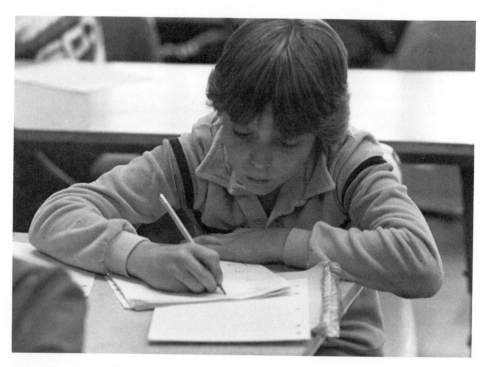

FIG. 13-1. The study of health can help elementary school children develop their basic skills of reading, writing, and locating information.
(Copyright 1983 by David Riecks.)

activity. Poster construction, puppet shows, and plays can be effective vehicles for health instruction, but when the poster, the puppets, or the play becomes the purpose of the experience, little in the way of health education is derived. Health instruction must be an effective experience, not a delightful diversion. An elementary school teacher should resolve to affect the health of each child favorably.

ORGANIZING FOR EFFECTIVE HEALTH INSTRUCTION

Once the health curriculum or course of study has been established, the next logical step is the organization of the implementation of the curriculum. Health instruction must be fitted into the total school schedule. More than time is involved. Effective instruction requires that all possible teaching opportunities be included in the class organization. The schedule for health instruction should allow for planned teaching, incidental learning, correlation, and integration. Although flexible, the schedule must be sufficiently definite to ensure effective health instruction. Certain current practices in education indicate the principles that will guide scheduling for health instruction:

1. A weekly schedule provides for extended time periods and allows for necessary flexibility.
2. A daily health period is not required for health instruction
3. Two fairly extended periods per week may be sufficient for health instruction in the primary grades, and three periods per week can serve the intermediate grades.
4. A flexible schedule allows for continuation of an activity that is particularly challenging.
5. Opportunities should be provided for the varieties of activities that health instruction entails.
6. When special health needs or interests require it, the schedule should be rearranged. Extra time invested in health instruction during one week can be followed by incidental instruction in the following week or weeks.
7. Opportunities for incidental and integrated health instruction should not be sacrificed to maintain a rigid schedule.
8. Correlation of health with other areas, to be effective, must be given a definite place in the organization for health instruction.

District health coordinator's role

The health director should be thought of primarily as a supervisor. Recent studies reveal the competent supervision more than justifies its cost in the added effectiveness that it gives to the school program. A supervisor who can help each teacher improve his or her services by 5% has made a considerable contribution.

The help of a supervisor enables teachers to do a more effective job. In helping teachers to organize their health instruction program, the coordinator may give them the benefit of his or her professional preparation and experience as well as knowledge of the total school health program. The health coordinator become the key to the grade-to-grade integration of health instruction and is also familiar with state requirements and resources. The health coordinator does not hand classroom teachers a schedule or plan for organization but instead works with them in developing or reviewing proposals for improving the program.

An experienced health coordinator recognizes individual differences in teachers and accordingly recognizes that each teacher organizes his or her teaching plan in a pattern that best fits his or her particular abilities. Variation from grade to grade in the organization of health instruction is an indication of a vital program.

During the course of the year the coordinator or supervisor may serve as a consultant with the teacher in working out problems or in developing approaches that might be introduced. The coordinator appraises the program both during the year and at the conclusion of the year.

Administrator's responsibility

If there is a health coordinator, the principal should serve as a resource person for organizing health instruction. Some elementary school principals have an excellent health background and can provide valuable health supervision. However, even principals with a very limited health background can be of assistance to the classroom teacher in resolving specific problems that may be particularly vexing.

School building health coordinator

Some elementary schools have regular staff members who serve as resource people in music, art, geography, health, and other areas. An elementary school teacher with a minor in health may well serve in these roles. This health resource person may serve as a consultant to other teachers in the building.

Classroom teacher's function

Minimal health preparation of the elementary school teacher should be course work in general hygiene, school health services, and health instruction. Further health preparation would be highly desirable, but the many competencies expected of the elementary teacher leave little room for electives in the college curriculum. However, in-service preparation could include such course work as the health of the school-aged child, physical growth and development, and mental health, as well as other courses.

Classroom teachers are the key persons in the organization and implementation of elementary school health instruction. Others may advise teachers and assist in various ways, but, because of their strategic location, only teachers are in a position to appreciate the total situation and the health implications inherent in it. Because they will direct children in learning, it is essential that they have a complete grasp of the health instruction plan and organization. If an inflexible plan and organization are handed to them, they are not likely to do an effective job of health teaching. On the other hand, if they have been prime figures in the development of a health instruction plan and organization, their familiarity with the *what*, *how*, and *why* of the program should make their contribution a more meaningful and more effective one.

When teachers are left to their own resources, they are justified in utilizing plans and programs that have been developed by others and then modifying and adapting them to their own classroom situations. Such curriculums should be treated as guides, and teachers should feel free and be encouraged to make adaptations to suit the needs of their students. The use of several sources may provide teachers with the substance from which to organize their own health instruction. Whatever the approach or source of reference, the health needs and interests of the children in a particular classroom should be the focal center from which the program emerges. The health concerns and outcomes in terms of the students are the vehicle that propels the program. The guiding motive in the organization of health instruction is to provide students with opportunities to explore health concerns and to solve vital health problems.

Certain universal health needs and interests of pupils make it possible for teachers to use available materials and to apply them effectively to the immediate situation. Yet each group of children has need for special health emphasis or the consideration of a different type of health program. For this reason, in a new situation an elementary schoolteacher might consider the organization of health instruction for a half year. A reappraisal at that time will indicate the strengths and weaknesses of the program and the modifications that are in order.

CLASSROOM INSTRUCTION

Motivating pupils sufficiently so that they want to establish desirable health practices is the basis for all health instruction. Motivation is the catalyst of all teaching, but it is most essential in health teaching.

Fundamental to motivation in elementary school health instruction is giving each pupil status in the classroom. A *team* concept — us, we, all of us — must permeate the atmosphere. This relationship within the groups should be supported by a strong teacher-pupil relationship. Active participation in health projects is needed for all pupils. Neither passive nor vicarious participation will establish health practices. Above all, an organic relationship of pupil to group and group to pupil must be maintained for effective health instruction.

Pride in oneself, in one's own accomplishments, and in one's own progress is basic to all of us. Developing this pride constitutes a most effective means for initiating a health practice and for continuing the practice until it becomes ingrained in pupil's mode of life. Appeal to pride in personal appearance can be as effective at the elementary school level as at adolescence if attention and praise are properly distributed.

Self-progress reinforced by an understanding of that progress motivates pupils in their quest for advancement. Competition with themselves can be wholesome motivation for pupils when realistic standards are guide and when counseling in appraisal of their advances, plateaus, and failures is offered. Achievements that are visible to children can stimulate them to further achievement. It may be necessary to help them see their achievements.

Unless children internalize health instruction themselves, the whole opportunity for education has been missed. They must be the center of action — the vital element of greatest consideration. Moreover, they should believe this and be stimulated by it. This, of course, is necessary for any teaching situation to be effective.

At all times the elementary school teacher should direct health instruction toward the establishment of certain desirable health practices. Knowledge and attitudes can grow out of the establishment of health practices, contributing to their formation and permanence. These practices should be related to recognized factors in health such as play and rest, vision promotion, hearing protection, care of the teeth, cleanliness, general appearance, use of the toilet, avoiding infection, work practices, sleep, safety at school, safety at home, going to and from school, bicycle safety, fire safety, water safety, courtesy, self-reliance, self-discipline, and social adjustment. Specific practices will be listed in units and other sources that follow, but the teacher with some degree of ingenuity can develop a list of practices suited to the particular group of youngsters in the room.

In a well-organized systemwide health program, certain specific health practices should be common to all elementary schools as a guide in health education. This common core of practices will provide continuity and intensification. It will ensure some measure of performance in health practices. In an elementary school where teachers agree on health practices to be established, the health program is assured of reasonably effective long-term results. Besides the reinforcing effect of such an established program, the likelihood of omissions is reduced, if not eliminated.

Various approaches to health instruction are in general use. Each has merit and can be used to advantage when adapted to particular needs and situations. Four approaches are of special interest:

1. Integrated living as health instruction
2. Planned direct formal and informal instruction
3. Incidental instruction
4. Correlated health instruction

Because all four approaches have special attributes and merits, the prudent elementary teacher uses all four in conducting an effective health instruction program. Together the four approaches tend to ensure the maximum in effective health instruction.

INTEGRATED LIVING AS HEALTH INSTRUCTION

Life is not cast in a mold of isolated islands or separate compartments. Interwoven in each child's daily activities are health implications, values, and factors. All adaptation that pupils make has implications for either mental or physical health. In some activities health occupies a prominent role, and in others it assumes a lesser role. Yet whether it occupies a major or minor role, if the opportunity for health instruction is fully developed, the resulting health education can be both effective and lasting. If learning is a meaningful and functional experience, it becomes an established, integral part of the mode of living of a child — the true goal of the school.

Pupil-teacher relationships

No one has objectively measured the specific influence of a particular teacher on a given pupil. Yet there is ample evidence that the teacher can modify the child in a beneficial way. Perhaps no phase of the school health instruction program can have a more beneficial, lasting effect than the teacher's interest in and encouragement of each child's health. The approval of the teacher can develop the self-interest in health that is necessary to the promotion of personal health. From such experiences will develop worthy health goals, which, because of self-esteem, each person will strive to maintain. Teachers make a lasting wholesome impression when they recognize and commend the child's cleanliness, appearance, dental care, posture, safety measures, dietary practices, courtesy, thoughtfulness, social adjustment, vitality, buoyancy, and general development. To the child, health truly becomes a matter of personal concern and gratification. It is the seed from which will develop a lifelong interest in personal health promotion.

Most teachers are interested in the well-being of schoolchildren. However, this interest should be expressed by interest in the child's health and his or her efforts in its behalf. Could there be a more worthy outcome of the total program of the school than students with a wholesome concern for their own health and with the necessary preparation to make the decisions that relate to their health and to that of their families? Pupil-teacher relationships provide the most effective means for motivating children to accept responsibility for the promotion of their own health.

School experiences

Many school activities with health aspects provide opportunities for effective education. At times the instructional opportunities are missed completely. Perhaps more frequently, the experience is given cursory treatment. An alert teacher not only uses the unusual event for instructional purposes but also recognizes opportunities for health instruction in the regular program.

There are many opportunities in daily school experiences to apply health knowledge. The acts of coming to school and going home involve problems in safety for pedestrians, for bicycle riders, for general traffic, and for bus riders. Within the school, safety is an ever-present problem. Lighting, ventilation, cleanliness, dental health, posture, activity, rest, lunchroom practices, and social problems provide a diversity of opportunities for learning and its application.

Unusual experiences can have health implications of instructional value. The illness of a child can have learning value for classmates if the teacher directs the learning into constructive channels. An appendectomy can be discussed in terms of early indications, the desirability of avoiding self-diagnosis and self-medication, the need for immediate medical care, the effectiveness of modern medicine, and the importance of relying on the physician to restore health. Thus the fact that it is the individual who promotes health and the physician who restores health can be reemphasized.

If a child in the class wears glasses because of a physician's advice, the wisdom of wearing glasses can be emphasized by a class study of the problem. If the situation is dealt with openly, the supposed onus that youngsters may associate with glasses is removed. The children can learn that wearing glasses is not a stigma, but the badge of a person who is wise enough to use the fruits of modern science, just as a wise person uses other modern inventions.

Occasionally sensitive circumstances that relate to health arise in the school. Discretion would indicate that the teacher consider the situation carefully. After extended deliberation a means of using the event for instructional purposes may be devised. Perhaps the solution will be to consider related problems rather than the specific event. If a child has been hospitalized with influenza, a discussion of the measures for control of communicable disea   rather than of influenza alone may be less disturbing but educationally just as valuable.

Many school experiences merit repeated consideration. A single discussion may create an interest but may not result in effective learning. Correlation of the factors in two or more experiences adds interest to the discussion and provokes thinking.

Community experiences

Events in the community may be a concern of schoolchildren. In the primary grades pupils have only slight community interest, which tends to develop as they reach the intermediate grades. Expansion of the municipal water facilities, construction of a sewage disposal plant, restaurant inspection, control measures for communicable disease, medical services, air pollution, safety programs, industrial health, recreation, and special health drives should be of interest to the future adults of the nation. Community health personnel can serve as a resource for stimulating the interest of children in community health.

Interest in local health can be projected to the state and nation. Children can acquire health understanding from epidemics, disasters involving health problems, new health experiments and discoveries, reports on the conquest of disease, extension of life expectation, and population growth. Indeed, international health can become interesting.

PLANNED DIRECT INSTRUCTION

With the elementary school program fragmented, as it tends to be, a scheduled time for health instruction is helpful. Doubtless a few teachers, highly skilled in incidental, correlated, and integrated health instruction, may do an effective job of health teaching without a scheduled period for health, but most teachers will need definite scheduled time to provide the necessary core instruction. A daily period is not necessary, but a fairly extended period of 30 minutes twice a week for primary pupils and three periods a week for intermediate children should serve as a minimum for core health instruction if supplementary health teaching makes a reasonably strong contribution. Such scheduling does not make an inordinate demand on school time.

Direct teaching is the core of the instructional program. Other procedures can supplement it advantageously, but the base of the instruction pyramid should be direct teaching. It serves many purposes and has definite advantages, such as the following:

1. Gives status to health as a subject area
2. Assures at least a minimum of emphasis on teaching
3. Provides an organized approach
4. Deals with realistic specific needs
5. Makes effective results possible for a teacher of average ability
6. Tends to emphasize the positive aspects of health
7. Can be applied even with incidental teaching
8. Can emerge from correlated teaching
9. Can be channeled into integrated and other approaches
10. Provides for outcomes in terms of interpretations, values, and other worthwhile attributes

The imaginative teacher can use direct teaching as an adventure in health education, as effective as it is interesting.

Allocation and gradation

Emphasis for areas of special teaching should be allocated in the overall plans for health instruction. The key must be the interests and needs of the children at each age level. Health instruction is effective when it begins with children and their concerns or problems. If they can identify with a health problem and associate themselves with it, it takes on a personal meaning. The most effective health education is achieved when it seems to emanate from children rather than to be imposed on them from above. Complexity of treatment is adjusted to the psychologic level of the pupils. Interests of the students indicate levels of maturity.

Areas of emphasis

Teachers can obtain an overview of the health needs, interests, and problems from observing the children; from their questions; from observing school, home, and community life; from statements of parents; from suggestions of health personnel; and from school records. Teachers will notice that children in their early years tend to be individualists, which is reflected in their health interests. Starting in about the fifth grade, the tendency toward gangs begins to be expressed in an interest in group and community health.

Several studies have revealed the almost universal health interests and needs of children at various levels. An elementary teacher can be guided by these studies if no other data are available. Where allocations of areas have been made on a school basis, results of these studies have frequently been used as a guide. Usually kindergarten and grades 1, 2, and 3 are grouped, and in grades 4, 5, and 6 individual assignments of areas are given. It will be noticed that the health of the individual is emphasized in the early years and community health is emphasized beginning with the fifth grade. Repetition and duplication are not necessarily objectionable. Certain duplications are inevitable, even desirable, but specific emphasis changes with the maturity of the pupil. Nutrition in the primary grades deals with a few simple dietary practices. In the intermediate grades an understanding of the *how* and *why* of certain nutritional needs is of interest to the pupils (Tables 13-1 and 13-2).

Motivation

A cue to all motivation in education is the natural human desire for self-status through attention, achievement, advancement, improvement, superiority, praise, and recognition. Motivation in health instruction should be relatively simple because health deals directly with a pupil's own welfare, but the whole experience must begin within the child if encouragement and direction are to be given him or her.

To promote self-identification in health, effort should be made to introduce each topic as a problem that is the concern of all who are present. By using a question as the vehicle, the problem should be launched with emphasis on *you, we, all of us,* or *you and I.* The question should include or imply self-improvement. How can *we* keep clean so that *we* always look nice? Out of this appeal to appearance and improvement will emanate subquestions of keeping the hair clean, having clean fingernails, and other specific activities. How can *you* keep *your* teeth healthy and looking nice? The approach can apply equally to *our* school, *our* community, and *our* nation.

Questions can serve various purposes in making the instruction effective, such as the following:

1. Arouse curiosity, stimulate interest, and develop purpose (Fig. 13-2)
2. Prepare pupils for learning by leading them to draw from their experiences what they need and are concerned about

TABLE 13-1. Areas of emphasis in kindergarten and primary grades and grade 4

Kindergarten and primary grades	Grade 4
Physical health	
Personal cleanliness	Vision and hearing
School cleanliness	Illumination
Rest and sleep	Ventilation
Eating practices	Clothing
Posture	Cleanliness
Play practices	Acitivity
Dental health	Dental problems
Lighting	Nutrition
Common cold	Preventing infection
Safety to and from school	Illness
Schoolroom safety	Avoiding poisons
Playground safety	Fire prevention
Home safety	Traffic safety
Body growth	
Mental health	
Sharing	Sportsmanship
Working together	Self-direction
Kindness	Confidence
Being friendly	Our friends
Orderliness	Being grown up
Depending on ourselves	Courtesy
Attaining goals	Accepting disappointments
Community health	
Home life	Family health
Sources of water and milk	Helping the neighborhood
Sunshine and health	Improving the neighborhood

3. Cause the student to think and evaluate
4. Understand the pupil's thinking
5. Help the student discriminate
6. Direct the pupil's attention to significant elements
7. Bring about new concepts
8. Lead the pupils to give expression to their thinking
9. Help pupils see the pathway that might be taken

Once the project is launched, guidance and particularly recognition are necessary. Because children are gratified by their achievements, they have something to live up to, something to improve. Self-status becomes a wholesome motivating force. Every child can achieve some degree of success in feeling well, in improving personal appearance, and in following recognized health practices.

TABLE 13-2. Areas of emphasis in grades 5 and 6

Grade 5	Grade 6
Physical health	
Appraisal of personal health	Bicycle safety
Personal health promotion	Safety patrol
Balanced diets	Health examination
Food preparation and care	Body function
Communicable diseases	Growth and development
Recreation needs	Grooming
Developing skills	Posture
Body development	Rest and sleep
Relaxation	Communicable diseases
Types of school accidents	Home and farm safety
Playground accidents	Emergency care
Fire prevention	First-aid procedures
Fire drills	Safety patrol
Mental health	
Family relationships	Interesting people
Peer groups	Personality
Loyalties	Emotional adjustment
Social status	Life goals
Emotional maturation	Self-improvement
Community health	
Home sanitation	Community disease control
Health advertising	Community water supply
Community safety program	Milk control measures
School sanitation	Community sanitation

Methods

The versatile teacher uses a diversity of methods and adapts teaching to the needs and purposes of the situation. Certain teaching procedures are especially adaptable to the elementary school level. These include group discussion, lecturette, counseling, construction, independent study, oral presentation, problem solving, project method, reports, demonstration, dramatization, exhibits, field trips, and audiovisual aids.

In kindergarten and the primary grades the health instruction program can be based effectively on the development of desirable health practices. "Things we do" is the theme:

1. Wash carefully each morning.
2. Wash hands before and after eating.
3. Wash hands before leaving the toilet room.
4. Keep the fingernails clean.
5. Wash hair at least once a week.

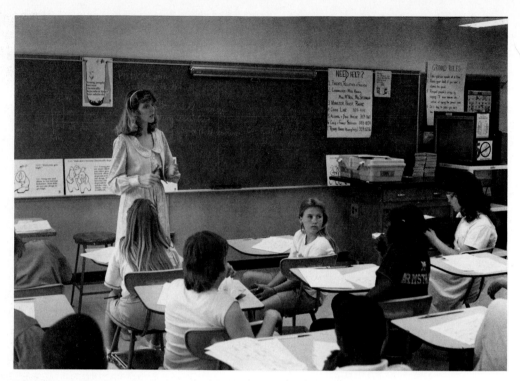

FIG. 13-2. The art of questioning requires skill in framing the question and sensitivity to the student's answer.

6. Keep the hair well groomed.
7. Bathe regularly.
8. Stand, sit, and walk tall.
9. Get to bed on time each night: kindergarten and first grade, 8:00 PM; second and third grades, 8:30 PM; fourth grade, 9:00 PM; and fifth and sixth grades, 9:30 PM.
10. Drink milk with each meal.
11. Eat fruit at least twice a day.
12. Eat green and yellow vegetables each day.
13. Include protein foods in each day's diet.
14. Brush the teeth after eating and floss before going to bed.
15. Visit the dentist regularly.
16. Keep fingers and other objects out of the mouth.
17. Use a clean handkerchief to cover a sneeze or cough.
18. Remain at home when ill.
19. Be alert for hazards that may cause accidents.
20. Follow all safety rules.
21. Use proper lights for all needs.
22. Keep things orderly.
23. Hang up wraps.
24. Play out of doors regularly if weather permits.
25. Work together with others.
26. Be friendly.
27. Accept disappointments cheerfully.
28. Finish tasks that are begun.

In the intermediate grades the health instruction program can be effectively incorporated into the general theme of daily living. This is functional instruction at its best.

The use of health texts or health readers and other written materials can be effective when these materials serve as a source of knowledge for pupils and do not constitute the total sum of the health instruction.

Materials

The busy elementary school classroom teacher must obtain instruction materials for a multitude of purposes. To assemble materials for health instruction poses an especially difficult task because of the diversity of topics encompassed by the term *health instruction*.

To assist the classroom teachers, several examples of health instruction units have been included in this chapter.

Two problems may be especially difficult for the elementary classroom teacher: What text should be used? Should commercially prepared materials for health instruction be used?

A textbook should be regarded as a reference. If textbooks are to be used in health instruction, certain standards in relation to health needs should then be met, in addition to the general criteria for all textbooks:

1. Primary emphasis should be on normal well-being.
2. Health principles should be stressed.
3. Discussion should be directed to the interests and needs of the pupils.
4. The topics of personal appearance, physical health, and mental health are important in the primary grades.
5. Community health should be included in the intermediate groups.
6. Basic anatomy and physiology are of interest to elementary school students, but health is more than anatomy and physiology.
7. An overview of each section can be of special value.
8. The literary style should be lucid and interesting.
9. Stimulating examples and original approaches add to the book's value.
10. Vocabulary should be adapted to the grade level.
11. A variety of suggested activities for pupils should be included.
12. Illustrations should be meaningful to the students.
13. Pupils should be able to understand and use the graphs and charts.
14. Suggestions for evaluation should be presented.

Commercial film makers, voluntary health organizations, and governmental agencies are producing an ever-increasing quantity of health education materials. Although the motivation in some instances may be to sell a product, much of this free and inexpensive material is of excellent quality. Because most schools have limited resources, it is important for teachers and curriculum coordinators to be aware of this potentially valuable source of instructional materials. However, it is essential that the teacher conduct a careful evaluation of such materials in order to determine their suitability for specific class needs. To aid the teacher in this effort, an evaluation form is included in Appendix A. The form has been adapted for use in the Office of the Superintendent of Public Instruction in the state of Washington. These general criteria can be readily adapted for use in health education.

Evaluation

In the final analysis, the effectiveness of the health instruction program should be measured in terms of improved health of the pupils. To a limited degree, this can be done both objectively and subjectively. The teacher can observe and measure the effect of health instruction in terms of the child's behavior. Health attitudes, health knowledge (Fig. 13-3), and health practices can be appraised in a practical way. Instruments for measurement are presented in Chapter 17. In considering specific evaluation of the health instruction, the teacher should ask one cardinal question: Is each child building a body of health knowledge and understanding that will enable him or her to make the decisions necessary for health?

ELEMENTARY SCHOOL CURRICULUMS: EXAMPLES

Several examples of health instruction materials for the elementary school have been selected to illustrate both subject matter and curriculum organization. Materials for the primary grades include the topic of sex education, which is illustrated by grade level units on human interrelationships. "Growing up healthy" illustrates a horizontal curriculum plan. It is designed as a year-long health teaching program composed of nine units to be taught by integration of the material with other basic subjects taught at the kindergarten level. The environmental health section illustrates the unit organization.

The Primary Grades Health Curriculum Project (PGHCP) has been included because it is an integrated part of a larger curriculum, a companion piece to be linked with the School Health Curriculum Project (SHCP) (see Chapter 12) for grades 4 to 7.

Thus the two projects, PGHCP and SHCP, provide an articulated health education curriculum from kindergarten to grade 7. An outline of the units for each of the primary grades is presented.

For the intermediate grades Unit 1, " Food Campaign," has been selected to illustrate the teaching of nutrition at the intermediate grade level. It is part of the National Dairy Council's comprehensive nutrition learning system. This sequentially planned curriculum includes instructional materials for preschool, the elementary grades, and the junior and senior high school levels.

The last example at the intermediate level is the level II oral health unit from the American Dental Association. The association has extensively field tested all of its health education materials. Both the teaching format and content organization should be useful to the teacher.

Sex education in the elementary school

Too many adults assume that the absence of formal sex instruction means that no sex education is occurring. However, the important question is not whether the child will receive sex education but rather what kind of sex education will the child receive. The reality of the home and parent relationship, how parents react to each other as sexual beings, the attitudes parents reveal toward their children's explorations of their bodies, the effect of parental efforts to establish the child's toilet habits, and family members' ability to give and to express love for each other all are factors that represent powerful forces shaping the child's sexual feelings and attitudes.

All too often sex education tends to be a narrowly based reproductive education or a kind of moralistic teaching. Children are very much interested in and curious about their bodies. Thus a study of the reproductive process can provide a good starting point from which to develop adolescents' understanding of their roles and relationships as men and women in the family context and in situations outside the family. Teaching about the anatomy and physiology of reproduction provides the teacher with a comfortable, objective, and impersonal approach to sex education. Eventually, such topics as dating relationships, sexual behavior, and moral codes must be considered. In these areas, students must be given a greater role and be encouraged to enter into open discussions and exchange of ideas—especially when questions such as standards of sexual behavior and the development of moral values arise. However, such discussions hold the potential for involvement in a school-community controversy. The teacher needs to be aware of the anxieties that many parents have about their child's sexual development. Such anxiety may be characterized as parental hopes that their child will grow up to lead a conventional life and will avoid "getting in trouble." However, there is also a kind of parental ambivalence, with some parents fearful that, on the one hand, children may *not* be getting the kind of education they need to become responsible adults and that, on the other hand, children may get the wrong kind of information, which may lead them into trouble.

Examples of instructional objectives for the primary student are as follows:
1. Develops a concept of self-worth and sexual identity
2. Recognizes that there are sex differences between boys and girls
3. Recognizes his or her role in the family
4. Accepts reproduction as a natural process of life
5. Develops an understanding and respect for the rights of others
6. Develops respect for the body and uses correct terminology in referring to parts of the body

Some instructional objectives for the intermediate student are as follows:
1. Continues to develop an understanding of the roles of each member of the family
2. Develops the self-image as a worthy member of society
3. Continues to develop an emotional acceptance of sex as a normal aspect of life
4. Develops an understanding of puberty and associated growth changes
5. Assumes more responsibility for his or her own care and for the care of others
6. Develops an ability to discuss sex objectively and in a dignified, unembarrassed manner

Human interrelationships: primary grades

The study of interpersonal relationships can provide an important vehicle for teaching sex education in the primary grades. Interpersonal relations are at the core of all sexual expression. Until about 10 years of age, a boy's output of male sex hormones (androgens) is but slightly greater than his output of female hormones (estrogens). In a 10-year-old girl the output of estrogens is little more than the output of androgens. At this stage of life children are neutral in sexuality and have no particular interest in anything of a sexual nature. Thus certain social conditioning must occur in order to help the boy and girl develop their roles as male and female.

AIM OF THE UNITS ON HUMAN INTERRELATIONSHIPS

Develops in children those qualities of personal worth that will command respect from others and will have a mutual respect for others.

OBJECTIVES

Develop in children attributes of:
1. Wholesome pride in self
2. Respect for parents
3. Respect for brothers and sisters
4. Respect for classmates
5. Respect for teachers
6. Respect for other people
7. Respect for authority
8. Respect for the rights of others
9. Respect for privacy
10. Respect for property
11. Thoughtfulness
12. Kindness
13. Fair play
14. Sharing
15. Obedience
16. Cooperation
17. Honesty
18. Courtesy
19. Responsibility
20. Consideration
21. Neatness

GRADE LEVEL UNIT TITLES

Kindergarten

Unit Title — Every Boy and Girl a Friend

Grade 1

Unit Title — Social Development

Grade 2

Unit Title — Social, Emotional Growth

Grade 3

Unit Title — Growth and Maturing

SAMPLE UNIT

The grade 3 unit has been selected to illustrate the unit format and the content.

Concepts and activities

    I. Life and growth
      A. Discussion
          1. All life has a beginning, grows, changes, matures, and eventually dies.
          2. In which ways are plants and animals alike and different?
          3. All life reproduces itself.
          4. How do plants reproduce themselves?
          5. What do plants need to keep alive, and where do these things come from?
          6. Plants grow, change, and carry on certain activities.
          7. How important are plants to the lives of all of us?

8. Animals have young that are hatched from eggs or are borne by the mother.
9. Care of the young is important for all animal species.
10. Care of their babies is important to our parents too.
11. Discuss the nature of human growth.
12. How do we change from babyhood through each stage to adulthood?
13. Discuss how boys and girls differ in their growth patterns.
14. All life needs nourishment for what purposes?
15. How does what we feed the baby differ from what children 8 or 9 years old are fed?
16. Discuss what is meant by a well-balanced diet.
17. How does the school lunch provide for growth?
18. Evaluate personal diets.

B. Construction
1. Have an aquarium or terrarium in the room to demonstrate the "web of life."
2. Grow plants from seeds and seedlings.
3. Make a chart of the four basic food groups.
4. Plan a single meal such as breakfast.
5. Plan a menu for a day.
6. Make a chart of stages of growth using cutouts as models.
7. Make a bulletin board or mural titled "What helps us grow?"
8. Make lists of how children differ: physical characteristics, manners, grooming, speaking, opinions, interests.

C. Dramatization and other activities
1. Get information from parents on family growth characteristics and report to the class.
2. Report on human growth differences throughout the world.
3. Using a veterinary resource, report on rate of animal growth over a period of several weeks.
4. Have a nurse, physician, or other resource person talk on human life, growth, and well-being.
5. Bring baby pictures to school and have children guess who each is.

II. Maturing
A. Discussion
1. How does maturing differ from growth?
2. What does it mean to act grown up?
3. What feelings or emotions do we have?
4. How do we control the emotion of anger?
5. How do we control selfishness or meanness?
6. Why do people dislike us if we cheat?
7. What is meant by:
   a. Happiness
   b. Honesty
   c. Courage
   d. Respect
   e. Forgiveness
   f. Responsibility
8. How do our thoughts about ourselves influence the way we think about others?
9. Why does self-respect promote respect for others?
10. Why should we always try to have more friends?
11. How do we get more friends?
12. What qualities do you like in others?
13. What do we mean when we say a certain third-grader acted like a first-grader?

14. What do we mean when we say a certain third-grader acted like a fifth-grader?
15. Notice individual differences and qualities.
16. How do we show others we value their friendship?

B. Construction
1. On the blackboard each week have a question relating to behavior asking if all students have exhibited a certain quality each day (e.g., "Am I courteous?" "Am I thoughtful?" "Am I dependable?").
2. Post pictures displaying desirable mature conduct.
3. Have children keep records of their good deeds.
4. Have children make an appraisal of their best qualities and those in which improvement is needed.

C. Dramatization and other activities
1. Read the book, *Laugh and Cry,* by Gerrold Beim, which explains that emotions are natural.
2. Tell stories to the class about people with exceptional courage, thoughtfulness, dependability, or other qualities
3. Have children report an exceptional case of helpfulness, courtesy, industriousness, or other qualities they have observed.
4. Have a skit that demonstrates courtesies of boys toward girls and of girls toward boys.
5. Demonstrate courteous conduct toward adults in various walks of life.
6. Have each of a panel of five give a description of some junior high youngster who is unusually mature and explain why he or she is regarded as unusually mature.

Evaluation

Observe class members regarding:
1. Interest in life about them
2. Concern for life
3. Interest in their own growth
4. Interest in children in other parts of the world
5. Interest in nutrition and nutritional practices
6. Concern about growth of others
7. Desire to improve relationships with other children
8. Interest in expanding friendships
9. Respect shown for adults and pupils
10. Increased sense of responsibility
11. Honesty
12. Obedience
13. Ability to make amends for mistakes

Growing Up Healthy: environmental health*

The President's Committee on Health Studies issued a special background paper entitled "Health Education of Preschool Children and their Parents" (1972) that stressed the need for health education throughout the entire program of early childhood education, with emphasis placed on the preschool and primary grades. *Growing up Healthy,* a health education

---

*The material in this section is from Hazlett, S.H.: Growing up healthy, 1983, Zellerbach Family Fund.

curriculum guide for the kindergarten level, provides an excellent example of an innovative response to this challenge. This curriculum project was supported by the Zellerbach Family Fund and was originally developed in conjunction with the San Francisco Unified School District. It is a multidisciplinary curriculum designed to enhance and reinforce the basic subjects of language arts, reading, and mathematics. These basic areas provide the avenues for the teaching of health. Materials included have been selected to illustrate the goals and one of the nine student behavioral objectives. Unit 8, "Environmental Health, " a unique topic for teaching health at this level, has been chosen to show how the unit is organized.

An inexpensive workshop leader manual that contains guidelines and procedures for conducting a short 2- to 3-hour workshop session is available. It is all that is required to prepare teachers to use the program. The curriculum is designed to cover one school year; each of the nine units covers approximately 1 month of instructional time. Another unique feature of the curriculum is its multilingual character. Parent letters are available in five languages: English, Spanish, Chinese, Tagalog, and Vietnamese. The curriculum has three major goals and one student behavioral objective for each of the nine units. To illustrate the program the goals and the student behavioral objective for Unit 8 are presented.

GOALS

1. To encourage kindergarten children to take an active role in developing and practicing good health habits
2. To improve compliance with Assembly Bills 2068 and 4284, which require children to have a physical examination before the third month of first grade
3. To assist parents and teachers in helping children make positive health habits an integral part of their daily lives.

STUDENT BEHAVIORAL OBJECTIVE

The student identifies ways to keep the environment safe and clean.

The *Growing Up Healthy* curriculum is organized into nine lesson units. The topics of these units are:

1. The physical examination
2. Cleanliness
3. Dental health
4. Nutrition
5. Safety
6. Foot health
7. Movement and relaxation
8. Environmental health
9. Mental health

Each lesson unit is divided into three major sections: preactivity, activity, and enrichment activities. The preactivity sections offer a variety of individual learning experiences. The activity section combines several learning experiences and offers suggestions for presentation of a half-hour lesson. Examples from Unit 8 are presented here.

Text continued on p. 321.

Growing Up Healthy

STUDENT BEHAVIORAL OBJECTIVE

The student identifies ways to keep the environment safe and clean.

Pre-Activities

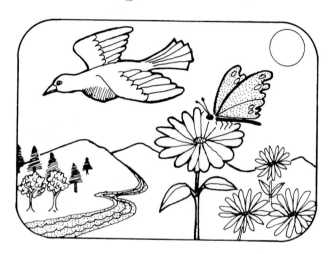

1. OUR BEAUTIFUL WORLD
   A. Read a book that presents our world as a beautiful environment to see, hear, enjoy. (One such book is: *Be Quiet Beside the Lake.*)

   B. View slides or pictures of forests, lakes, birds. Variation: take a field trip to a park, lake, or forest

   C. Discuss:
      (1) Our world gives us many beautiful sights, sounds and scents to enjoy.
      (2) What are some of the beautiful sights? (butterflies, blossoming trees, wildflowers, hills, birds, squirrels)
      (3) What are some of the beautiful sounds? (raindrops dropping, birds singing)
      (4) What are some of the beautiful scents? (flowers, fresh air)
      (5) How can we keep sights and sounds in our world healthy and beautiful? (by not littering, by not writing on walls, by being quiet in quiet places, by taking care of natural resources)

PRE-ACTIVITIES (cont.)

2. PAINT YOUR BEAUTIFUL WORLD
   A. Ask students to imagine that they are in the most beautiful place in the world. Imagine:
      (1) What your special, beautiful, clean place looks like and smells like.
      (2) That you are exactly where you would like to be in your beautiful environment.
      (3) How you feel in your beautiful environment.
   B. Ask students to paint or draw a picture of themselves in their special place.

3. HEAR YOUR BEAUTIFUL WORLD
   A. Discuss:
      (1) All places can be beautiful. The city, country, our homes, and schools have beautiful sights, sounds and scents.
      (2) Our own classroom is a beautiful place with beautiful sights and sounds.
      (3) What are beautiful sights in our classroom?
      (4) What are beautiful sounds in our classroom?
      (5) What are beautiful scents in our classroom? (flowers, food we prepared)

4. A NEW WORD: ENVIRONMENT
   A. Discuss:
      (1) Our environment includes all the sights and sounds in the world around us.
      (2) What are some things that are in our environment? (plants, people, buildings, animals)
      (3) When at school, our environment includes the classroom, school building and school yard.
      (4) When at home, our environment includes our apartment or house and neighborhood.
      (5) Our environment includes everything in the air, water, and on land.
   B. Ask children to identify animals that live in one of the three areas of the environment: land, water, or air.
   C. Discuss: We want to take care of our environment so animals, plants, people can live there well.

5. TREATING PETS RIGHT
   A. Show pictures of pets: cats, dogs, birds, etc.
   B. Discuss:
      (1) Part of keeping care of our environment is taking proper care of our pets
      (2) How do we treat our pets right?

Activity

PREPARATION/MATERIALS

1. Cans (i.e., soup) that have been covered with cloth and sealed with a rubber band
2. A non-toxic "smellable" substance in each can. (i.e., vinegar, lemon slice, pickle, perfume, coffee, orange slice, peppercorns)
3. Two large sheets of paper, one labeled "It smells good!" with a drawing of a happy face and the other labeled "It smells bad!" with a drawing of a frowning face

DESCRIPTION OF ACTIVITY

Each child smells the content of each cloth-covered can, identifies if the smell is pleasant or unpleasant, then places the jar on the appropriate sheet of paper.

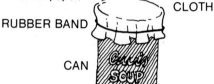

CLOTH

RUBBER BAND

CAN

ACTIVITY

1. INTRODUCTION
   A. Discuss the fact that our environment includes everything that we see, hear, and smell.
   B. Tell children that some things in our environment smell good, while other things smell bad.
   C. Explain that each child (or group of children) will smell a mystery substance and decide if it smells good or bad. (You may wish to add that the children will not taste or touch the substances, only smell them.)

2. SCENT INVESTIGATION
   A. Children individually smell each cloth-covered can.
   B. Each can is placed on the "happy face" paper if it has a pleasant scent, on the "sad face" paper if it has an unpleasant odor.

3. DISCUSS:
   A. Scents and odors make the air, which is part of our environment, smell good or bad.
   B. We can keep our air clean and sweet-smelling by not putting bad odors into it.
   C. How can we keep our air clean? (properly disposing of garbage; wearing clean clothes; wiping and washing spills such as spilled milk)
   D. Tobacco smoke in the air is not good for you. It can be harmful when you smoke the cigarette or cigar; it can be harmful if you breathe the smoke from someone else's cigarette or cigar. When you can, avoid breathing smoke from someone's cigarette or cigar.

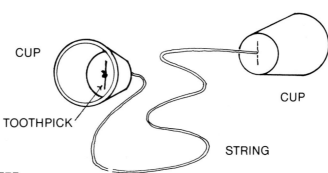

1. SOUND TRANSPORTER
   A. Discuss:
      (1) When the sounds in the air are quiet, we can hear what we want to hear.
      (2) When the air is filled with loud noises, it is very hard to hear what we want to hear.
   B. Have each child make a string and paper cup telephone from a string, two toothpicks and two styrofoam or paper cups, by:
      (1) Using a pencil to poke a small hole in the base of each paper cup.
      (2) Threading a string through the hole in each paper cup.
      (3) Tying the end of each string to a toothpick.
   C. Direct each pair of children to pull taut the string linking the two cups.
   D. One child talks softly into one cup while the other listens in the other.
   E. Ask children to find out how well or poorly the cup-telephone works in quiet and noisy environments.
   F. Discuss:
      (1) It is easier to hear what we want to hear in quiet environments.
      (2) How can we keep our environment from being too noisy? (by talking softly; placing items down gently)

2. IT'S UP TO ME!
   A. Discuss:
      (1) Our environment includes things that we see as well as smell and hear.
      (2) The world we see may be clean and beautiful or it may be unkempt and dirty.
      (3) How does our room look when it is clean? (equipment is put away; coats are hung up; the floor is clean)
      (4) How does our room look when it is dirty? (pencils, crayons, materials are left on the floor; clothing is not hung up)
   B. Ask children to look for things in their classroom environment that look good.
   C. Ask children to:
      (1) Look for things in their classroom environment that do not look good.
      (2) Discuss how those places could be improved.
      (3) Carry out a plan for improving their classroom environment.

ENRICHMENT ACTIVITIES (cont.)

3. USE IT ALL
   A. Discuss:
      (1) We use up many things in our environment.
      (2) What are some things that we use? (water, paper, food, clothes).
      (3) We can run out of some things (water, paper).
      (4) It is important to not be wasteful in using some things.
      (5) How can we be more careful in using up things our environment gives us? (taking only as much food as we can eat; using both sides of a piece of paper; not letting the water run while brushing our teeth)
   B. Identify a way to conserve the use of some item in the classroom.
   C. Practice conserving at least one item in the classroom.
   D. Identify ways to conserve the use of water at home and at school. Some responses include: not running water while brushing teeth; filling the bathtub only part way full, taking a short shower.

4. LESS LITTER
   A. Children can search for and pick up litter in their school yard.
   B. They may then draw and paint posters which tell children to put litter in trash cans and waste baskets.
   C. Children can recycle aluminum pop cans and newspaper as a money-earning class project. Some stores pay 5¢ each for all-aluminum pop cans.

5. LANDFILL FIELD TRIP
   Note: Children may be surprised to learn that today's landfills are very different from yesterday's dumps. Current methods of solid waste disposal are often highly mechanized, scientific, and technical.
   A. Children may visit a landfill and learn how the city disposes of their waste materials, then discuss:
      (1) Why is it important to dispose of used-up items properly, instead of littering?
      (2) What would the world look like if everyone tossed their used items, food scraps, wastepaper into the street?
      (3) How is your garbage taken from home (or school) to the landfill?

6. HEALTH WORD
   Children may learn this lesson's health word, "environment," in five languages. You may simplify this activity by having the children learn this lesson's health word in two languages.

Vietnamese	Chinese	English	Spanish	Tagalog
khoảng-chùng	環境	environment	ambiente	kapaligiran
(kooahng joŏng)	(hwán-jìng and wāan-gíng)		(äm-bǐ én-tay)	(kä-pä-lee-gee-rän)

Primary Grades Health Curriculum Project*

The Primary Grades Health Curriculum Project is organized around the theme "Me, my feelings, my senses, and my body."

> Health is a feeling
> Health is an experience
> Health is a habit
> Health is a way of life
> Health is personal

This curriculum project, like its predecessor the School Health Education Curriculum Project, is developed according to a common unit format for each topic and grade level. The following outline is the framework for the content material of all grade units.

Introduction	Curiosity arousal and motivation of students
Phase I	Overview of the feelings and the five senses (grades K-2) or the body systems (grade 3)
Phase II	Appreciation of specific senses (grade K-2) or body systems (grade 3)
Phase III	Structure and function of the senses (grades K-2) or body systems (grade 3)
Phase IV	Diseases and problems of the senses (grades K-2) or body systems (grade 3)
Phase V	Care of the body and prevention of disease
Culmination	Synthesis of previous phases

The pattern of development is to present the overall interrelationships among the systems of the body, then to focus in each grade unit on specific sense organs of the body, and finally to return to a concept of the interdependence of all body systems. The factors that change from unit to unit are the body senses or body systems studied in depth. This same outline is the framework for grades 4 to 7 of the School Health Curriculum Project, a complementary curriculum. The first grade unit "Super Me" is selected to illustrate the five-phase organizational structure.

Food — Your Choice: A Nutrition Learning System†

The lesson selected to illustrate the intermediate level curriculum is taken from the National Dairy Council's comprehensive nutrition learning system. It is designed for the fifth- or sixth-grade student. As illustrated by the learning activities, the psychologic and sociologic dimensions of food choices are introduced to clarify students' values and to make them aware of the factors that influence their choices. The unit for this grade level comprises 14 different learning activities, each of which is related to a specific learning outcome. An interdisciplinary content chart is provided in which each of the 14 learning activities is correlated with the traditional subject matter areas taught at this grade level.

---

*The material in this section is from the primary grades health curriculum project. DHEW Pub. no., (CDC) 80-8382, Atlanta, 1980. U.S. Department of Health, Education and Welfare, Public Health Service, Centers for Disease Control, Bureau of Health Education.

†From Food—your choice, Rosemont, Ill., 1981, The National Dairy Council. Courtesy National Dairy Council.

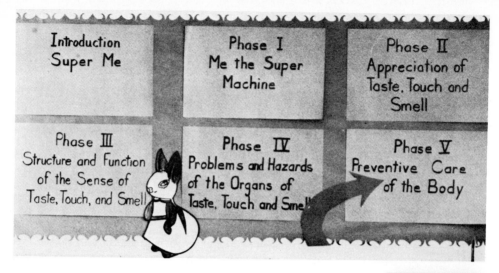

First Grade: "Super Me"

The first grade unit elaborates some of the concepts introduced in kindergarten and focuses on three senses: taste, touch, and smell.

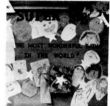

Major Concept Development

Introduction: Each person is unique and important at the same time that each person shares common needs with others. The special quality of being human is to cherish and take care of one's self and one another.

Phase I: The body is a super machine of many identifiable parts which work together in wonderful ways. The children learn the names of body parts, how they function, and the motor skills that use these body parts, such as skipping, hopping, tying shoes, and riding a bike. They express what they feel about their own body features.

Phase II: Taste, touch, and smell communicate information about the human body and its environment and can contribute to safe and healthful living.

Phase III: The structure and function of the tongue, skin, and nose bring experience of the world through taste, touch, and smell. Students learn (1) the specific sense organs of taste, touch, and smell; (2) the function of the nerves and the brain in relation to these organs; (3) the major structures of the skin and the functions of each; (4) the major functions of the nose, and (5) the major structure and functions of the tongue.

Phase IV: Diseases and environmental hazards can affect the senses of taste, touch, and smell. Diseases have symptoms and causes (virus, germs), and some diseases, communicable diseases, can spread (for example, colds, flu, pneumonia, mumps, measles, chicken pox, polio). Medicines can be helpful or harmful, depending on how they are used.

Phase V: The spread of disease can be prevented by health habits such as covering a sneeze, washing hands, caring for cuts, and being immunized. Overall health of the super machine is promoted through sleep, exercise, good nutrition, safety, good decisions about substance use and abuse, and relationships with others.

Culmination: In group activities, the children express what they have learned about taking care of their bodies, especially the senses of taste, touch, and smell.

The elementary school program of *Food — Your Choice* is divided into three levels. Each level is packaged in its own box.

Level 1, for kindergarten and first and second grades, introduces 5- to 7-year-old students to basic nutrition concepts.

Level 2 builds on and extends the concepts introduced in Level 1. Level 2 serves students in the third and fourth grades. It provides 8- and 9-year-old students with opportunities to manipulate materials as they acquire additional knowledge about nutrition.

Level 3, designed for fifth and sixth grades, introduces students to the economic and sociologic ramifications inherent in nutrition. It broadens the scope of the earlier programs and moves 10- to 12-year-old students from a personal and family food orientation to a more global one.

This material includes a list of 14 learning activities and shows how these activities are related to learner outcomes. Finally, the interdisciplinary content chart is an example showing how the content of this curriculum has been developed to correlate to all subjects of the school curriculum.

Learning About Your Oral Health, level II: 4-6

The following unit illustrates another way in which the subject matter (content) of health education can be organized. The unit on human interrelationships or sex education for kindergarten through third grade presents a grade-by-grade progression of the social, emotional, and physiologic aspects of sex education. The oral health unit, however, presents a horizontal structure emphasizing a particular sequence of topics — integrating dental health with other school subjects such as art, drama, language arts, science, history, and social studies. The unit offers an in-depth study of dental health, focusing on preventing dental disease by controlling of plaque in the mouth through oral hygiene (flossing and brushing), use of fluorides, and proper diet. In addition to the benefits afforded by integrated learning, the unit provides some classroom activities designed to stimulate student interest and understanding of the importance of dental health to total health.

When curriculum materials such as the American Dental Association's oral health program are used, teachers must make special adaptations for the particular school system and give careful study to the materials in order to understand the guiding philosophy of the developers. This unit is designed as a health instruction resource for children in the intermediate grades (4 to 6). The teacher must decide which grade level is most appropriate for teaching the unit. Regardless of the grade level selected, experience indicates that the oral health program should be taught as a unit and that the topics covered should be presented in the sequence suggested by the guide.

Research experience at the University of Illinois has demonstrated that fifth-grade teachers with a minimum of preparation can use this program to achieve effective results with their fifth-grade students.

The material from the *Learning About Your Oral Health* curriculum* has been selected to illustrate certain unique features. The design of each grade-level guide in the curriculum has been developed to serve as a complete teaching package. For example, the sections "Forward to the Teacher" and "Dental Health Facts for Teachers" provide the teacher with the essential background information needed to teach the unit. A section of the teaching guide has been selected to illustrate the horizontal or parallel column structure of the teaching unit. This structure shows the interrelationship of the behavioral objective content, suggested learning activities, and finally the related activities that provide for the correlation of dental health learning to other school subjects.

---

*Material that follows is from Learning about your oral health, Chicago, 1980, Copyright by the American Dental Association. Reprinted by permission.

Text continued on p. 331.

LEVEL 3
UNIT ONE: FOOD CAMPAIGN
UNIT OVERVIEW

Table of contents

*Indicates advance preparation for the teacher.

LEARNER OUTCOMES

Learner outcomes, with a description of behavioral indicators expected at the completion of Unit One, are listed below. Activities are indicated by number after the learner outcome to which they most clearly relate. The sequence for instruction in the classroom is suggested by the table of contents for each unit.

The learner will:

Explain how advertising affects food choices of self and others as shown by the ability to analyze advertisements for appeals and participate in the planning, conducting, and evaluating of a class publicity campaign.
Activities 1, 2, 3, 14

State the major nutrients and their functions as shown by the ability to cite the nutrients provided by food and state their contribution to energy, growth, and health.
Activities 4, 9, 14

Describe the digestive process as shown by the ability to explain the digestive system and label its organs.
Activity 5

State factors that influence nutrient allowances as shown by the ability to tell that age, sex, size, and activity influence nutrient allowances.
Activities 6, 11

Explain nutrition information panels on food packages as shown by the ability to state the two conditions in which nutrition labeling is required and recognize the correct format of nutrition labeling.
Activities 7, 8

Explain the U.S. RDA and how to use it as shown by ability to locate and transpose nutrition information from food packages and make bar graphs using the percentages of the U.S. RDA from a food package.
Activities 7, 8

Classify food on the basis of nutrient content as shown by the ability to classify foods as to food group and plan and evaluate a day's food intake by using the recommended number of servings from the Four Food Groups.
Activities 8, 12, 13

Test for the presence of specific nutrients in food as shown by the ability to separate milk into its proteins, administer iodine-water solution to foods to see if starch is present, and to burn several foods to see if minerals are present.
Activity 10

Evaluate eating patterns in terms of energy, growth, and health as shown by the ability to analyze a lunch menu to see if it meets the Type A Lunch Menu Pattern and classify foods as being orally safe or orally hazardous.
Activities 11, 12

Prepare a variety of foods as shown by the ability to participate in a snack-tasting party.
Activity 12

Plan and evaluate meals and snacks as shown by the ability to analyze a lunch menu to see if it meets the Type A Lunch Menu Pattern, classify foods as being orally safe or orally hazardous, and plan and evaluate a day's food intake by using the recommended number of servings from the Four Food Groups.
Activities 11, 12, 13

Support eating patterns that enhance energy, growth, and health as shown by the ability to plan and evaluate a day's food intake and cite the nutrients provided and their contribution to energy, growth, and health.
Activity 13

Choose foods that result in a nutritionally adequate diet as shown by the ability to plan and evaluate a day's food intake.
Activity 13

INTERDISCIPLINARY CONTENT

Correlations with other subjects

Activities	Math	Language arts	Science	Social studies	Arts	Health	Food preparation
1. Clarifying our values		×		×			×
2. Naming factors that influence food choices		×		×			
3. Analyzing advertising appeals		×		×			
4. Introducing nutrients, functions, and food sources		×	×			×	
5. Focusing on the human fuel system		×	×			×	×
6. Investigating energy	×		×			×	
7. Hunting for nutrition information	×			×			
8. Classifying comparison cards	×	×			×		×
9. Scoring the servings	×		×			×	
10. Experimenting with food	×		×			×	×
11. Looking at breakfast and lunch	×	×				×	
12. Controlling the snacks	×		×			×	×
13. Planning and supporting a day's intake	×	×	×			×	
14. Publicizing food	×	×	×	×	×	×	

FOREWORD: TO THE TEACHER

As an elementary school teacher, you are in a unique position to help prevent oral disease among your students. Your guidance and motivation can establish effective oral care habits that will benefit them all their lives.

This is of major importance because oral disease is one of the most prevalent health problems in America today. It is the exceptional person who possesses a full complement of 32 teeth, none of which is either filled or decayed. Statistics reveal that by the time the average child is 6 years old, three primary teeth have been attacked by decay at least once. By age 21, the average young adult has 11 decayed, missing or filled teeth. While neglect of daily personal oral care during early years takes a heavy toll in tooth decay, many people do not realize that it also sets the stage for periodontal (gum) disease. Although periodontal disease is regarded as a disease of older persons because it becomes more severe with age, early stages of the infection can usually be seen in children. The most frequent sign is swollen gums which bleed easily (gingivitis). This illustrates vividly the need for education of our country's children in methods of preventing dental caries and periodontal disease.

The overall goal of classroom instruction is the prevention of oral disease. To accomplish this goal, students need to develop appropriate knowledge, skills, and attitudes as well as assume a greater responsibility for their own oral health. Within the classroom, instruction in flossing and brushing is essential to ensure proper habit development and positive behavioral change. However, this is only one component of a total preventive instructional program. To strengthen awareness and appreciation for oral health, it is important to study the relationship of other factors that affect it. Subjects that can be integrated with daily classroom brushing and flossing activities include diet and nutrition, use of fluorides, professional dental care and safety/first aid. This teaching packet has been designed to assist you with your program.

Many local dental professionals (dentists, hygienists, assistants), and women's auxiliary groups are interested in assisting with prevention-oriented dental health education in the schools. These groups are useful resources and you may wish to contact them for assistance in program planning.

BASIC CONCEPTS

The underlying philosophy of the program is summarized by the following statements:

1. Health education focuses on the total person. According to the World Health Organization, "Health is a state of complete physical, mental and social well-being, not merely the absence of disease and infirmity."
2. Optimal oral health is an integral part of total health.
3. Optimal oral health in part depends on acceptance of oral health information, practices, and services.
4. Optimal oral health in part depends on knowledge of the structure and function of oral tissues, and the causes and treatment of various oral diseases.
5. Optimal oral health in part depends on a positive attitude toward oneself, oral health practices and products, as well as professional dental health services.
6. Optimal oral health in part depends on each individual's acceptance of the responsibility to promote programs of community dental health.
7. Developing and maintaining optimal oral health is the responsibility of:
   a. the individual
   b. the family
   c. the dentist and the dental professional team
   d. the community
8. Most oral disease is preventable by:
   a. use of fluorides
   b. correct, thorough, and consistent daily personal oral care
   c. proper diet
   d. professional care at appropriate intervals
9. Many oral injuries are preventable through observance of safety precautions.
10. Oral diseases and problems should be treated promptly to restore the optimal function of oral structures.

TABLE OF CONTENTS:

                    Printed in U.S.A.

Dental Health Facts for Teachers

Important Notice: Please review this section prior to teaching the dental health unit

So much knowledge is now available about dental health that one might ask "Why haven't individuals accepted more responsibility for their oral health?" If we could simply answer this question or if we knew the actual reasons why people neglect their oral health, then we could readily develop more effective educational programs. The question, however, is not easy to answer. We do not know all of the factors that influence behavior. Some of the more important deterrents to good oral health have been identified as: (a) lack of knowledge and practice of proper oral care techniques; (b) poor nutrition; (c) fear of dental visits; and (d) economic considerations.

Most dental problems *can* be prevented if children and parents are well-informed of the causes of dental disease and practice proper methods of prevention. This can be accomplished through sound dental health education programs within the schools. The establishment of positive dental health habits, attitudes, and behaviors is best accomplished during childhood. To assist you in teaching your dental health unit, we have prepared background information on oral disease, its causes, and how it can be prevented or controlled effectively.

PLAQUE: WHAT IS IT?

Plaque is a soft, sticky, colorless layer of bacteria and bacterial by-products that is constantly forming on the teeth. The bacteria are most harmful when they have had a chance to organize into colonies, a process that takes about 24 hours.

The acids and irritants produced by the bacteria in plaque are recognized to be the primary cause of the two most common dental diseases: (1) dental caries (tooth decay), the major cause of tooth loss in children, and (2) periodontal (gum) disease, the major cause of tooth loss in adults.

THE RELATIONSHIP OF PLAQUE AND DENTAL CARIES

The most widespread dental disease in children is dental caries. It is almost as prevalent as the common cold. Dental caries should not be considered just a hole in the tooth. It is the result of a bacterial infection. For caries to occur, there must be plaque, sugar, and a tooth susceptible to acid attack.

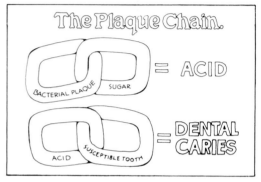

The Plaque Chain.

BACTERIAL PLAQUE + SUGAR = ACID

ACID + SUSCEPTIBLE TOOTH = DENTAL CARIES

The decay process begins with colonies of bacteria (dental plaque) that stick to the teeth. When food containing sugar is eaten, the bacteria break down the food and change the sugar to acid. The sticky bacterial plaque then holds the acid to the tooth surface, allowing it to attack the enamel on the teeth. These acids may act on the tooth for at least 20 minutes after food is eaten. Whether or not the enamel will be destroyed depends on the hardness of the tooth enamel, the strength of the acids, and the length of time the acids are allowed to remain on the teeth. After repeated acid attacks, the enamel is broken down. Once this happens, the bacteria gain access to the body of the tooth and a cavity results. A partial solution to this decay producing acid is to limit the number of times per day sugar is consumed. However, the problem is not simply the *amount of sugar eaten.* The **frequency** of eating sugar-rich foods, the **length of time** the sugar stays in the mouth, and the **physical form** of the food (such as sticky sweets) are all important factors in producing cavities.

The decay process is as follows:

1. Sugar combines with bacterial plaque; acid is formed as a by-product. This is the beginning of the decay process.
2. ENAMEL, the hard outer protective covering of the tooth, is etched by the acid.
3. The decay spreads into the DENTIN, a slightly softer layer that forms the bulk of the tooth.
4. If the decay penetrates to the PULP, the soft center tissue containing blood vessels and nerve tissue, an abscess may form at the root of the tooth.
5. If not treated by endodontic (root canal) therapy, the tooth may be destroyed.

While caries can be arrested and corrected at most points of its progress, it is best to have early diagnosis and treatment to stop the decay process before irreparable damage is done.

THE RELATIONSHIP OF PLAQUE AND PERIODONTAL DISEASE

Periodontal disease is a disease of the gums and other supporting structures of the teeth. It is the greatest single cause of tooth loss in adults. Early signs of periodontal disease such as bleeding of the gingiva (gums) during brushing can be observed even in children as young as 5 or 6 years of age. Although severe stages of this disease are found less often in children than in adults, it is believed that a large percentage of periodontal problems in later life are due to neglect of oral care during childhood and adolescence. The disease usually progresses over a long period with little or no pain. Unless measures are taken to prevent it, periodontal disease can, in time, destroy the gingiva, bone, and other structures that support the teeth.

The most common type of periodontal disease begins as gingivitis (inflamed gums) and, if not treated, progresses to periodontitis (involving the supporting bone tissue as well as gums). The first stage of periodontal disease begins when harmful bacteria and irritants infect the tissue which surrounds the teeth. As bacteria multiply, they form an invisible layer (plaque) on the teeth. Plaque accumulation along the gum line causes the gum tissue to become red, puffy, and sore, and it is likely to bleed. In many cases, people carelessly accept bleeding and swollen gums as a normal condition because they experience little discomfort. As a result, gingivitis is often neglected until it has reached an advanced stage, making treatment more complicated and more expensive.

Periodontitis, often incorrectly referred to as pyorrhea, usually begins as gingivitis. If gingivitis is not treated, the inflammation spreads along the roots of the teeth. As the gums separate from the teeth, pockets are formed which become filled with food particles, calculus (mineralized plaque), bacteria, and, sometimes, pus. As the disease progresses, the bone supporting the teeth is destroyed. The affected teeth eventually become very loose and drift from their normal position. Finally, unless the individual receives treatment, the teeth are lost because of the destruction of the supporting bone and other tissues.

There are other factors that may also contribute to or aggravate periodontal disease. They include:

— inadequate nutrition (a balanced diet is needed to provide the nutrients not only for general health but also for the health of the gums and the bones that support the teeth);
— "plaque traps" (such as worn-out fillings, the broken edges of badly decayed teeth, ill-fitting bridges or partial dentures, and maloccluded, crowded, or missing teeth);

— smoking and tobacco chewing;
— bruxism (the continual or repeated clenching and grinding of teeth); and
— improper use of dental floss, toothbrush, and toothpicks.

Many individuals are not familiar with the warning signs of periodontal disease. If your students notice any of the following symptoms, advise them to see the dentist at once:

1. Gums that bleed when brushing or flossing.
2. Persistent bad breath.
3. Soft, swollen, or tender gums.
4. Pus from the gum line when pressure is applied.
5. Loose permanent teeth.
6. Gums shrinking away from the teeth.
7. Any change in the way the teeth come together.

NOTE: The best time to prevent periodontal disease is early in life. Individuals can help accomplish this goal by controlling the plaque on the teeth.

METHODS OF PLAQUE CONTROL

DISCLOSE

The thorough removal of dental plaque can be taught more easily if the plaque can actually be seen. Since plaque is colorless, it can be "disclosed" or colored with the aid of a disclosing agent (tablet or solution). Disclosing agents are harmless vegetable dyes that show where plaque exists on the teeth. When the disclosing agent is swished in the mouth, it colors the plaque. If any color is left on the teeth after brushing and flossing, the individual should clean those areas again.

For your assistance, the following is a suggested classroom disclosing technique:

1. Chew a disclosing tablet or swish a disclosing solution around in the mouth.
2. Empty the mouth (spit out or swallow the solution — it's harmless); rinse with water.
3. Examine the teeth with a mirror in a good light. The color seen on the teeth shows the plaque that must be removed by flossing and brushing. When the color is no longer visible on the teeth, the plaque is gone. (Note: The disclosing agent may color the tongue and gums for a short while.)

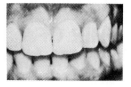 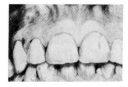

(before disclosing)   (after disclosing)

Teaching Units for Grades 4-6

PLAQUE ATTACK

Goals: To develop the knowledge, skills, and attitudes needed for the prevention of oral disease.

To develop an awareness of the relationship of the oral structures to diet and nutrition, sensory perception, speech and expression of emotion.

To develop an understanding of the cause of most oral disease.

To develop an awareness that most oral disease is preventable.

To develop an acceptance of personal responsibility for daily plaque removal.

Behavioral Objectives	Content	Suggested Activities	Related Activities in Other Classes
The student can list functions of the mouth as the first organ of digestion.	**Why Teeth?** Eating food. The mouth is the beginning of the digestive system. The teeth and tongue prepare food for swallowing. Salivary glands secrete a digestive juice, saliva, which is mixed with food to start the digestive process. Muscles in the tongue, cheeks, and palate move the food along to be swallowed.	Ask students what they would like to know about their oral health. List their questions on the chalkboard. Retain a copy for reference during the unit. Give each student a copy of the spirit master entitled "The Mouth" to study and discuss. Have the class discuss ways in which oral structures of various animals are adapted to their particular diets. How do these structures and diets differ from man's? Examples — cow, duck, dog, squirrel, shark, tiger. Have the class consider the question, "If there were no saliva to be mixed with food, what could still be swallowed easily? Which would be very difficult to swallow? How would this affect nutrition?"	**Special Project:** With teacher assistance, have a small committee of class members develop a bulletin board display of parts of the body involved in the digestion process. List the function of each respective part. **Art:** In small groups, have students develop a clay model of the teeth and gums. Have them compare their model with the spirit master entitled, "The Mouth." **Science:** Have students select one of their favorite animals. After studying their animal through a variety of sources, have students construct a clay model of the animal's teeth and gums. Compare it to the human model.
The student can describe how oral structures contribute to enjoyment of eating and to protection.	**Tasting and Feeling Food** The tongue has taste buds which can taste sweet, sour, bitter, and salt. The lips and tongue have many nerve endings to tell whether food is too hot and might burn the mouth, or if there are foreign objects (bones, etc.) which should not be swallowed. The tongue and roof of the mouth (palate) feel the texture of foods.	Ask the class to compile a list of things they like to taste — ice cream, hot corn on the cob, cold watermelon, sour pickles, salty potato chips, etc. Ask the class to consider the way a cold can distort the sense of taste. What favorite foods lose their appeal when perception of taste (smell) is altered? Bring to class sample foods paired for similar consistency and different taste. Blindfold students and have them hold noses as they are given sample foods. Have them try to identify each food according to taste. (Examples — mustard and catsup, apple and raw potato, cider and vinegar, custard and mayonnaise, salt and sugar, melon and cucumber.) Ask the class to consider ways of checking food for foreign objects other than feeling with lips and tongue.	**Art:** Using construction paper, scissors, and a marking pen, have students make a diagram of the tongue and map out the taste buds. Ask students to list one food in each taste bud area that best represents the sense of taste (i.e., sour pickles in the sour taste bud area, sunflower seeds in the salty taste bud area, etc.)

INCIDENTAL INSTRUCTION

Opportunities and a need for casual or incidental health instruction arise naturally in the course of a school day. Some phases of health teaching may best be handled by such incidental instruction. Problems that are of deep personal concern to a particular pupil or particular types of pupils may be dealt with most effectively by incidental treatment. However effective such instruction may be for certain purposes, if the teacher relies entirely on incidental health instruction, a decidedly limited health instruction program results, regardless of how skillful the teacher may be.

Pupil-teacher conferences and counseling frequently include incidental health instruction. When a teacher discovers the particular needs and problems of a child, the person-to-person relationship promotes a clarifying discussion of the problems. The conference may proceed beyond the original problem and explore related problems of interest and importance.

In class a pupil's question on a health matter may be an occasion for the whole class to learn. At times a discussion of a question considerably removed from health may gradually shift to its health aspects. An alert teacher uses expressed class interests and explores a whole area of health, perhaps leaving the class with several questions to ponder over, and concludes the discussion at a later date.

Simple incidents in school can have meaning in health terms, and the teacher can make effective use of such realistic teaching situations. Health terms occasionally are used in areas aside from health instruction, and opportunities are presented for the pupils to expand their vocabulary. Examinations usually offer opportunities for incidental health instruction. This is particularly true during the review of the examination after the tests have been scored and returned.

Daily newspaper, radio, and television reports frequently have health topics of interest to the pupils. A new health discovery, an epidemic, a person who has reached 100 years of age, and a physician who has practiced for 50 years are examples of news items that provide both the opportunity and necessity for consideration in the classroom.

Opportunities are plentiful for the alert teacher who utilizes incidental instruction to fortify and amplify planned health instruction (Fig. 13-3). Spontaneous live instruction is usually most stimulating to the pupils.

CORRELATED HEALTH INSTRUCTION

Correlation is a reciprocal relationship, and a kindred relationship or alliance exists between health and other cognate areas, which provides opportunities for effective instruction. Health aspects can enrich other fields and make experiences more stimulating and rewarding for the child (Fig. 13-4). There are many opportunities in health for instruction in the basic academic skills as well as in the field of life experiences. In health instruction, diction, pronunciation, spelling, coherence, and clarity are important. In a very real sense health involves history, art, and the people of other lands.

Reading

Health readers are available at various levels. They are interesting, are written with regard for comprehension by children, and can be used to encourage general supplementary reading.

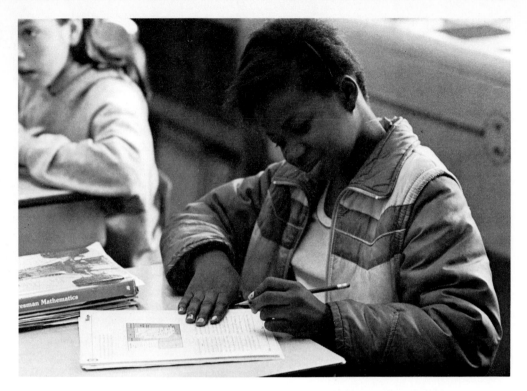

FIG. 13-3. Health knowledge is an important aspect of health education evaluation. *(Copyright 1983 by David Riecks.)*

For the teacher who seeks to enrich the curriculum of the superior pupil, health readers as well as health projects offer a fertile field of exploration.

Language arts

In writing and speaking assignments, health topics are a frequent choice of pupils. Reports on special health topics, field trips, and health experiences are used. Articles on health in the school may be written for newspapers. Letters asking agencies for health materials and requests to the health department provide correlated health and writing experience.

Spelling also can be included. Of the 2000 basic words in common usage, which are the core of instruction in elementary school spelling, many are in health literature. From classroom health study an instructor can find ample material for spelling purposes.

Art

Paper cutting, crayon fill-in, and free drawing can deal with health topics. Paste-on or original posters can be health posters. Health report cards can be a health project.

Music

Implications of mental and physical health in vocal and instrumental music are of interest. Many musical compositions have references to health. Health parodies on recognized songs should be avoided.

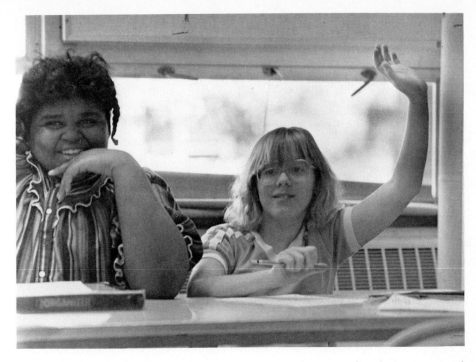

FIG. 13-4. Classroom strategies that attract attention and interest of students are essential to effective learning.
(Copyright 1983 by David Riecks.)

Arithmetic

Keeping records of changes in height and weight, attendance, and illness provides problems in arithmetic. Calculation of sleeping time and the amounts of certain foods consumed in a given period of time can be interesting experiences in arithmetic. The intermediate grades may be interested in rates for various health factors.

Geography

Health customs, life span, health problems, and dietary practices of peoples of other lands can be of interest to pupils. How other people live usually interests children.

History

The influence of health and disease on history challenges the imagination of youth. Health problems of different periods in history and health problems of famous historical figures are of special interest. Celebrated men and women health heroes live in historical perspective.

Nature study

The life and habits of lower animal forms have health implications. Feeding habits are particularly germane. The interrelationships that exist between humans and the plant and animal world are concepts that children should acquire as fundamental education.

Children must be helped to see relationships in life. Especially important are the relationships of health to the many aspects of everyday living.

SUMMARY

This chapter is introduced with a general discussion on the conditions necessary for establishing an effective health instruction program in the elementary school. Although local school curriculums will vary in pattern and the details of their curriculums, experience has shown that certain organizing conditions contribute very importantly toward achieving an effective health education experience for children. To this end, a list of eight suggestions for scheduling the health motivation program is included.

In this regard the role of school district health education coordinators can be an invaluable asset to the program. Typically the coordinator is a specialist in health education with a strong preparation in the content and instruction materials of health education.

As such the coordinator oversees and monitors the overall program reporting directly to the associate superintendent for instruction on the status and progress of the health education program. The coordinator becomes an important support person to the busy classroom teacher by providing assistance when needed, consulting, giving demonstrations, and conducting special in-service workshops for teachers. Experience has shown that school districts with a health educator coordinator have superior programs.

The four patterns of instruction traditionally employed in the elementary schools are discussed; in addition the pupil-teacher relationships, school experiences, and community experiences are discussed as rich resources for creative classroom teaching in making health teaching both interesting and vital in the lives of children.

Because of the scope and varied nature of health interests and health needs of children, organizing a curriculum that is both flexible and organized to assure appropriate progression of learning experiences becomes a challenging task. To assist the classroom teacher and curriculum coordinator in this task, subject matter topics of interest at the various grade levels are suggested along with the normal school day activities that can become effective teaching methods. Goodlad's (1979) conceptual framework (see Chapter 12, p. 273) for organizing the curriculum can be readily adapted to the local school curriculum. Sex education in the elementary school is discussed, and examples of objectives for this instruction are provided.

This chapter concludes with several examples of health teaching units at both the primary and intermediate grade levels.

STUDY QUESTIONS

1. How is health instruction presented under an integrated, correlated, and direct teaching plan?
2. What are the functions of a school health coordinator?
3. What criteria should be considered in evaluation of health textbooks and other health education materials?
4. In terms of curriculum planning what is meant by terms such as *scope, sequence progression,* and *articulation*?
5. What are the sensitive and controversial aspects of teaching sex education?
6. Assuming you have the responsibility for planning a primary level health instruction program what five high-priority health units would you include?
7. How does the Primary Grades Health Curriculum Project differ in its curriculum organizational scheme from that of the American Dental Association's Oral Health Level II Program?
8. How might the effectiveness of a health instruction program be determined?

REFERENCES

Allendorff, S., Sunseri, A.J., Cullinan, J., and Oman, J.K.: Student heart health knowledge, smoking attitudes, and self-esteem, J. Sch. Health **55**:5, 1985.

Allensworth, D.: Teaching materials on world hunger and other international health problems, Health Educ. **18**:41, 1987.

American Dental Association: Learning about your oral health: preschool, level I: K-3, level II: 4-6, Chicago, 1980, the Association.

Cornacchia, H.J., Olsen, L.K., and Nickerson, C.J.: Health in elementary schools, ed. 6, St. Louis, 1984, The C.V. Mosby Co.

Cvetkovich, G., and others: Child and adolescent drug use: a judgement and information processing perspective to health-behavior intervention, J. Drug Educ. **17**:295, 1987.

Frank, C., and Goldman, L.: Growing up healthy in New York City, Phi Delta Kappan **69**:454, 1988.

Hazlett, S.H.: Growing up healthy: health education curriculum guide for kindergarten, ed. 4 (developed in the San Francisco Unified School District), 1983.

Health education of preschool children and their parents: a background paper prepared for the President's Committee on Health Education, New York, 1972, Xerox Corp.

Hufford, A., and Lipnickey, S.: Promoting self-responsibility using the school nurse in a health awareness program for primary students, J. Sch. Health **57**:195, 1987.

Mayshark, C., Shaw, D.D., and Best, W.H.: Administration of school health programs: its theory and practice, St. Louis, 1977, The C.V. Mosby Co.

Mental Health Materials Center, editor: Education-for-health: the selective guide. Health promotion, family life and mental health audiovisuals and publications. A publication of the National Center for Health Education in association with the Mental Health Materials Center, New York, 1983, National Center for Health Education.

Nagy, C., and Nagy, M.C.: Administrative perceptions of health education in the special education curriculum, Teacher Education and Special Education **10**:131, 1987.

National Dairy Council: Food — your choice: a nutrition learning system. Rosemont, Ill., 1981, the Council.

Oei, T., and Fea, A.: Smoking prevention program for children: a review, J. Drug Educ. **17**:11, 1987.

Pollock, M.B., and Middleton, K.: Elementary school health, St. Louis, 1984, The C.V. Mosby Co.

Raper, J., and Aldridge, J.: What every teacher should know about AIDS, Child Educ. **64**:146, 1988.

Roberts, S.W.: Food first, educating our children, Health Educ. **18**:17, 1987.

Shupe, S.D., and Sandoval, W.M.: Nutrition education: from the lunchroom to the classroom, J. Sch. Health **57**:122, 1987.

Steinberg, V. and Fry, T.: The writing process in the health class, Health Educ. **19**:50, 1988.

Tucker, A.W.: Elementary school children and cigarette smoking: a review of the literature, Health Educ. **18**:18, 1987.

U.S. Department of Health, Education and Welfare: The primary grades health curriculum project, Pub. no. (CDC) 80-8382, Atlanta, 1980, Public Health Service Centers For Disease Control.

U.S. Department of Health and Human Services: Better health for our children: a national strategy. The report of the Select Panel for the Promotion of Child Health, Pub. no. 79-55071, 1981, Public Health Service.

Health Instruction in Secondary Schools

OVERVIEW   Although controversy over the goals of secondary education has always existed, there appears to be less disagreement among today's critics than in the past. The arguments over the school's role tend to polarize between the so-called compassionate critics, who argue that the curriculum should be focused on the needs of the student, and the "back to basics" critics, who argue that the school should confine its efforts to teaching fundamental skills and those subjects that prepare the student for entrance to a college or university.

This chapter describes the departmental structure of the secondary school and its separate course (subject matter) orientation. Although the study of subjects from a separate course perspective offers certain advantages, the pattern of separate courses tends to create an isolated and unrelated approach to teaching that may make learning more difficult for the student. Several different curriculum patterns, including correlation, integration, and a broad fields approach, are presented in relation to this problem. Modular scheduling, which divides the curriculum into smaller units or modules, offers the promise of more flexibility in class schedule and the hope of improving student learning.

The recommended schedule and the health content for a comprehensive health education program are presented. Also given is an illustration showing how the Teenage Health Teaching Modules program organizes a comprehensive curriculum. A summary review of some of the most important health problems facing the nation is provided together with a list of suggested health education objectives.

Materials from three innovative approaches to teaching health at the secondary school level are included. The handling of controversial topics is discussed. Several different types of controversies are examined, and suggested guidelines are offered to help schools handle controversies. Recent developments in professional preparation for health education are reviewed including the minimum competencies required of all health educators. An example of teacher certification standards and undergraduate preparation in school health education is presented.

OBJECTIVES   After reading this chapter, the student should be able to:

1. Identify the controversies over the purposes or goals of secondary education
2. Explain the organizational patterns that are typical of most secondary schools
3. Identify the health education curriculum content recommended by the education commission of the state
4. Identify the characteristics of the secondary school student that have important implications for the health instruction program
5. Identify several major adolescent health problems that have important implications for the health education curriculum

6. Explain several different types of controversies that need to be recognized by the school health educator

7. Distinguish between a moral and moralistic perspective in teaching a topic such as human sexuality

8. Identify several responsibilities and competencies that have been identified by the National Task Force and that are common to all health educators

9. Explain teacher certification requirements for health education teaching

10. Discuss the code of ethics for health educators proposed by the Society of Public Health Education

GOALS OF SECONDARY EDUCATION

Secondary schools are the principal vehicle for youths' transition into adulthood. As such there is general agreement that the major purpose of American secondary education is to define and establish education for American contemporary life. Although there is general agreement on this broad purpose or goal, there have always been a variety of interpretations. The differing conceptions of what constitute desirable goals of secondary education persist. The broad general direction in which education is going is toward a useful education for all American youth, stressing individually and socially significant learning. The exact nature of such education continues to be a matter of controversy. However, as Van Til (1978) has observed, the areas of agreement appear to be expanding and the swing back and forth between extreme positions of critics seems to be narrowing. The extremes of these differences are between the critics of secondary education characterized by the compassionate critics, who are calling for a youth-centered school stressing the needs and interests of the individual, and the back-to-basics critics, who are calling for emphasis on the three R's and solid content courses to assure the graduates successful entrance to college.

The reaffirmation of the cardinal principles of education is perhaps a good indication of this larger consensus that is developing in regard to the purposes of schooling. Because of the historical significance of this statement, the National Education Association (1976), as part of the bicentennial celebration, appointed a panel of nationally prominent leaders and asked them to reexamine the cardinal principles. The panel reaffirmed the validity of these principles and their value as goals for all secondary schools. However, the panel chose to restate and to reinterpret each of the goals in order to make them more relevant in terms of the needs of today's society. For example, the panel's interpretation of the goal of health was as follows, "The scope and importance of health as an educational objective has become even more important than it was in 1918."

ORGANIZATION OF THE SECONDARY SCHOOL CURRICULUM

Frequently, secondary schools have a departmental structure that is organized by subject matter or disciplines. A typical schedule for the secondary student would include courses such as English, mathematics, science, social studies, health, art, music, and physical education. Other characteristics that are typical of secondary education in the United States center around the school day, class schedules, and the role of teachers and students. Typically the school day begins at 8:30 AM and concludes about 3:30 PM. Students usually attend school starting after Labor Day and continuing until the first week of June. The pattern of secondary schooling has become so standardized that it is assumed that students will study certain distinct and separate subjects. Moreover, the knowledge gained from some of the subjects will not be for practical purposes or immediately useful but instead will be of value in its own right. Classes in secondary schools are usually taught by a teacher who specialized in that subject matter. Typically classes will have approximately 30 students, and the class functions as a group with the teacher playing a dominant role in the classroom. Students are usually assigned homework to be carried out between classes, which includes assigned readings in the class textbook in addition to other class activities or study materials provided by the teacher.

One of the problems of departmental organization is that in the horizontal structure of disciplines, the subject matter tends to become isolated and compartmentalized. Moreover, when several subjects are taught simultaneously, they may not be well coordinated and are taught separately and unrelated to other subjects in the curriculum. When this occurs, it becomes difficult for the student to assimilate the information. To overcome this difficulty, secondary schools have experimented with several different patterns of course organization. Such an example is the teaching of two courses according to a correlated plan, for instance, the teaching of U.S. history and English, the teaching of mathematics and science, and, to a lesser degree, the teaching of biology and health as correlated subjects.

The broad fields approach represents still another attempt to integrate and to show the relationships between subjects. An example is social studies, which combines history, geography, economics, and political science; language arts is another example in which elements of English, speech, literature, spelling, reading, and grammar are combined. In this regard some educators have advocated a broad fields approach for the teaching of health-related topics under a title such as health and physical fitness, which would include aspects of health, exercise, physical development, safety, and recreational activities.

Still another approach is that of the core curriculum, which is also designed to establish meaningful relationships between subjects. This interdisciplinary curriculum seeks to bridge broad fields of study by designing courses or study themes such as the study of an American city or the family or the study of problems such as community health, consumer spending, and social problems.

> The quest for better organization of the secondary school program goes on. Sometimes it takes the form of core or common learning programs, team taught or community-oriented. Through such programs, students can work together on interdisciplinary problems encountered by young people in our society. Sometimes it assumes the form of individualized instruction through contracts, learning packages, learning centers, technology, and independent study (Van Til, 1978).

In an effort to overcome the disadvantages of rigid subject matter categories and school scheduling, a modular plan for class scheduling has been developed. The major objective of this approach is to provide a more flexible plan for individualizing instruction. This objective is accomplished by allowance for greater variability in the scheduling of time, space, staff, and students. The conventional seven-period day of 55-minute modules is changed to a series of 21-minute modules each day, or a total of 105 such modules in a weekly cycle. The advantages of this plan include the varying of class size to allow for small-group seminars, large lectures, or laboratory classes of predetermined size. Moreover, the time length of a class can be varied to accommodate differing instructional needs. By use of the computer a variety of scheduling configurations can be developed.

Traditionally the recommendation for health instruction in secondary schools has called for a 1-year or two-semester health course to be offered at both the junior and senior high school levels with the minimum for such instruction being a one-semester course at each level. However, with the creation of more flexible scheduling patterns has come the development of health education curriculum modules. The module is a smaller version of the traditional instructional unit. It allows for greater flexibility in scheduling as well as the teaching of health. The Teenage Health Teaching Modules (THTM; Education Development Center, Inc., Newton, Mass., 1982) are a good example of this development. The THTM, a health education curriculum, is composed of 16 modules, each comprising 4 to 15 hours of instruction. The modules are designed so they can be taught independently or be taught as part of a larger course of study.

During the past 15 to 20 years investigators have studied several different patterns of health instruction including the core course concept, integrated health instruction, correlated instruction, and several patterns of scheduling health instruction. Unfortunately the results of most of these experiments are not at all clear and are lacking in careful documentation and evaluation. On the other hand, studies have sought to determine the comparative effects of different scheduling patterns such as the teaching of health on an alternating-day schedule with physical education or the teaching of health on a block-of-daily-time schedule. The latter approach, namely, direct teaching, is preferred by most health educators. Also, as McClendon and Tayeb (1982) have pointed out, when health instruction is offered as a separate semester course, students have been found to achieve higher health knowledge and application test scores.

A pattern of alternating 9-week blocks of class time between health instruction and physical education has become a fairly widespread practice in secondary schools. Although such a plan does offer the advantage of a concentrated time period for instruction and subject matter continuity, there are certain other disadvantages. All too often, this pattern results in a single teacher having responsibility for teaching the two courses without being adequately qualified in both areas. A further disadvantage of this arrangement stems from combining of classes that are not compatible in terms of scheduling class size, use of facilities, and course evaluation.

JUNIOR HIGH SCHOOL HEALTH INSTRUCTION

Junior high or middle school is a transition from the self-contained classroom in the sixth grade to departmentalized instruction in the seventh grade. It represents a change in the relationship between students and teacher. Junior high school teachers often do not have the opportunity to establish the degree of rapport with students possible in the elementary grades. However, when the seventh-grade curriculum is modified by large core areas, the transition for the students is easier, and teachers have a better change to establish a close relationship with students. Health instruction, as all other instruction at this stage in school, must recognize the factors that motivate students and account for their interests and conduct (Fig. 14-1).

Students between 12 and 15 years of age include children who are in the homophilic,

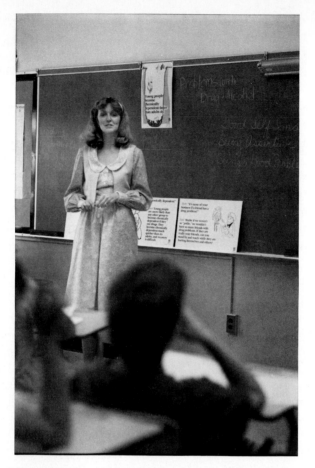

FIG. 14-1. Accepting the individuality of each student helps to give him or her a greater sense of self-worth and interest in school.

or gang, period, a few who have not yet reached that stage, and perhaps one fifth who can be classed as adolescents. To complicate the picture, physiologically and socially a 12-year-old girl is almost 2 years ahead of a boy.

During the homophilic period girls are arm-in-arm with girls and boys tend to gang up with boys. Group loyalty is exceedingly important. The teacher should capitalize on the strong desire for approval by their associates and the tendency toward united action by directing health instruction into channels of group approval and action. Group interest can mean group accomplishment and community interest.

Health instruction goals for junior high school

Health practices previously established will continue to be fortified in the junior high school, and new practices, particularly those associated with group health responsibility, will be established. Knowledge to promote understanding of health measures and procedures will be provided in the junior high school. However, greatest attention should be given to the development of attitudes that are essential to provide the necessary intensity to health practices and to assure the fullest use of health knowledge.

Many health attitudes, in terms of ideal personal and community attainments, will prove to be the most lasting and valuable in terms of the individual's lifelong health measure. Among these will be attitudes that are directed toward the following:

1. Resolution to attain a high level of health
2. Pride in a high quality of well-being
3. Application of reasoning to health problems
4. Conviction that only established health principles should be used
5. Acceptance of responsibility for the health of others
6. Ideals of citizen responsibility
7. Cooperation with community health efforts
8. Insistence on high community health standards
9. Pride in community assets

The knowledge of health that the junior high school students should acquire is expressed in the areas of primary interest at this level.

SENIOR HIGH SCHOOL HEALTH INSTRUCTION

Health schools of today encompass at least three broad purposes that seek to provide the student with (1) the skills and knowledge that are needed to continue further study at the higher education level, (2) basic preparation needed for a vocation, and (3) preparation for accepting the responsibilities of adulthood. Health education at the senior high level is most often considered to be one of the essential requirements in this preparation for adulthood.

To be effective, health instruction must be adapted to the distinctive characteristics of the high school age. At times the individual displays the consistency of maturity and at other times the inconsistency of immaturity. Youth is a period of transition from the dependence of childhood to the independence of adulthood. Self-assertion, determination, and independence reveal the desire of all young people for emancipation from adult domination and for recognition as competent, self-reliant persons in their own right. They want to know the *how* and *why* as well as the *what*. High school students are imaginative, enthusiastic, sensitive, and idealistic. They seek status within their group and try to merit the respect of their instructors. They need to develop a mature standard of values that will provide a basis for positive motivation. Gaining self-esteem that grows out of successful and satisfying participation is essential to their ultimate well-being.

At the high school level, teachers are working with students who have virtually attained their maximal level of native intelligence. They will gain a great deal more knowledge from experience and from instructors who can challenge these young people by providing stimulating opportunities for learning. Their experiences can be most meaningful when students have a role in planning and implementing the instructional program. In education, as in self-growth, the individual must participate actively in the process whether the learning involves memorization, analysis, or creativity. Effective learning must develop as growth from within. The teacher guides this growth by providing motivation through wholesome experiences. Although students will learn something about health without a teacher, a well-designed health instruction program increases both the quantity and quality of student learning (Fig. 14-2).

ORGANIZING FOR HEALTH INSTRUCTION

Health instruction is a recognized area in the curriculum of the junior high school, and there are very few junior high schools that do not offer formal classroom instruction in health. The scheduling of health instruction follows a variety of patterns. Unfortunately in some junior high schools health instruction has not been given enough attention and care in planning to ensure its effectiveness. In such schools there is an urgent need to apprise the responsible administrators of the importance of health and what an effective health instruction program can do for students.

Few subject areas offer the student as much in a functional way as does health. Several factors determine the schedule and emphasis assigned to health instruction. The traditional background of the school, state requirements, community demands, the general pattern of the curriculum, the understanding of the administrators, and the competence of the health teachers all affect the nature of health instruction programs.

Correlation of health and other subject fields

Because of the departmentalized organization in the junior high school, there is difficulty in correlating health and other subject areas. In the self-contained classroom of the elementary

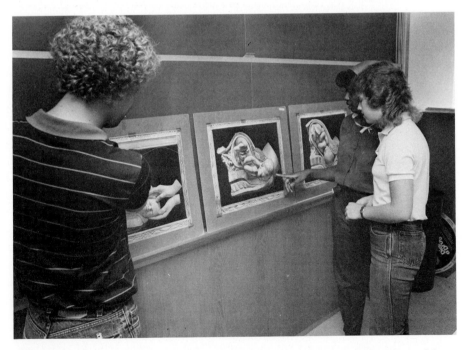

FIG. 14-2. Adolescent girls studying models depicting the anatomy and physiology of the reproductive process during pregnancy and normal delivery.
(Mary E. Allen.)

grades it is both easy and natural for the teacher to recognize and use these correlations for more effective teaching. Because correlated instruction is also important at the secondary school level, health instruction should be done through other subject fields. The following discussion applies to junior and senior high schools alike.

Integrated and incidental health learning

The daily experiences of junior high school students are rich in health implications. Opportunities for integrated health instructions are plentiful, but usually only the health instructor capitalizes on them. However, if the organized health class does its work effectively, the students will be alerted to the health significance of everyday occurrences. If students are stimulated and challenged by a competent health instructor, a considerable amount of integrated health learning will go on.

In-service preparation of all the school staff in the possibilities and value of integrated health instruction is an ideal that rarely becomes reality. Yet the health coordinator or the health teacher may enlist the cooperation of other staff members, particularly those who have some background in health education or health related preparation.

Incidental health instruction arises from student-teacher conferences, questions from students in the classroom, injuries to students, news reports, and tests and as an outgrowth of some topic outside the health field. Incidental instruction should not be superficial teaching. Any topic under consideration should be developed sufficiently so that the students understand and appreciate it.

Various activities in the regular program of the school provide health learning opportunities. Assemblies, lunchroom service, projects of the student council, announcements on the bulletin board, safety drives, and health examinations all contribute to the understanding, appreciation, and practice of health.

DETERMINING THE CONTENT OF HEALTH INSTRUCTION

Initiating a course of study through a survey of student health interests illustrates an important principle in curriculum planning, relevance of the instruction. This principle recognizes that (1) learning is more efficient when the subject is of interest to the student and (2) information is more likely to be applied when it is of interest to the student. However, if the health education curriculum is to include the health content of greatest value to the student, it must draw on at least two additional sources of information. The foundation of the modern school health education curriculum should rest on (1) the health needs and interests of the student, (2) the health needs of the larger society, and (3) the body of health knowledge or the discipline of the health sciences. Examples of health topics identified from each of these sources include the following:

I. Health topics identified by a study of the individual student
  A. Growth and developmental characteristics
    1. Junior high school level
      a. Sexual development causes student to be very aware of body changes
    2. Senior high school level
      a. Interest in opposite sex provides incentive for developing responsible adult roles in preparation for marriage

       b. Growing interest in adult consumer role and many existing misconceptions about medications

  II. Health needs of society

    A. Morbidity and mortality data reveal need to prevent such problems as deaths caused by cardiovascular diseases and accidents

    B. Need for early detection and treatment of cancer

    C. Disease effects caused by smoking

    D. Disease and suffering caused by misuse of drugs

  III. Data from health knowledge or the health sciences

    A. Human experiences and scientific research have created a body of information that has been organized into broad categories such as nutrition, environmental health, mental health, communicable and chronic diseases, family health, and dental health

Two important publications illustrate the full scope of the content topics that may be treated in a comprehensive health education curriculum. the two examples are the 10 content areas recommended by the School Health Education Task Force of the Education commission of the States (1981) and the Teenage Health Teaching Modules program components (Education Development Center, Inc., 1982) prepared by the Education Development Center of Newton, Massachusetts. The latter program was developed for the Center for Health Promotion and Education, formerly the Bureau of Health Education, which is located at the Centers for Disease Control in Atlanta.

Content areas recommended by School Health Education Task Force*

The 10 content areas recommended by the task force as minimal elements of a comprehensive school health education program are given below. After the title of each is a brief list of topics that might be included in teaching this content area. It should be noted that this section is meant to provide *examples* and thus is not all inclusive.

1. *Personal health:* physical fitness and lifetime physical activities, cardiovascular health, sleep, rest, relaxation, recreation, growth and development, nutrition, oral health, vision and hearing, prevention and control of disease, safety, body systems and their functions, aging, coping with death and dying

2. *Mental and emotional health:* Positive self-concept, personality, emotional stability, responsibility, motivation, independence, mental disorders, coping with stress, mental health services.

3. *Prevention and control of disease:* contribution of early scientists, causes of disease, preventive measures, chronic disease, degenerative disease, communicable disease, immunization, personal health practices, community efforts

4. *Nutrition:* food choices, elements in food that contribute to good nutrition, factors influencing choices, individual nutritional requirements, food groups and nutrients, food sources, weight control, effects of nutrition on growth and activity, nutritional challenges, food preparations and protection, consumer protection

---

*Modified from Guidelines for improving school health education K-12, Columbus, 1980, Ohio Department of Education.

5. *Substance use and abuse:* personal goals, individual responsibility, substances beneficial to humans, classification of substances and their effects on the body, implications of use of substances, how habits are formed and influence health, use and misuse of tobacco, alcohol, and other drugs, treatment and rehabilitation programs, respect for self and others

6. *Accident prevention and safety:* attitudes toward safety, causes of accidents, home and school safety, traffic (automobile, bicycle, school bus) safety, fire prevention, survival education, environmental hazards, accident prevention — potential hazards, first-aid and emergency health care, safety personnel, resources, and agencies, individual safety precautions, recreational safety, occupational safety, safety rules, laws, regulations, legislation

7. *Community health:* individual responsibility, healthful school, home, community environment, community health resources and facilities, official and nonofficial health agencies, health service careers, pollution control (clean air and water), occupational environments, safety hazards and natural disasters, community involvement — a shared responsibility (health planning)

8. *Consumer health:* individual responsibility, propaganda in advertising, social and economic factors, laws for consumer protection (food labeling), protection agencies, health agencies, and organizations, health insurance, selection of medical services, quackery, reliable sources of health information, evaluating health products and services, use of trained medical personnel

9. *Environmental health:* environmental pollution, effect of environment on health (radiation, pollution), environmental protection agencies, population density, world health

10. *Family life education:* family composition and roles, life cycles (human growth and development), the reproductive process, heredity, marriage, selecting a compatible life partner, family relationships, parenting

Teenage Health Teaching Modules*

The Teenage Health Teaching Modules (THTM) program consists of 16 teaching modules. Each module is a complete teaching kit for a unit on a designated topic and includes a teacher's guide with pages designed to be duplicated for student handouts. Many modules also include student materials, such as information sheets, posters, educational games, and, in some cases, student booklets. Each module provides 4 to 15 hours of instruction. Many are suitable for grades 7 though 12; some are recommended for either junior or senior high.

Taken as a whole, the set of modules can constitute an introductory survey course on health. Used independently, modules can be selected to supplement materials already in use. There is no prescribed sequence or required number of modules, so that teachers can, if they choose, introduce one module one year and others later on. Activities are designed to be implemented by teachers from a variety of subject areas, for example, health, home eco-

*From Teenage Health Teaching Modules Project, Education Development Center, 55 Chapel St., Newton, MA 02160. Used with permission.

nomics, social studies, science, language arts, and physical education.

Table 14-1 has guided THTM module development and illustrates the ways in which the program reconciles the concern for a comprehensive approach with the need for attention to commonly acknowledged health topics.

Adolescence is a period of rapid and varied physical cognitive, and psychosocial development. Psychologists have identified many developmental tasks individuals in our culture confront as they move from adolescent to adulthood. In an effort to combine the principles of developmental theory with those behaviors that are believed to be health promoting, THTM has developed the concept of *health* tasks. Health tasks are those physical, mental, emotional, and social tasks adolescents need to resolve in order to develop to their full health potential. The project has identified 16 critical health tasks and developed modules that focus on each one. The health tasks, which are also the titles of the modules, are listed down the left side of Table 14-1.

In addition to addressing the very special concerns of adolescence, the modules also involve students in a exploration of the traditional health content areas generally recommended for comprehensive school health education programs. The health content areas recommended in the Education Commission of the States publication. *Recommendations for School Health Education: a Handbook for State Policy Makers,* appear along the top of Table 14-1. The *X*'s indicate which content areas are covered in each module. Although each module focuses on a specific adolescent health task and includes explanations of priority health content areas, all modules are carefully constructed to develop skills in five basic areas: (1) self-assessment, (2) communication, (3) decision making, (4) healthy self-management, and (5) health advocacy.

ADOLESCENT HEALTH AND THE NATION'S OBJECTIVES

Healthy People: the Surgeon General's Report on Health Promotion and Disease Prevention (U.S. Department of Health and Human Services, 1979) recognized that the control and prevention of the major health problems affecting Americans today, especially the chronic diseases and accidental injuries, call not only for changes in life-style but also for changes in the environment. Moreover, it was stated that disease prevention and health promotion activities must necessarily play a key role in the effort to improve the future health status of Americans. AS such, it is also evident that if healthful and safe patterns of living are to be established early and maintained throughout the life span, health education of schoolaged children and of the public must be given increased emphasis.

After the establishment of five general health goals for the 1980s by the surgeon general's report there were issued two subsequent volumes, *Promoting Health, Preventing Disease: Objectives for the Nation* (U.S. Department of Health and Human Services, 1980) and *Implementation Plans for Attaining the Objectives for the Nation* (U.S. Department of Health and Human Services, 1983e). These publications have provided both the framework for planning and the specific action steps from improving the health of all Americans.

Two of the five goals for the nation have major implications for the school health program. They are as follows:

> To improve child health, foster optimal development, and by 1990 reduce the deaths among children ages 1 to 14 years by at least 20% to fewer than 34 per 100,000

TABLE 14-1.   Teenage health teaching modules

Health tasks* of adolescence and program introduction	Priority health content areas									
	Personal health	Mental and emotional health	Prevention and control of disease	Nutrition	Substance use and abuse	Accident prevention and safety	Community health	Consumer health	Environmental health	Family life education
Health Is Basic: An Introduction to THTM	X	X	X	X	X	X	X		X	X
Understanding Growth and Development	X	X	X	X	X	X	X			X
Being Fit	X	X		X	X					
Eating Well	X	X	X	X				X		
Communicating in Families	X	X							X	X
Promoting Health in Families	X	X	X	X						X
Having Friends	X	X		X						
Living with Feelings	X	X	X	X	X					X
Handling Stress	X	X		X	X	X				
Protecting Oneself and Others	X	X		X	X	X				
Preventing Injuries	X	X			X	X				
Improving Health and Safety in the Workplace	X	X	X		X	X				
Locating Health Resources	X	X	X	X	X	X	X	X		X
Using New Health Research	X	X	X	X	X		X	X		
Acting to Create a Healthy Environment	X	X			X	X	X	X	X	
Planning a Healthy Future	X	X	X	X	X	X	X	X	X	X

From Teenage Health Teaching Modules Project, Education Development Center, 55 Chapel St., Newton, MA 02160. Used with permission.

*Understanding sexuality is a key health task of adolescence. The project plans to develop a module *Sex Education: Deciding What's Right for Your Community*, which would include an annotated bibliography of available materials and guidance for educators and parents to help them decide which approaches and materials on sexuality are appropriate for their community.

To improve the health and habits of adolescents and young adults, and by 1990 to reduce deaths among people ages 15 to 24 years by at least 20% to fewer than 93 per 100,000

After the issuance of the surgeon general's report of 1979, some 500 persons representing a broad spectrum of interests and organizations from both the private and public sectors came together to develop the objectives for the nation. From these deliberations the following 15 priority areas were identified and implementation plans (U.S. Department of Health and Human Service, 1983e) were developed for each area:

1. High blood pressure control
2. Family planning
3. Pregnancy and infant care
4. Immunization
5. Sexually transmitted diseases
6. Toxic agents and radiation control
7. Occupational safety and health
8. Accident prevention and injury control
9. Flouridation and dental health
10. Surveillance and control of infectious diseases
11. Smoking and health
12. Prevention of misuse of alcohol and drugs
13. Improved nutrition
14. Physical fitness and exercise
15. Control of stress and violent behavior

A careful analysis of the objectives and priority areas reveals that there are many areas in which the school health education program can make an important contribution to the attainment of the nation's health objectives. As stated in the implementation report (U.S. Department of Health and Human Services, 1983e), "Success will depend heavily on a sustained commitment from Americans at every level of society. . . ."

School officials and curriculum coordinators are encouraged to examine carefully these three major reports in order for the schools to contribute importantly to the attainment of the nation's health goals for the 1980s. An analysis of the 15 priority areas has revealed the following nine special needs of the adolescent. To assist the school in carrying out its responsibilities to students and to the nation's goals the following objectives are offered:

HIGH BLOOD PRESSURE CONTROL

The problem

There are approximately 60 million people who have high blood pressure that increases their risk of illness and premature death. Although the National High Blood Pressure Education Program has helped to bring high blood pressure under control, there are still many people who are not sufficiently aware and informed about the importance of accurate diagnosis and the appropriate care needed for its control (U.S. Department of Health and Human Services, 1983e) (Fig. 14-3).

Objectives

1. Increase students' knowledge of the nature of high blood pressure and its effect on the body

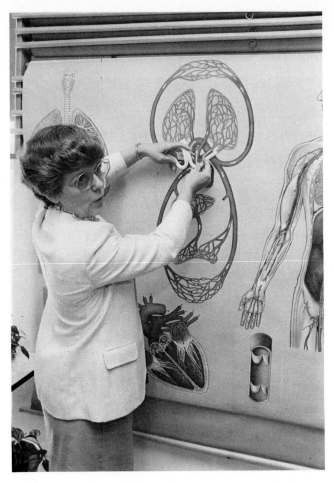

FIG. 14-3. High school health instruction must give greater emphasis to the study of the cardio-vascular system and the prevention of heart and blood vessel disease.
(Mary E. Allen.)

2. Increase students' knowledge and acceptance of treatment for high blood pressure and the necessity of complying with the prescribed medical care in controlling high blood pressure
3. Increase students' knowledge of the relationship between sodium in the diet as a contributing factor and high blood pressure
4. Increase students' acceptance of the necessity for reducing the amount of sodium in the diets of most Americans
5. Increase students' awareness of the sodium levels of various foods and recipes

FAMILY PLANNING

The problem

Of the approximately 3½ million births each year it is estimated that 1 million are unplanned. More than 1 million pregnancies are terminated by legal abortions each year. There is a disproportionately higher risk of unplanned pregnancies among the poor, among black women, and among teenagers. The proportion of women 15 to 19 years residing in metropolitan areas of the United States who have had premarital sexual experience increased from 30% in 1971 to 49% in 1979. Over 56% of the unmarried 17-year-old men in metropolitan areas have had sexual intercourse (U.S. Department of Health and Human Services, 1981; U.S. Department of Health and Human Services, 1983e).

Objectives

1. Increase students' knowledge and acceptance of the risks of premarital sexual relations and the social, economic, and personal costs of adolescent pregnancy and parenthood
2. Increase students' knowledge and acceptance of the proper uses of fertility control and the appropriate alternatives
3. Increase students' knowledge and acceptance of community family services including education, counseling, and medical services
4. Increase students' ability to explain the various contraceptive methods, natural family planning, and their relative effectiveness and safety
5. Increase students' knowledge and acceptance of the importance of prenatal visits and prenatal care to the health of the unborn child and to the mother
6. Increase students' knowledge of the ways of protecting and promoting health during adolescent pregnancy and parenthood
7. Increase students' knowledge of adolescent reproductive behavior, pregnancy, and parenthood that will protect and promote the health of the adolescent mother and the child
8. Increase students' knowledge of the importance of choosing foods wisely, the dangers of cigarette smoking, and the uses of alcoholic beverages and other drugs during pregnancy and lactation
9. Increase students' knowledge and acceptance of their roles as parents in participating in primary health care for their children including well-child care, growth and development assessment, immunization programs, screening, and diagnosis and treatment of special conditions
10. Increase students' knowledge and acceptance of the importance of using appropriate child-restraining devices in autombile travel

SEXUALLY TRANSMITTED DISEASES

The problem

Most recent estimates indicate that some 10 million cases of sexually transmitted diseases occur annually. A large proportion of these diseases (86%) occur among the 15- to 29-year-old age group. The most common of these diseases are trichomoniasis, gonorrhea, nongonorrheal urethritis, genital herpes, and syphilis. Among the more serious complications of these diseases are pelvic inflammatory disease, sterility, infant pneumonia, infant death, birth defects, and mental retardation (U.S. Department of Health and Human Services, 1983e).

Objectives

1. Increase students' knowledge of sexually transmitted diseases including knowledge of how these diseases are contracted and passed to others
2. Increase students' knowledge and acceptance of the importance of early medical diagnosis and treatment of these diseases
3. Increase students' knowledge of the serious complications of these diseases such as infant death, birth defects, and mental retardation

ACCIDENT PREVENTION AND CONTROL

The problem

More than 153,000 Americans die annually from accidents, with nearly half of these relating to motor vehicle deaths. Fifty-five percent of fatalities for the 15- to 24-year-old age group are the result of accidents. The cost of accidents from injuries, damage, and lost productivity for the nation amounted to approximately 832 billion dollars (U.S. Department of Health and Human Services, 1983e). Boys are more likely to incur an injury from accidents than are girls. For the age group of 12 to 17 years the leading causes of accidents were recreational sports including football, basketball, bicycles, baseball, and skateboards.

Objectives

1. Increase students' knowledge and appreciation of the problems arising from adolescent drinking as a factor in automobile accidents
2. Increase students' knowledge of the various causes of accidents
3. Increase students' knowledge and acceptance of using seat belts and child safety restraints in preventing injuries relating to motor vehicle accidents

SMOKING CONTROL

The problem

Cigarette smoking is the largest single preventable cause of illness and premature death in the United States. It is the major cause of lung cancer death in the United States, and it is a causal factor in coronary heart disease and other blood vessel diseases. It is the most important cause of chronic obstructive lung disease. Each year cigarette smoking is associated with 300,000 premature deaths. Maternal smoking during pregnancy causes retarded fetal growth, increased risk for fetal abortions, fetal deaths, and neonatal deaths (U.S. Department of Health and Human Services, 1983e). The most recent national survey of adolescent smoking (U.S. Department of Health and Human Services, 1979) indicated that girls are more likely to smoke than boys.

Objectives

1. Increase students' knowledge of cigarette smoking as one of the major risk factors for heart disease
2. Increase students' knowledge and acceptance of cigarette smoking as a major cause of lung cancer and as a contributing factor in other forms of cancer including laryngeal, esophageal, and bladder cancers
3. Increase students' knowledge and acceptance of cigarette smoking as a major cause of chronic obstructive lung disease including bronchitis and emphysema
4. Increase students' knowledge and acceptance of the special risks of cigarette smoking for women who are pregnant

ALCOHOL AND DRUG MISUSE PREVENTION

The problem

The alcohol consumption for all persons older than 14 years has increased by 10% over the last 10-year period (U.S. Department of Health and Human Services, 1980). Drinkers 14 to 17 years of age are estimated to be more than 3 million, or approximately 19% of this age group. Ten percent of all deaths in the United States are alcohol related. Alcohol is related to several diseases including cirrhosis of the liver and cancer of the liver, pancreas, and mouth. In addition, alcohol consumption during pregnancy is related to a variety of harmful effects to the fetus including decreased birth weight, spontaneous abortion, and physical and mental defects. The drug misuse problem appears to be increasing. Currently there are 16 million marijuana users, and 10 million people have tried cocaine. It is estimated that 1 million persons misuse barbiturates and 30,000 persons are addicted to barbiturates (U.S. Department of Health and Human Services, 1983e). Recent reports show a decline in cirrhosis mortality. The 1990 goal of a mortality of 12 per 100,000 should be attained (National Center of Health Statistics, 1986). Based on a 1982 National Institute for Drug Abuse household survey and a 1984 high school survey, alcohol use and drug use continue to decline among youths.

Objectives

1. Increase students' knowledge and appreciation of the risks associated with alcohol abuse
2. Increase students' knowledge about drugs and the nature of their effects
3. Increase students' knowledge and appreciation of the risks associated with regular cigarette smoking, marijuana, and barbiturate use
4. Increase students' knowledge of the social problems that result from alcohol and drug misuse such as family disruption and crime (Figs. 14-4 to 14-6)
5. Increase students' knowledge of the health consequences of drug misuse such as addiction, disability, and automobile accidents

IMPROVED NUTRITION

The problem

There is a substantial proportion of Americans 20 to 74 years of age who have an inappropriate nutritional status. About 14% of men and 24% of women are classified as obese. Good nutritional status is essential for the adolescent to ensure optimal growth and development, physical activity, reproduction, lactation, recovery from illness and injury, and the maintenance of health throughout life. Iron and folic acid deficiencies are common among pregnant and lactating women. The average American needs to reduce the amount of daily sodium ingestion.

Objectives

1. Increase students' knowledge of an optimal diet and its relationship to healthy growth and development, to physical activity, to successful reproduction and lactation, and to the maintenance of health
2. Increase students' knowledge of weight control through an appropriately balanced diet and physical activity
3. Increase students' knowledge and acceptance of the U.S. dietary goals (below) and their relationship to disease prevention and health promotion
4. Increase student's knowledge of sodium, calories, fat, and refined sugar as factors in cardiovascular disease
5. Increase students' knowledge and acceptance of the importance of providing appropriate nutrition for infants and young children (Fig. 14-7)

PHYSICAL FITNESS AND EXERCISE

The problem

Only about 35% of U.S. adults exercise regularly and only 33% of U.S. schoolchildren participate in a daily physical education program. Most people do not exercise enough or in a manner to achieve the maximal benefits. Exercise as a therapeutic regimen should be increased (U.S. Department of Health and Human Services, 1983e).

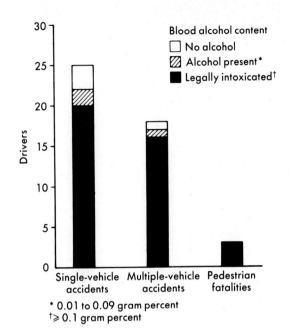

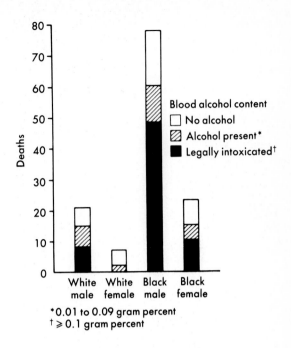

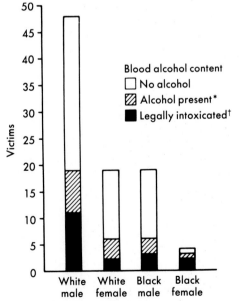

FIG. 14-4.   Blood alcohol content of drivers involved in fatal motor vehicle accidents in Fulton County, Georgia, 1982.
(From U.S. Department of Health and Human Services: Morbidity and Mortality Weekly Reports **32***(47):Nov. 11, 1983.)*

FIG. 14-5.   Alcohol use among homicide victims by race and sex in Fulton County, Georgia, 1982.
(From U.S. Department of Health and Human Services: Morbidity and Mortality Weekly Reports **32***(47):Nov. 11, 1983.)*

FIG. 14-6.   Alcohol use among suicide victims by race and sex in Fulton County, Georgia, 1982.
(From U.S. Department of Health and Human Services: Morbidity and Mortality Weekly Report **32***(47):Nov. 11, 1983.)*

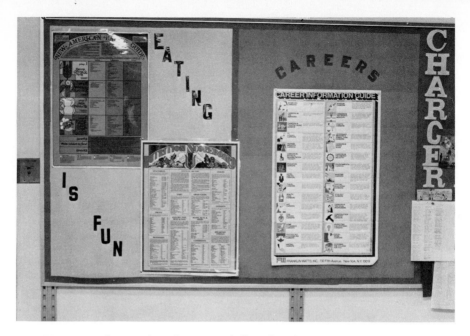

FIG. 14-7.   Providing timely and attractive bulletin boards serves to raise student awareness of current developments and also to reinforce important classroom learnings.
(Mary E. Allen.)

Objectives

1. Increase students' knowledge of the role of physical fitness and exercise in maintaining and promoting health
2. Increase students' knowledge of the importance of regular participation in physical activity

---

Dietary goals for the United States

1. To avoid overweight, consume only as much energy (calories) as is expended; if overweight, decrease energy intake and increase energy expenditure.
2. Increase the consumption of complex carbohydrates and "naturally occurring" sugars from about 28% of energy intake to about 48% of energy intake.
3. Reduce the consumption of refined and processed sugars by about 45% to account for about 10% of total energy intake.
4. Reduce overall fat consumption from approximately 40% to about 30% of energy intake.
5. Reduce saturated fat consumption to account for about 10% of total energy intake and balance that with polyunsaturated and monounsaturated fats, which should account for about 10% of energy intake each.
6. Reduce cholesterol consumption to about 300 mg per day.
7. Limit the intake of sodium by reducing the intake of salt to about 5 g per day.

3. Increase students' knowledge and acceptance of the *type* and *duration* of exercise that promotes cardiovascular fitness
4. Increase students' knowledge of the benefits of cardiovascular fitness in relation to mental health
5. Increase students' knowledge of the role exercise plays in a weight control program
6. Increase students' knowledge of the different types of exercise needed to develop general physical fitness including cardiovascular fitness, flexibility, strength, and coordination

CONTROL OF STRESS AND VIOLENT BEHAVIOR

The problem

Improperly controlled stress is believed to contribute to various forms of physiologic and psychologic dysfunction, such as depression, fatigue, obesity, coronary heart disease, suicide, and violence. Each year there are many thousands of premature deaths from homicides and suicides. It is estimated that there are 2000 deaths and up to 4,000,000 injuries inflicted on children each year by abusing parents. Abusive behavior of parents is believed to be partially caused by stress. Groups such as males, teenagers, the elderly, and the economically disadvantaged appear to be more vulnerable to stress. The suicide rate for 15- to 24-year-old males increased by 41% between 1970 and 1978 (U.S. Department of Health and Human Services, 1983b), but there has been a modest downward trend in the suicide rate in this age group since 1983 (National Center for Health Statistics, 1986).

Objectives

1. Increase students' knowledge of stress including the psychologic and physiologic factors giving rise to stress
2. Increase students' knowledge of the various forms of physiologic and psychologic dysfunction, such as depression, fatigue, obesity, heart disease, suicide, and violence, that are believed to be related to stress
3. Increase students' knowledge of the injuries and deaths of children inflicted by abusing parents
4. Increase students' knowledge of the factors and conditions believed to be related to stress among teenagers, the elderly, and the socially disadvantaged (Figs. 14-8 and 14-9)

DEALING WITH CONTROVERSIAL SUBJECTS

A realistic assessment of the nature of education indicates that controversy will always surround the educational process. This is a direct result of the role education fulfills in our society. Viewed one way, the role of education is to prepare young people to function effectively within society. Accordingly, education provides young people with the skills that are important for responsible citizenship and effective participation in family and community affairs. Viewed another way, the role of education is to prepare young people to deal with changes in society and to stimulate thinking, creativity, and interpretive skills that may lead to changes within the society. This tension between the role of education as a stabilizing force and the role of education as a vehicle for change often results in controversy.

Controversy presents a useful challenge to school personnel to interpret clearly to the public what they are doing and the value of such action. A community controversy about school-related issues presents a challenge to school personnel to do what they should be most effective at doing: interpreting information in such a way that others can understand and use that information.

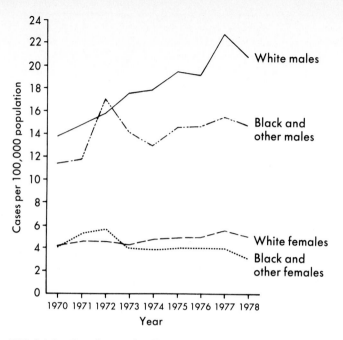

FIG. 14-8. Suicide rates for all persons 15 to 24 years of age by race and sex in United States, 1970 to 1978.

*(From U.S. Department of Health and Human Services: Morbidity and Mortality Weekly Report **32**(35):Sept. 9, 1983.)*

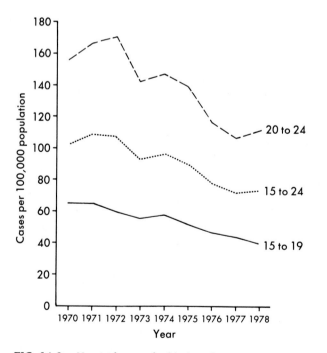

FIG. 14-9. Homicide rates for black males 15 to 24 years of age by age group in United States, 1970 to 1978.

*(From U.S. Department of Health and Human Services: Morbidity and Mortality Weekly Report **32**(35):Sept. 9, 1983.)*

Nature of controversy

Controversy occurs for many reasons. At least three different types of controversy can be identified.

Scientific controversy. With mass communications the public receives a great deal of conflicting information concerning health-related issues. As new knowledge develops and scientists refine existing knowledge, quite often points of contention occur. One group of scientists will discover the health implications of a particular medicine, food, or personal habit, and another group of scientists will find contradicting information. This is the nature of science: to find the truth through repeated searching and questioning. Scientists anticipate disagreement, but the public does not. Nutrition, for example, is full of topics for which the scientific findings are not yet clear. For the teacher this type of controversy presents a challenge to help students understand the scientific method and the reasons that there are so often contradictions in science. However, until there is clear scientific evidence on a particular point, it would be unwise for a teacher to take sides.

Conflicts of science and religion. Scientific controversy differs greatly from the controversy that pits the findings of science against religious beliefs. For example, there is scientific evidence that fluoride added to public drinking water reduces tooth decay among young people and accordingly enhances health, reduces health care costs, and improves nutrition.

However, some communities hold religiously based beliefs that chemicals, such as fluorides, which can be poisonous in large quantities, should not be added to the water. A community's referendums to fluoridate water supplies can often be defeated by these groups. This type of controversy, between religion and science, can be especially costly to a community. In the case of water fluoridation, the first cost is in depriving young people of an effective dental decay prophylaxis and the second is in the dissension and distrust caused within the community.

Philosophic controversies. Scientific controversy results from different interpretations of scientific findings; controversies involving science and religion contrast the findings of science and the beliefs of religion. Personal philosophies may be based neither on science nor on established religion. Philosophic controversies may surround issues of teaching methods, hiring practices, discipline, and educational philosophy. Today the notion of values clarification as a teaching technique is likely to provoke objection from some and support from others, arousing controversy. The report of the National Commission on Excellence in Education (1983) on the quality of education in the United States, entitled *A National at Risk: the Imperative for Educational Reform,* reflects the greatly differing philosophies on how schools should be managed. One example of such a controversial area is seen in the differing values placed on extracurricular activities. Some persons believe that these activities encroach unnecessarily into school time for instruction, whereas others believe that the informal learning resulting from these activities far outweighs the value of the time lost to formal instruction.

Knowledge as a basis of controversy

In our educational system, knowledge is basic. Without knowledge decisions cannot be made, problems cannot be solved, and relationships cannot be established. First and foremost, schools teach facts and information and the methods to derive factual information, the basis of knowledge. The scientific method is the generally accepted method of deriving information or facts and has as its aim the discovery of "truth." A collection of factual information constitutes knowledge.

Knowledge and facts, however, do not represent wisdom. Wisdom is how knowledge is applied and comes with experience and the development of values.

Despite these well-accepted principles of education, the argument is widespread that knowledge about some topics, such as sex, is dangerous. Why should knowledge about sex encourage promiscuous sexual behavior when knowledge about anarchy is not equally feared for encouraging students to become anarchists? In fact, the earlier a person engages in sexual relationships, the less he or she is likely to know anything about sex. Gordon (1981) points out that informed students are most likely to postpone sexual relations until they are emotionally ready, or, when and if these students are sexually active, they act appropriately to avoid pregnancy or sexually transmitted diseases.

To suggest that access to knowledge should be denied because it would foster inappropriate use of that knowledge contradicts the basis of our educational system and the principles of democracy (Fig. 14-10).

Controversy and values

Most often the basis of controversy in a school centers on the issue of values. Questions about what should be taught and who should teach it are an extension of the concern about whose values will be presented to the student along with the factual content material. No teaching is value free regardless of how much teachers may attempt neutrality in their presentations.

Because most teaching is value laden, there is a concern among parents, school board members, and administrators that the values that are taught, directly and indirectly, have a basis in fact and fall within the range of values of the larger society. A history teacher does not teach the various political systems of communism, anarchy, democracy, and fascism and then suggest that they all have equal merit and that students should select the one they will follow. By word, attitude, and practice the teacher will clearly show a preference for a political system. Similarly the nutrition teacher does not teach about foods without telling students which are the better selections.

In sex education it is clear that it is better for teenagers not to become pregnant for both physiologic and psychologic reasons. Any teacher who teaches about contraception and does not also present some basic guidelines about the values of avoiding pregnancy is in a sense practicing educational malpractice. However, when a teacher describes contraceptives as a means of avoiding pregnancy, that teacher may still be at odds with some groups in the community who do not accept contraception because it violates religious dictates. Others may believe that giving knowledge about contraception implies tacit approval of premarital sexual intercourse.

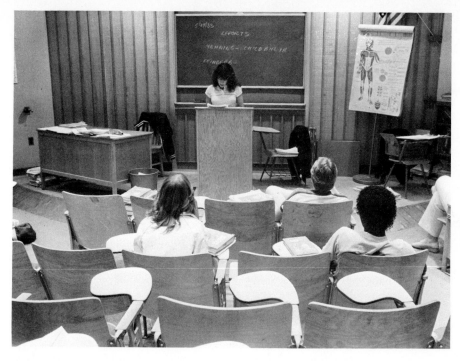

FIG. 14-10. Giving a formal report in the health education class provides opportunities for the students to improve their communication skills while gaining self-confidence and greater maturity.
(Mary E. Allen.)

Moral and moralistic perspectives

Education takes place in a moral context, not a moralistic context. A moral perspective encourages the accpetance of the aspirations of society but maintains the right of individual liberty. A moralistic context imposes a personal perspective in a persistent and dogmatic way. Gordon (1981) points out that it would be appropriately moral to tell a student that sex before marriage is against the principal teachings of organized religion. It would be moralistic and inappropriate to say that if students participate in sex before marriage they risk damnation. Such a statement, though inappropriate in the public school, may be appropriate in some parochial schools.

The distinction between moral and moralistic perspectives is important when dealing with issues of controversy. The teacher who does not clearly make this distinction is likely to irritate unnecessarily some students or parents. Implicit here is the ability to separate personal values and interpretations from those that represent the views of the larger society. However, it is possible that any specific community may not endorse the views of the larger society, and on some issues there is not a clear position of the larger society. Teachers therefore should be aware of the moral and moralistic perspectives of controversial topics.

When teachers work in areas of controversy, they must be well prepared and knowledgeable about all aspects of the subject. Of course, this is true in all areas of teaching, but it is especially critical in areas that are likely to come under public scrutiny. Fortunately most teachers who are willing to teach in areas of controversy realize this point.

An evaluation of student knowledge gains in selected health education topics taught in a sample of Nebraska schools showed that few schools taught about sex, but in those that did, student knowledge gains, compared with those of students who had not had similar instruction, were significantly higher. Further analysis suggested that teachers willing to teach about this topic prepared themselves especially well. The quality of their teaching and their sensitivity to issues of possible controversy increased, and in so doing they reduced the likelihood of possible community reaction (Newman et al., 1978).

Respecting the rights of all parties

Kirschenbaum (1982) points out that probably as many as half of the school districts in the United States have no clearly stated procedure for dealing with controversy. Kirschenbaum suggests that the following points should serve as guidelines for planning ways to deal with the resolution of controversial situations:

1. Clarify relationships between the school and the community with respect to curriculum and instruction
2. Avoid unnecessary conflict
3. Handle legitimate complaints and controversies in a way that respects democratic principles and professional practice

Relations between the school and community are best clarified with a specific statement on the community's role in the governance of the schools. Obviously this relationship begins with the school board as the community policy-making organization for the schools, but many more forms of relationships can be established by the school board. Advisory panels, expert panels, textbook selection committees, and grievance review panels represent examples of roles for community involvement and relationships between the school and community.

Clearly stated policies that stipulate the responsibilities of these groups will improve their effectiveness and avoid possible confusion.

Conflict can be avoided by administrators who are sensitive to the needs of individuals and who quickly identify and deal with potential conflict situations. Conflict may also be avoided by having ample opportunity for community input and dialog in the planning of new school programs or proposed changes in existing programs. For example, a revision in the school's physical education goals from one of recreation activities to aerobic fitness activities could benefit from public hearings concerning the advantages and disadvantages of the existing programs compared with those of the proposed programs. In this way all sides of an issue can be heard before a final decision is made concerning the proposed change. Even if the change is objected to by some, they will have been given a chance to express their views. Of course, this does not preclude any chance of later conflict, but it reduces the likelihood of such and brings the important issues to the public's attention.

If conflict develops that cannot be dealt with informally, clearly established means to resolve the conflict should exist and be known to those involved. These means of conflict resolution should guarantee the rights of due process and include clear appeal options. A complaint about a curriculum item or teaching method may be dealt with as an administrative matter by the principal or whoever is in charge of curriculum matters. Failure to resolve the issue informally may lead to the issue being referred to a faculty panel. If the issue is still not resolved, a right of appeal may exist to the superintendent, who may appoint a joing school-community review group. Failure at this level may lead to an appeal to the school board. Variations on this hierarchy of conflict resolution steps could be many, but every school board should have a clear and specific set of policies.

Based on his work with the National Coalition for Democracy in Education, Kirschenbaum (1982) suggests that the rights and privileges of parents, school members, professional teachers on the school staff, and students all be considered judiciously in dealing with matters of controversy and disagreement.

Parents and community members.   Parents are a single group of taxpayers who share, along with other taxpayers, the burden of paying for the schools. Because parents have children participating in the education process, their voices are more clearly heard than other taxpayers and community members in general. However, all citizens share the tax burden of supporting the schools, and so all have the right to participate in the school's governance.

Community members have the right to elect members to the school board and thereby directly participate in the establishment of community education policy. Community members can attend meetings of the school board, express opinions, visit and observe the school in operation, and serve on advisory groups within the school.

Parents have the right to be informed about their children's educational progress, to know of the content of their child's educational experience, and to request that special needs for their children be met. If certain parts of the curriculum are in conflict with the parents' values, they can request that their children be excused from these units. They do not have the right, however, to prevent other children from participating in these units.

School board.   School boards serve as the community's representatives to establish goals, set policies, and hire competent professional staff, who in turn will carry out the day-by-day operations of the school and implement the school board's policies. If controversial issues cannot be resolved by the professional staff, the school board will become involved as the final arbitrator. The board's rights and responsibilities include establishing and imposing educational policy, but the board cannot infringe on or impose its will in matters that are not distinctly educational.

Professional staff.   The school's professional staff works within the bounds of the policies established by the school board. They are expected to maintain communication with the school's community. The professional staff are expected and have the rights and responsibilities to establish curriculum, determine teaching methods, and revise, replace, and maintain the teaching resources necessary for optimal learning by their students.

Students.   Students have the right to expect well-trained and competent teachers, adequate educational resources to facilitate learning, and a broad-based curriculum with a variety of subject matter area. At the same time, students have the right to develop their own opinions, to voice their opinions in appropriate ways and settings, and to choose among a variety of educational opportunities provided by the school. Students also have a right to privacy and due process.

Handling controversy

Controversy is not necessarily bad. Simply put, controversy is a discussion of contrary opinions. Out of controversy may come new agreements, positive ideas, and new energies to solve old problems. Out of controversies may also come dissension, disagreement, and disunity. Each year, hundreds of school districts face controversy and channel the contradictory energies in a positive manner, whereas other districts fail to resolve contrary positions, and accordingly programs, students, teachers, parents, and the communities suffer.

The basic points in dealing with controversy are (1) understanding the nature of the controversy and (2) having a procedure for handling controversial topics. This procedure must have its foundation in a clear recognition of the legitimate interests and rights of the parties involved. Similarly these established procedures should be known to all who are interested and involved in the quality of education and the conduct of their community's schools.

INNOVATIVE HEALTH INSTRUCTION: SOME EXAMPLES

Three examples of recent innovative approaches to health instruction are presented. The materials were selected not only because they represent certain innovations but also because they concern topics that have been identified as important to the nation's health objectives and to the health needs of adolescents as well. Also, because of the controversial nature of sexually transmitted disease, it was believed to be of use to both teachers and school officials to learn something of the scope and approach to teaching about these diseases as defined in the California project.

The materials selected represent two state projects, "Decisions about Alcohol and Other Drugs," sponsored by the Nebraska Division on Alcoholism and Drug Abuse, and "Teaching about Sexually Transmitted Diseases," a project of the California State Department of Education, and also an individual self-learning, self-care project, "Willpower? Skillpower!" an outgrowth of an experimental study conducted by Schindler (1982).

The materials were selected to illustrate differing aspects of health teaching in today's schools. The Nebraska project offers some important guidelines for teaching secondary school students about alcohol using a decision-making approach. Included is the introduction to the guide, which calls attention to the alcohol problem in American society and the importance of an educational approach to deal with the serious problem of teenage drinking and driving. The guide offers a unique approach to this problem. Traditionally alcohol education has adopted a fear approach that points to the consequences of violating the law or the tragedies resulting from the inexperienced driver and drinker. Increasingly, behavioral scientists are stressing the importance of teaching decision-making skills. Their approach goes beyond the giving of facts about alcohol and helps the student to become aware of the emotional and psychologic as well as the social forces that are shaping the teenager's behavior.

Helping teenagers to become more aware of these influences is a first step in the decision-making process. Helping them to know when more information is needed, to examine carefully the options, to evaluate the consequences of their choices, finally to commit themselves to the decision—living with the decision—is an essential step toward becoming a truly healthy person.

The material on sexually transmitted diseases represents an area of the health education curriculum about which very little has been written. In addition to defining the subject, the information for the teacher should be of value in teaching this topic.

The Willpower? Skillpower! program represents an adaptation of behavior modification and social learning theory. Students are taken through a series of steps designed to help them learn techniques of self-monitoring, self-reinforcement, and self-evaluation. Selected excerpts from this program have been included to illustrate several of the steps in this process. The aim of the program is to help students gain the understanding and the skills necessary to undertake successfully personal health behavior change.

Decisions about alcohol and other drugs*

WHY TEACH ABOUT ALCOHOL AND OTHER DRUGS?

Alcohol and other drugs are an almost inescapable part of life in the United States today. Over 80,000,000 Americans drink socially; the vast majority of Americans have taken or will take over-the-counter or prescription medicines at some time; and a rapidly growing percentage of Americans, particularly young people, have used controlled substances for nonmedical purposes.

Because drugs are powerful substances, with significant and often unpredictable effects on the mind and body, use of drugs is often accompanied by problems. Alcohol, in particular, causes major problems for many people. It has been estimated that more adults are directly or indirectly affected by alcohol-related problems than by any other single health problem.† Other drugs, too, pose serious risks to health and safety. The nature and extent of drug problems vary greatly from community to community, but almost everywhere we see:

- Traffic accidents and fatalities associated with drinking drivers;
- Interaction effects resulting from using drugs in combination (particularly mixing alcohol and other drugs);
- Negative effects resulting from drug experimentation, particularly by young people; and
- Problems caused by alcoholism or other drug dependency, affecting not only the drug-dependent person, but those close to him/her as well.

Parents and teachers, while recognizing that these problems must touch young people as well as adults, may not be aware of the full extent of alcohol/other drug use among teens, or of the very real decisions that even elementary and junior high students must make.

Given the problems arising from alcohol/drug use in the society as a whole and the pressure on young people to drink and use drugs, it is important that young people be adequately prepared. They must be ready to handle the experiences they are likely to encounter as teenagers and to anticipate the problems they may encounter as adults.

---

*The material in this section is from Decisions about alcohol and other drugs: a curriculum for Nebraska schools, 1982, The Nebraska Prevention Center for Alcohol and Drug Abuse.

†Cited in Peter Finn and Jane Lawson: A teacher manual for use with Jackson Junior High, 1982.

A measure of the importance of alcohol/drug education to young people is the eagerness with which they seek out information about these substances. Young people are hungry for information about the effects of drugs; they want to discover what others think about drug use, and what the actual consequences of a choice to use alcohol or other drugs will be. A school-based alcohol and other drug education program can meet this need for information with *facts* rather than *myths*. But such a program should do more than simply inform. Information alone will not prevent problems. A successful drug/alcohol program must do more. It must help young people to form positive attitudes about themselves and about their ability to make their own decisions, whatever the pressures may be. It must foster a sense of personal responsibility for the consequences of decisions, and encourage the development of the ability to cope successfully with life problems. It must, in short, help build the kind of inner strength and sense of self that can make informed, conscious decision-making a reality.

CURRICULUM GOALS AND OBJECTIVES

In line with the assumptions above, the major goal of this curriculum is to help young people make informed, conscious decisions about their personal use of alcohol and other drugs, and hence ultimately to help reduce the incidence of problems associated with the use of these substances. More specifically, students will be able to:

- Identify and practice decision-making skills;
- Recognize drugs that they are likely to encounter or use;
- Understand the effects of such drugs alone and in combination, and understand the possible consequences of misuse or abuse;
- Understand and respect the body's natural functioning and the effects of alcohol and other drugs on that functioning;
- Understand and weigh the influence of family, media, and the law on drug/alcohol and other drugs on that functioning;
- Recognize the importance of standing up to peer pressure when it conflicts with personal principles and goals;
- Weigh the consequences of a decision to drink and drive, and make informed decisions based on that knowledge;
- Identify and practice alternatives to the use of alcohol or other drugs that satisfy human needs in positive ways;
- Develop techniques for handling stressful social situations involving drugs or alcohol;
- Recognize when alcohol/drug behavior creates problems for others; and determine appropriate interventions;
- Recognize and, if necessary, seek out resources available to help persons with alcohol/drug problems and their families; and
- Make decisions governing prsonal alcohol/drug behavior in line with personal principles and goals.

This curriculum was developed in a systematic fashion based on the goals listed above. In addition to these broad goals, specific student-oriented learning objectives were developed to aid the formation of each activity. A review of the objectives within this curriculum will be helpful in the development of a specific alcohol and other drug education unit.

CURRICULUM ORGANIZATION

The activities and content information that compose this curriculum are organized into seven major sections or clusters. Each cluster concentrates on a different facet of the overall decision-making process. The first cluster, "Introduction to Decision-making," helps students discover why decisions are important and what elements are involved in making informed, conscious decisions. A five-step decision-making process is introduced, and students have the opportunity to practice working through the process to arrive at a decision. The five steps of the decision-making process are listed below and are presented for use in graphic form throughout the curriculum.

1. Defining the problem
2. Looking at influences
3. Identifying alternatives
4. Looking at risks and results
5. Deciding, acting, and evaluating

The process is discussed in more detail in the introduction to Cluster I.

Subsequent clusters expand students' comprehension of the various steps in decision-making and provide ongoing practice in making decisions in difficult situations. At the same time, students' understanding of the nature and effects of chemical substances is also enhanced.

As previously mentioned, each section of this curriculum is referred to as a cluster. Each cluster consists of a *Cluster Summary, Activity Summaries,* and, if needed, supplementary *Teacher and Student Information.* The Cluster Summary is found at the beginning of each cluster and is an overall review of the content covered within the cluster. The summary states the concepts of the cluster and reviews what student objectives, activities, and resources are used within the cluster. In observing the Cluster Summary, it should be noted that the objectives, activities, and resources are read from left to right. An objective may have one or more activities that relate to it, or there may be more than one objective that relates to only one activity.

The activities within each cluster are described in the Activity Summary. The Activity Summary is an actual outline of the "steps to learning" that have been identified for each activity. Within the summaries can also be found a synopsis of the activity followed by the student objective(s) that are addressed in the activity. A listing of the resources needed for the activity are found in the left margin of the summary. These resources include handouts for the students, visuals to aid the teacher, films, Student/Teacher Information, and an Evaluation Component.

The handouts intended for use within the activities are duplication masters and are included directly in the activity. The visuals listed are transparency masters, also found in the activity, that may be utilized by the teacher. Films mentioned within this curriculum are available upon request from the sources identified within the Activity Summary. Additional Student Information is provided and may be reproduced at the teacher's discretion. Supplementary Teacher Information is included in a few activities and will provide the teacher with an immediate resource. It is suggested that the teacher review each activity in advance of the class period in order to have the appropriate materials produced.

An "Evaluation Component" is included in each cluster to help the teacher evaluate student learning performance. The component consists of a set of test items that are matched with the objectives for each cluster. The objectives which do not have actual test questions may be assessed as students complete an activity or handout. Teachers will have to observe students working or collect and assess responses on the handouts to assess the objectives. If a teacher would like to construct a pre-test to assess students' entry levels, the test items could be combined into one examination. After analyzing the results, the teacher could then select the clusters or specific activities where students have the greatest needs. In a similar fashion, test items from two or more clusters could be combined into a post-test administered at the end of the drug/alcohol unit. Student responses to such a test would provide the teacher with an accurate assessment of the objectives which students have mastered.

An addendum entitled "Drugs and Pregnancy" is included following Cluster VII. This section was prepared to supply educational material dealing with the effects of drug use during pregnancy. The addendum is organized along the same lines as the previous clusters.

A Resource Section is the final unit in this curriculum. This section provides the teacher with immediate information and acts as a reference for much of the content material discussed within the activities. The Resource Section comprises the following components:

- Teaching strategies
- Suggested films

- Sources for drug and alcohol instructional material
- Helping children with alcoholism in the family
- Directory of Nebraska Alcoholism and Drug Abuse Services
- Nebraska alcohol and drug laws
- Glossary
- Bibliography of materials used in developing this curriculum

THE DECISION-MAKING PROCESS

The following example illustrates how the decision-making process can be applied to decision-making dilemmas that teenagers must face.

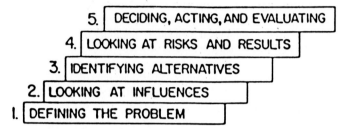

5. DECIDING, ACTING, AND EVALUATING
4. LOOKING AT RISKS AND RESULTS
3. IDENTIFYING ALTERNATIVES
2. LOOKING AT INFLUENCES
1. DEFINING THE PROBLEM

Situation: Jane is at a party. She drove there with Jim and Jerry in Jim's car. It is getting late. Jim has been drinking heavily all night. His speech is slurred, and he weaves as he walks.

Now Jim wants to leave. "Come on, Jerry and Jane, we're going." Jerry suggests that Jim let him drive. "No way! I'm fine! Come on—*now!*"

Step 1: Defining the problem. Jane definitely sees a problem here. On the one hand she needs to get home—she promised her parents to be back by 12:30. On the other hand, it doesn't look like Jim's in much shape to drive. Deciding whether to drink and drive is Jim's problem, but since he's clearly bent on driving, the problem becomes hers as well. She must decide whether to go with him, or if not, what to do. She must also decide whether or not to attempt to influence Jim's decision.

Step 2: Looking at influences. Jane's parents want her home. She likes Jim a lot when he's not drinking and doesn't want to alienate him. Both of these are strong influences that Jane must weigh.

Step 3: Identifying alternatives. Jane has several alternatives:
Go with Jim;
Call her parents to come get her;
Stay overnight;
Call a cab;
Find another ride.
In terms of influencing Jim's decision, she can:
Do nothing;
Steal the car keys;
Try to get Jim so drunk he passes out;
Mobilize group pressure to influence Jim.
In identifying the alternatives she realizes she needs more facts. Is there someone else she can ride with? She asks, and discovers that Barbara is going her way and would be willing to drop her off.

Step 4: Looking at risks and results. To go with Jim means a risk of a serious accident. Jane would call her parents, but then they'd know that drinking had been going on, and they would probably be angry. Staying overnight might also create parental worry. She could call a cab, but that would take most of her spending money for the month. Probably her best bet would be to accept the ride with Barbara.

But what about her feelings about Jim? Jane would prefer not to see him hurt. She could steal the car keys so he couldn't drive, but that would surely anger Jim. She could try to get him so drunk, he'd pass out, but it might not work and besides, she really needs to get home soon. Mobilizing group pressure might not work, and might anger Jim as well, but it could influence him to let Jerry drive.

Step 5: Deciding, acting, and evaluating. Jane decides that the risk of alienating Jim is more than outweighed by the danger of drunk driving. She will not ride with Jim. Her concern for Jim outweighs the risk of angering him by getting the group to pressure him, so she figures she'll try that. Perhaps he'll then let Jerry drive. If not, going with Barbara seems the best bet. Jane talks to several people, including Bob, a person Jim respects highly. Bob and several others reason with Jim. Gradually, Jim is won over. He agrees to let Jerry drive home. After Jane is home, she thinks about what transpired. She's safe, Jim's safe, she's home only a little after 12:30. All in all, it seems like a good decision.

Teaching about sexually transmitted diseases*

INTRODUCTION

The following pages contain suggestions for structuring classroom activities for a 5-day VD education unit. Since students in junior and senior high schools are at so many different levels of understanding and skill development, a wide variety of learning activities are offered here from which the teacher may choose. Some of these may be more appropriate to junior high school students, others to senior high school students. The activities were designed, at any rate, to provide both the teacher and the students the kind of flexibility that will maximize learning opportunities and minimize the need for sophisticated skills or knowledge of the topic beforehand.

The unit was designed to be implemented over a period of 5 days in periods approximately 45 minutes long. Individual teachers may wish to depart from this suggested pattern, however, and should feel free to use any parts of the unit that they find helpful. Other teachers may choose to follow the unit exactly as it is outlined. If so, all they need to do is choose the activities they intend to implement and prepare the materials described for those activities. In many cases student worksheets are provided in order to facilitate completion of the activity. These worksheets are referred to by number, and they begin on page 40. They were designed to be copied or displayed via overhead projector.

Although the teacher is encouraged to use the recommended activities and materials in any way he or she wishes, these materials are based on a particular instructional approach that the teacher should clearly understand before beginning the unit.

Too often the primary focus of venereal disease education has been on facts through the heavy use of films, outside health experts, and health pamphlets. This approach assumes that information about VD alone will influence behavior. In reality, a combination of affective and cognitive learning is better suited to the kinds of long-term behavioral changes that VD education attempts to bring about. Therefore, the recommended activities for VD education in this unit include opportunities for communication, discussion, consideration of alternative procedures and points of view, and exercising of decision-making skills.

GOAL: To encourage an awareness among adolescents about the nature and extent of sexually transmitted diseases, ways of preventing them, and the need to seek medical diagnosis or assistance whenever their presence is suspected.

AN OVERVIEW OF SEXUALLY TRANSMITTED DISEASES

Concept 1   Sexually transmitted diseases may have immediate and long-range effects on individuals and society

---

*From Teaching about sexually transmitted diseases: a curriculum guide and resources for grades 7-12, Sacramento, 1980, California State Department of Education, pp. 6, 12, 28, and 31.

Concept 2   Ten specific sexually transmitted diseases are a serious health problem because of their incidence or their effects

Concept 3   Sexually transmitted diseases can be treated and prevented

Concept 4   Individuals have a personal and social responsibility to assist in the prevention and control of sexually transmitted diseases

A NOTE ON TERMINOLOGY

Until relatively recently the term "venereal disease" referred to five specific diseases only. The two most commonly known are gonorrhea and syphilis. The others, extremely rare, are chancroid, lymphogranuloma venereum, and granuloma inguinale. Since all are communicated through intimate sexual relations, they were subsumed under the term "venereal," which takes its root from Venus, the ancient Roman goddess of love. Aside from the mode of transmission, these five diseases are completely separate and distinct.

In recent years many other diseases that are spread primarily through sexual contact have been added to the list. These include nongonoccocal urethritis (NGU), herpes simplex virus 2, trichomoniasis, and several others. Because these "new" conditions have expanded the original definition of venereal disease, clinicians now use "sexually transmitted diseases" and "sexually transmissible diseases" as the equivalent of "venereal diseases."

In this publication the terms "VD" and "venereal disease" are used interchangeably with the more current terminology. Teachers who offer instruction about sexually transmitted diseases should be acquainted with all the various terms. They should also emphasize throughout the VD education unit that "VD" refers to a wide variety of different and distinct sexually transmitted diseases.

TO THE TEACHER

In many ways sexually transmitted diseases are still cloaked in an aura of secrecy. Sexually transmitted diseases are essentially a health problem, however, not a moral problem. Consigning these diseases to the realm of guilt and shame (the traditional attitude) makes them diseases that people are less likely to discuss openly and then do something to control.

The main role of the teacher in a VD education unit is to create a classroom atmosphere in which sexually transmitted diseases can be talked about openly and comfortably. Therefore the teacher must feel comfortable with these kinds of discussions before initiating them with students. Students may ask direct and specific questions about the use of condoms, sexual intercourse, homosexuality, and similar topics. Moreover, the teacher must feel comfortable not just with the topic, but with informal student discussions in general.

Some tips on making VD instruction effective

Although the basic classroom atmosphere is paramount, teachers should not overlook several other principles of effective instruction that can help to make a VD education unit lively and interesting:

Involve all the students. Even when the teacher has succeeded in creating a comfortable atmosphere for discussion, students may be reluctant to express themselves on what they consider a potentially embarrassing topic. Some students may even suspect that they have a venereal disease and may, therefore, be unwilling to betray their anxiety. While the teacher should not force students to participate in discussions, every effort should be made to elicit input from all the students in the class. This can be accomplished through classroom activities that use writing in addition to discussion and through occasional small-group activities.

Don't do all the talking. When presentation of facts is required, lectures may be the most efficient technique. If the teacher does too much of the talking, however, he or she will risk creating one-way communication.

Listen to the students. If a teacher avoids doing all the talking, he or she may still not be listening to the students. Listening, in this context, means being responsive to the students' concerns and questions without judging them — in short, structuring the class so that students feel free to ask questions and volunteer their thoughts and opinions.

Vary the pace and style. Mixing different kinds of activities within a single class period will help to sustain the students' interest. Although the five-day unit in this book offers several different options, the teacher should avoid relying on any one particular technique. The use of different techniques and activities will provide variety and texture to the class.

Avoid the use of slang. Some students have probably already acquired "street knowledge" about venereal diseases. The kinds of attitudes and misinformation commonly associated with street knowledge are counter to the purpose of an effective VD education unit. Therefore, from the beginning the teacher should avoid slang and encourage the correct use of terms. (On the other hand, a stilted classroom atmosphere emphasizing *only* the use of proper terminology should also be avoided. Students should be able to feel comfortable discussing this subject.)

SECOND DAY: COMMUNICABLE DISEASES

Rationale

The purpose of this lesson is to begin exploring the content of the unit. Since many students may already be familiar with the communicable disease cycle, the teacher may decide simply to review this information and proceed to the content designed for the following lesson.

Objectives

The teacher will determine whether or not the students are familiar with the communicable disease cycle and, if not, present this information so that it is clearly understood.

The students will:
- (Objective 1A) Describe the infectious disease cycle.
- (Objective 1B) Identify common reportable communicable diseases.
- (Objective 1C) Explain why sexually transmitted diseases are a serious health problem.

Activity 5: handshake (10 minutes)

Explain that this is an activity designed to offer a concrete illustration of how a communicable disease spreads through a population. Assign a number to everyone in the class. Then tell all the students in the class to shake hands with two other students. After the handshaking, pick two numbers out of a hat and explain that the students who have these numbers are designated as having a communicable disease. Then, in a class discussion, figure out who in the class may have "contracted" the disease through the handshake. The percentages may be made more realistic by figuring the odds of contracting a disease like gonorrhea — 20% to 50% for men, and over 50% for women.

Activity 6: the infectious disease cycle (20 minutes)

Draw the diagram of the infectious disease cycle on p. 16 on the chalkboard, and explain the cycle to the students. Ask for student volunteers to assist in the explanation. Duplicate and hand out copies of the infectious disease cycles for measles, syphilis, and gonorrhea from p. 16 (or display them on an overhead projector) and, after making sure that the students understand this material, ask the class to discuss the similarities and differences of the three diseases. Emphasize during this discussion that while measles creates its own immunity, syphilis and gonorrhea can be contracted through reinfection over and over again. Also emphasize that most other sexually transmitted diseases follow cycles that are similar to those of syphilis and gonorrhea.

Willpower? Skillpower!*

INTRODUCTION (FRAME 1)

Willpower? Skillpower! is a program to help you learn two important life skills: how to change your own behavior, and how to help others change theirs. This program teaches you methods that have been proved effective in helping people lose weight, stop smoking or drinking, improve physical fitness, or modify other personal habits. While other programs may teach you to handle only one problem, *this course teaches you the skills of personal problem solving that can apply to changing most personal habits.* Skill power is the emphasis of this program.

Willpower? Skillpower! does not emphasize the use of personal "willpower" to change personal habits. The idea of "willpower" is very vague and doesn't help explain success or failure when attempting to change. Imagine the following conversation:

Cathy: "I heard that Bill is going to stop smoking so he can compete better for a position on the wrestling team."

Jason: "Well, he shouldn't have any problem. He has lots of willpower."

Cathy: "How do you know that?"

Jason: "Bill lost 10 pounds last month to get into a lower weight class for wrestling, and I'm sure that took lots of willpower to do!"

The above conversation shows that the idea of "willpower" is often used in circular arguments. What allows Bill to stop smoking or lose weight? Willpower! but how do we know whether Bill has this willpower? Because he can stop smoking or lose weight! This kind of thinking is limited and often self-defeating. Too often "weak willpower" is given as an excuse for not changing bad habits into good ones, or why temptations get the best of us. *Willpower? Skillpower!* will teach you that it doesn't take "willpower" to change your habits. All you need to do is learn, practice, and apply the skills of self-change to your own behavior.

PROGRAM OUTLINE (FRAME 2)

Over the course of the seven sessions in the *Willpower? Skillpower!* program you will learn the techniques of self-monitoring, self-reinforcement, and self-evaluation that behavioral scientists use to help people change. By becoming your own behavioral scientist, you can apply these same skills to improve your own health. Briefly, here is a listing of the sessions in the program:

    I. Introduction and problem acceptance
    II. Self-monitoring: the why and how of who, what, when, and where
    III. Choosing a good goal for self-change
    IV. Individual methods for self-change
    V. Community programs for self-change
    VI. Selecting your program
    VII. Checking program results (evaluation)

The program is designed to last for seven weeks—the minimum time needed to show small changes in behavior. This may seem a long period of time for such small results, but remember that some habits have been with you for years!

CHANGE TAKES TIME, AND HEALTHY CHANGE TAKES EVEN MORE TIME.

Remember this line when you or someone else you are helping change expects results overnight or within too short a period of time.

SELF-MONITORING AND SELF-AWARENESS (FRAME 2)

Self-change is not an easy process. For each program of self-change that is successful, there are many attempts at self-change that fail. Why does this happen? For one reason, too often people make

---

*The material in this section is from Willpower? Skillpower! © 1982 by Jay and Jane Schindler, La Crosse, Wisc.

careless assumptions about what their problem really is. Most people jump into a program that they quickly designed for themselves, not giving much careful thought to the underlying reasons for their problem. What results is a program that might seem appropriate, but doesn't get at the real solutions to the problem. For example, let us assume that Cathy has a problem of obesity that may be linked to one major difficulty: Cathy consumes more calories than she expends, or burns up. But does this mean that she should eat less, or exercise more? Does Cathy snack too much between meals, does she eat too much at her meals, or does she simply not burn off enough calories through vigorous exercise?

If Cathy can't answer these questions and others like these, how can she really come up with an effective diet program that will help her lose weight? But suppose Cathy had taken the time to collect information on her eating and exercise habits for a short period of time, say 10 days. At the end of these 10 days Cathy could examine her personal habits carefully and determine what factors seem to be important in her weight control. By becoming a *behavioral scientist* and collecting information on herself, Cathy could now study the situation much more carefully and completely. Not only may the causes become more obvious, but possible solutions could be discovered. Also, by collecting this objective information accurately, Cathy could discover if her habits are really as bad as she thinks they are. This is important because people sometimes exaggerate how terrible their habits are, often making it difficult for them to get motivated enough to change.

By becoming more aware of the personal habits that we participate in — the *what, when, where, with whom,* and *why* of self-change — we can focus our energies for self-improvement more efficiently and effectively.

PROBLEM ACCEPTANCE (FRAME 3)

Everyone has problems, and we must face and resolve them every day. But, as suggested by the above quote, usually the most difficult part of helping people change is having them realize that a problem does exist in the first place. Accepting the fact that one has, or "owns," a problem is half the battle toward helping people change. Have you ever been in the situation where you just couldn't help a friend or family member recognize the problem that they faced? It might have made you feel frustrated, helpless, or angry that you couldn't reach them. Motivating people to accept that they have a problem is never easy, but some important principles for motivating change are listed below. Use these principles wisely.

Principle 1: Honestly express your concerns about your friend's problem situation. Help them to feel and know that your concerns are in *their* best interest, not your own. You might want to carefully present the short-term and long-term effects of not accepting the problem but keep in mind that they may already know what's in store for them if they don't change. Don't assume that you are going to "enlighten" them, or that you are "better" than them because you saw the problem that they face.

Principle 2: Carefully listen to and understand their position, and let them know that *you* understand it. Helping people change usually takes more careful listening than talking. After all, how can you help someone if you do all the talking and don't let them explain their position to begin with.

Principle 3: Do not make the problem your own. It's kind to be helpful as someone tries to change, but it's not appropriate to resolve a problem that belongs to someone else. Do not take responsibility for their success or failure; they may blame you if they don't reach their goal. Or, if they do reach their goal, they may become dependent upon you for success in the future.

In summary, problems are a fact of life for everyone, and people are often measured in our society by how well they handle the problems they face. Learning to recognize a situation as a problem is the first, and often the most difficult, step toward reaching goals. Helping other people accept the fact that they have a problem requires honest and open communication that carefully expresses your concerns, yet leaves the responsibility to accept the problem and solve it with them.

FRAME 3

Take a look at the personal health habit information in Cathy's Self-Awareness sheet below, and see if you can discover what factors influence her eating habits the most.

Date: Feb 10, 1983 Problem Event: EATING HABITS ID: STC2CLB						
Before	During	After	When	Where	With whom	Comments
	(Urges-thoughts-moods)					
really wasn't hungry	breakfast 2 pcs toast, cereal	Blah! School!	7:30	kitchen	Mom	sometimes skip breakfast
donuts looked so good!	3 powdered donuts	felt like a pig!	9:40	locker	Chris & Mary	they gave them to me!
determined not to eat alot	pizza, milk yogurt, salad	Good! Controlled my eating	12:30	lunch room	Patties Mary, Joan	
depressed about flunking math test	2 baloney sandwiches, milk, cookies	blew it! mad at myself	3:00	kitchen	alone	I use food to feel good!
Jim didn't talk to me	3 brownies & juice	day can't get worse!	4:30	Mary's house	Mary, Mary's mom	was visiting Mary
I will control myself	1 hamburger, chips jello, milk	Good! Didn't overeat	6:00	kitchen	family	dinner, quiet at home
Hungry! School worries	cheese sandwich cookies, milk	here I go again!	8:30	kitchen	alone	snack

HOW TO SELF-MONITOR (FRAME 4)

Self-monitoring of personal habits is not difficult, but it does require increased awareness on your part. This increased self-awareness of a particular health habit can actually change the health habit in a positive way (called "reactivity"). This change doesn't always occur, however, and it sometimes will disappear after monitoring your own habit for a while, so don't depend on it to completely change you. We'll learn other self-change tactics in the next session of *Willpower? Skillpower!*

Self-Awareness sheets are a quick and easy way to jot down important information about your personal health habits. You should write down your feelings, thoughts, and information immediately after your problem event occurs, because memories of personal problems often disappear quickly or become confused. Remember, the more complete and accurate your Self-Awareness records are, the more easily you can discover the factors that influence your habits.

It is helpful to monitor *when, with whom,* and *where* you are when your problem event occurs, because these facts could give important clues to your habits. We saw this was true with Cathy's problem. Also, for each specific problem there are specific clues that occur *before, during,* and *after* the problem event. These clues are very helpful when attempting to change. Look at Cathy's chart and circle those clues that you will look for when you fill out your own Self-Awareness charts.

SELF-CHANGE STRATEGIES (FRAME 1)

Willpower? Skillpower! emphasizes three major approaches to self-change: intrapersonal strategies, interpersonal strategies, and environmental change strategies.

Environmental change strategies focus on how you can modify your physical and social surroundings to help you succeed in changing personal habits. Interpersonal strategies draw on the help and encouragement of close friends, parents, and others who are willing to help aid you in reaching your self-change goals. Finally, intrapersonal techniques have you look at the mental comments you think about yourself, modifying those comments that are self-destructive, and have you use your creative mental abilities to help you continue in your attempts at change.

All three self-change strategies are helpful, and those people who use all three strategies simultaneously when attempting to change personal health habits are usually much more successful than those who try using just one or two of the strategies listed above.

ENVIRONMENTAL CHANGE STRATEGIES (FRAME 2)

Our surroundings usually have a strong influence on our health habits. Just imagine the following situation and see what you would do:

You are working part-time in a candy store after school to make some extra money for yourself. The store manager sometimes gives you candy for free to eat in the store, but he doesn't like you taking the candy home to eat. This afternoon business is a bit slow, and the store manager is talking to you as he munches on some new brand of candy. He offers you some pieces of it to eat. You're not really hungry, and you have told yourself before that you've got to cut down on "junk food," but this candy smells so delicious!

DO YOU ACCEPT THE CANDY AND EAT IT?

Obviously, one way to help reduce temptations is to modify the environment so that giving in to temptation is not so easy, or not possible. There are three general ways this can be done: (1) situation modifications, (2) making the behavior difficult, and (3) reminders.

Situation modification: The easiest way to refrain from temptation is to avoid the tempting environment to begin with! If you're a sucker for fresh donuts, stay out of the donut shop. Don't go in there with your friends, and don't hang around your friends when they're eating donuts. It's that simple.

If one place gives you lots of trouble, for example, the kitchen at home, stay away as much as you can from that place. In fact, if the kitchen gives you too much trouble, get out of the house if possible. Don't feel you have to resist temptation to be successful at self-change — it's much easier if there is no temptation to begin with.

INTERPERSONAL TECHNIQUES (FRAME 3)

Modeling: Do you have a friend who can easily handle the problem situation that is troubling you? For example, maybe Jason can't get through lunch time without running outside to smoke a few cigarettes, but Paul, a friend of Jason, has learned how to handle the situation. Maybe Paul's secret is chewing gum, but obviously he can handle lunch hour better than Jason. Jason should take the time to observe Paul during the lunch hour to see how his friend does it.

In the same way, if you have a friend who can get through a situation that you find difficult, take the time to observe and try on your friend's behaviors. This doesn't mean that you must maintain these behaviors for a long time, just until you discover whether they work for you.

Contracting: One of the most powerful techniques of behavior change today is interpersonal contracting. By bringing close friends, parents, or other important people into your self-change strategy, you gain their support and encouragement as you attempt to change. Also, your desire to do well is strengthened when you know these important individuals are concerned about you and the results of your program. Involve those individuals who are genuinely interested in helping you improve and are able to encourage you when the going gets tough. Explain to them what you are going to do and how they can help you reach your goals. Then fill out a contract with them so that both you and your "support team" are committed to improving your health habits. Take the contract seriously, and try your best to fulfill it. . . .

TEACHER PREPARATION IN HEALTH EDUCATION

The field of health education has developed rapidly over the recent past. Together with the increasing number of states that have begun to implement comprehensive school health education programs there has also been an increased demand for the health education specialist. According to a recent survey conducted by the Education Commission of the States (1981) 41 states reported employing health education specialists. This development has also been paralleled by a rapid rise in the number of colleges and universities offering professional preparation in health education. For example, in 1967 there were only 58 institutions offering preparation, but by 1981 this number had increased to 261, representing an increase of about 450% in 15 years.

Impressive as this growth has been, the results of the 1978 Role Delineation Conference and subsequent actions of the National Task Force on the Preparation and Practice of Health Educators may lead to even more significant developments. The work of the task force has helped to define the role of the practicing health educator. Moreover, members of the profession have accepted the definitions, responsibilities, and competencies that are considered basic to the functions of all health educators (see box on next page). Also it is anticipated that this development will lead to some general form of awarding credentials for the field, which in turn should lead to the establishment of standards and national recognition of the preparation and training required of all health educators, regardless of whether they work in community health departments, hospitals, or schools. With the rise of school health education, many state departments of education have adopted certification standards for the health education teacher. The box on p. 376 outlines the requirements for the Standard High School Certificate established in Illinois. According to these requirements, to be certified as a high school health education teacher, one must have at least 32 semester hours of preparation in health education (area of specialization). Those teachers who already hold a teacher certificate in another specialty may qualify to teach health as a second field by satisfactorily completing at least the 20-semester-hour-minimum program (see box on p. 377). Since the state certification standard is defined as the minimum, colleges and universities offering a major in the field usually establish requirements that go beyond those of the state standard.

SUMMARY

The chapter begins with a discussion of the purpose of secondary education and the controversies that had existed over the years. With one group arguing for a "back-to-basics" approach emphasizing the traditional subject-matter curriculum — math, science, english, and art — to prepare students for entrance to college. The other view in this debate holds that the curriculum should serve the needs of the adolescent. The departmental structure of secondary schools clearly reflect a subject matter orientation. Subject areas represent the departments, the formal course offerings, and the teachers themselves, who are prepared as subject matter specialists.

This period of the child's schooling experience between elementary and senior high school is one of transition from the self-contained classroom-integrated learning experience of the elementary school with a single teacher to multiple classrooms, teachers, and special subject departmental organizations of the secondary school. Such a transition can be stressful to the student. As a consequence, today's health education curriculum is placing less emphasis on learning the facts about health and more emphasis on helping students develop new academic and social skills that will help students adjust to the challenges of secondary education.

Curriculum patterns for offering health instruction are reviewed, including the separate health course and the teaching of health in correlation with science. A common curriculum pattern of offering health instruction at the senior high school is the one or two semester course or scheduling health education and physical education into four 9-week

Guide for the development of a competency-based curriculum for entry level health educators

Responsibility I: assess the need for health education

Terminal competency   A: Identifies needed health-related data about social and cultural environments, growth and development factors, needs and interests of defined populations

B: Analyzes information to determine areas of need of defined populations

C: Identifies potential targets for educational intervention

Responsibility II: plans health education programs

Terminal competency   A: Participation in the planning process

B: Gains support for the program

C: Develops program objectives

Responsibility III: coordinates planned health education programs

Terminal competency   A: Carries out designated administration activities for the educational program

B: Maintains support of other staff for health education programs

C: Acts as a facilitator

D: Assists other staff and volunteers responsible for carrying out health education activities

E: Advocates for health education

Responsibility IV: provides direct health education services

Terminal competency   A: Skillfully uses educational methods

B: Monitors education activities

C: Serves as a resource person

Responsibility V: evaluates health education

Terminal competency   A: Designs plans to assess educational methods and achievement of education/program objectives

B: Implements evaluation plan

C: Interprets results of evaluation

Responsibility VI: promotes organizational and social development

Terminal competency   A: Works with others to modify policies of institutions, agencies, and groups to more effectively meet identified needs

Responsibility VII: continues to develop professionally

Terminal competency   A: Implements career plans

B: Improves professional competencies

Established by the National Task Force on the Preparation and Practice of Health Educators. From Henderson, A.C.: The refined and verified role for entry-level health educators, Eta Sigma Gamma Mongr. Series, vol. 1, no. 1, Sept. 1982.

Standard high school certificate for State of Illinois

The Standard High School Certificate is valid for 4 years for teaching in grades 6 through 12 of the common schools. This certificate may be issued to graduates with a bachelor's degree from a recognized college who present certified evidence of having earned credits as follows:

Semester hours

A. General education 42
    1. Language arts 8
    2. Science and/or mathematics 6
    3. Social science (including a course in American history and/or government) 6
    4. Humanities 6
    5. Health and physical education 3
    6. Additional work in any above fields and/or psychology (except educational
       psychology) to total 42
B. Professional education 16
    1. Educational psychology (including human growth and development) 2
    2. Methods and techniques of teaching at the secondary level or in a teaching
       field 2
    3. History and/or philosophy of education 2
    4. Pre–student teaching clinical experiences equivalent to 100 clock hours* . . . .
    5. Student teaching (grades 6-12)† 5
    6. Electives in professional education may be taken from the above fields and/o
       guidance, tests and measurements, methods of teaching reading, and in-
       structional materials to total 16

If the grade level of your student teaching was not on the high school level, it will be necessary for you to submit a letter of verification of successful teaching experience from the appropriate school district official where you were employed. This letter should state all employment dates, the schools in which you were employed, your assignment, and the type of teaching certificate held. Verification of Chicago, Illinois, teaching experience should be obtained from the Director of Personnel of the Chicago Board of Education. These official letters must be submitted to the office of the Regional Superintendent of Schools of the Illinois county in which application is being made

C. One major area of specialization‡ 32
    or
   three minor areas of specialization (24 each) 72
D. General electives to make a total of 120

*Applicants with successful teaching experience at the 6-12 level need not complete pre–student teaching clinical experiences.

†Applicants presenting the required credit in student teaching and evidence of successful teaching experience need not complete another student teaching experience.

‡If your area of specialization is the same as one of the general education categories, then the same courses may be used for both requirements.

State Board of Education Document No. 1 (Oct. 1977)

Health education

20 semester hours in the field

Required health education component

One course from each of the following areas to total 10-14 semester hours:

1. Advanced concepts of health
2. Programs in school health
3. Programs in community health
4. Curriculum development and evaluation in health education

Additional health education components

One course from at least three of the following areas to total 6-10 semester hours:

1. The growing and developing organism
2. Ecological relationships
3. Disease control
4. Human sexuality and family life
5. Food practices and eating patterns
6. Consumer health sources and resources
7. Safety
8. Mood-modifying substances
9. Personal health practices
10. Mental/emotional health

---

alternating time blocks. A new curriculum for secondary school health education, Teenage Health Teaching Modules (THTM), is introduced together with a scope and sequence chart illustrating its modular teaching plan.

The nation's 1990 objectives for health are examined for their curricular implications relating to adolescent health. Health topics emphasized includes controlling high blood pressure, family planning, sexually transmitted diseases, accident prevention, smoking control, alcohol and drug misuse, nutrition, physical fitness exercise, and stress control.

The chapter concludes with selected curriculum examples and a discussion on the teaching of controversial subjects.

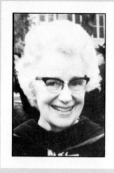

Ruth Grout

BORN   October 4, 1901, Princeton, Massachusetts

EDUCATION   B.S., Mt. Holyoke College, 1923; M.P.H., Yale University, 1930; Ph.D., Yale University, 1939

Ruth Grout's love of nature and her intellectual curiosity were channeled into the areas of zoology-physiology and sociology-economics at Mt. Holyoke College. This broad interest in the physical and social nature of humanity found its outlet in the field of health education. While teaching biology at New Haven High School, she worked with Dr. Reginald Atwater on the School Health Education Study in Cattaraugus County, New York. As director of the study, the information gained formed the basis of her doctorate thesis at Yale.

Her professional career included a stint with Tennessee Valley Authority and the U.S. Office of Education, but the heart of her work was done during her 24 years as professor of health education at the University of Minnesota. From 1952 to 1956 she served on the Joint Committee of the National Education Association and American Medical Association. Her text *Health Teaching in Schools* is widely used.

Her interest in health education broadened worldwide as a World Health Organization consultant in Europe, southeast Asia, Africa, and Jamaica. She evolved four basic principles of health education, which she espouses today in her busy retirement:

1. People should be actively involved in making health decisions that affect them.
2. Health education must be part of health programs, such as personal, community, and political programs.
3. Health education is a function of *all* health and education personnel who deal with the individual, family, school, and community.
4. Health education is of universal importance.

STUDY QUESTIONS

1. What is meant by the term *broad fields approach* when it is applied to organizing the secondary school curriculum?
2. What advantages does a modular scheduling plan offer for health instruction?
3. What is recommended for health instruction at the secondary level, in terms of credit, amount of time, class schedule, and so on?
4. What criteria might the health educator use in determining the content to be included in a high school health course?
5. Given the nation's health priorities, what three major health problems might the health educator include in the high school health course?
6. What are some of the major health and social consequences of teen-aged alcohol abuse?
7. What different kinds of controversies is the health educator likely to encounter in his or her teaching?
8. What guidelines might the teachers and school officials use in handling controversies?
9. What abilities or competencies should the practicing health educator be able to demonstrate?
10. What discrepancies or potential areas of weakness are apparent when the competencies identified in the box on p. 375 are compared with the Standard High School Certificate for Illinois presented in the box on p. 376?

REFERENCES

Adeyanju, M., Creswell, W.H., et al.: A three-year study of obesity and its relationship to high blood pressure in adolescents, J. Sch. Health **57**(3):109, 1987.

Better health for our children: a national strategy. The report of the Select Panel for the Promotion of Child Health to the United States Congress and the Secretary of Health and Human Services, vol. III, a statistical profile. DHHS-PHS Office of the Assistant Secretary for Health and the Surgeon General, Washington, D.C., 1981, U.S. Government Printing Office.

Blum, R.: Contemporary threats to adolescent health in the United States, JAMA **257**:3390, 1987.

Cissell, W.B.: Teaching about international health in United States public schools, Health Education **18**(1):10-11, 1987.

Decisions about alcohol and other drugs: a curriculum for Nebraska schools, 1982, The Nebraska Prevention Center for Alcohol and Drug Use.

DiPesi, L.: Focus on the positive: the campaign for child survival, Health Education **18**(2):13-15, 1987.

Education Commission of the States: Recommendations for school health education: a handbook for state policy makers, Denver, 1981, Education Programs Division.

Education Development Center, Inc.: Teenage health teaching modules, Newton, Mass., 1982, the Center.

Framework for health instruction in California public schools, Sacramento, Calif., 1978, Office of State Printing.

Gill, D.G.: Illinois State Board of Education, State Superintendent of Education, State Teacher Certification Board, 100 N. First St., Springfield, IL 62777.

Gordon, S.: The case for a moral sex education in schools, J. Sch. Health **51**:214, 1981.

Gordon, S., Scales, P., and Everly, K.: The sexual adolescent: communicating with teenagers about sex, ed. 2, North Scituate, Mass., 1979, Duxbury Press.

Greydanus, D.: Risk-taking behaviors in adolescence, JAMA **258**(15):2110, 1987. (Editorial.)

Hirschenbaum, H.: Handling school-community controversies over health education curriculum, Health Education **13**:7, Nov.-Dec. 1982.

Horrocks, J.E.: The psychology of adolescence, ed. 4, Boston, 1976, Houghton Mifflin Co.

Hughes, L.W., and Ubben, G.C.: The secondary principal's handbook: a guide to executive action, Newton, Mass., 1980, Allyn & Bacon, Inc.

Johnston, L.D., O'Malley, P.M., and Bachman, J.G.: Use of licit and illicit drugs by American high school students, 1975-1984, DHHS Pub. no. (ADM) 85-1394, Washington, D.C., 1985, U.S. Government Printing Office.

McClendon, E.J., and Tayeb, R.M.: Studying the school health program: a review of the findings, Kent, Ohio, 1982, American School Health Association.

Miller, L., and Downer, A.: AIDS: what you and your friends need to know, a lesson plan for adolescents, J. Sch. Health **58**(4):137, 1988.

National Commission on Excellence in Education: A nation at risk: the imperative for educational reform. A report to the nation and the secretary of education, U.S. Department of Education, April 1983.

National Education Association: The cardinal principles revisited, Today's Education **65**:59, Sept.-Oct. 1976.

Newman, I., et al.: Adolescent health knowledge revisited, Neb. Med. J. **63**:406, 1978.

Ohio Department of Education: Guidelines for improving school health education K-12, 1980, the Department.

O'Rourke, T., Smith, B., and Nolte, A.: Health attitudes, beliefs and behaviors of student grades 7-12, J. Sch. Health **54**:210, 1984.

Petosa, R., Hyner, G., and Melby, C.: Appropriate use of health risk appraisals with school-age children, J. Sch. Health **56**:52, 1986.

Schindler, J., and Schindler, J.: Willpower? Skillpower! La Crosse, Wisc., 1982 (unpublished).

Scott, H.D., and Cabral, R.M.: Predicting hazardous lifestyles among adolescents based on health-risk assessment data, Am. J. Health Prevention **2**(4):23, 1988.

Slaby, A.: Prevention, early identification, and management of adolescent suicidal behavior, R.I. Med. J. **69**:463, 1986.

Teaching about sexually transmitted diseases: a curriculum guide and resources for grades 7-12, Sacramento, 1980, California State Department of Education.

U.S. Department of Health and Human Services: Guidelines for effective school health education to prevent the spread of AIDS, Morbidity and Mortality Weekly Report, vol. 37, no. S-2 (suppl.), Jan. 29, 1988.

U.S. Department of Health and Human Services: Healthy people: the surgeon general's report on health promotion and disease prevention, Washington, D.C., 1979, U.S. Government Printing Office.

U.S. Department of Health and Human Services: Promoting health/preventing disease: objectives for the nation, Washington, D.C., 1980, U.S. Government Printing Office.

U.S. Department of Health and Human Services: Food for the teenager during and after pregnancy, DHHS Pub. no. (HRSA) 82-5106, Washington, D.C., 1982, U.S. Government Printing Office.

U.S. Department of Health and Human Services: Morbidity and Mortality Weekly Report, vol. 32, no. 35, Sept. 9, 1983b.

U.S. Department of Health and Human Services: Morbidity and Mortality Weekly Report, vol. 35, no. 44, Nov. 11, 1983c.

U.S. Department of Health and Human Services: PHS health education focal points, Atlanta, 1983a, Center for Health Promotion and Education, Division of Health Education, Centers for Disease Control.

U.S. Department of Health and Human Services: Prenatal care. USDHHS HHS-396, Rockville, Md., 1983d.

U.S. Department of Health and Human Services: Promoting health/preventing disease: Public Health Service implementation plans for attaining the objectives for the nation, USDHHS PHS Office of the Assistant Secretary for Health, Office of Disease Prevention and Health Promotion, Washington, D.C., Sept.-Oct. 1983e (suppl.), U.S. Government Printing Office.

Van Til, W.: Secondary education: school and community, Boston, 1978, Houghton Mifflin Co.

Yarber, W.L.: AIDS: what young adults should know, instructor's guide, Reston, Va., 1987, American Alliance for Health, Physical Education, Recreation and Dance.

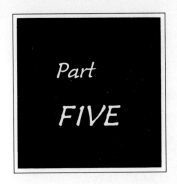

Part

FIVE

Healthful School Living

15

Policies and Practices in Health Teaching

OVERVIEW   *The focus of this chapter is on the role of school policies and their importance to the conduct of an effective health education program. Policies, in the context of schools, represent the agreements and official position of school authorities regarding a particular issue or issues. As such, policies serve as the basis for communication and understanding. Once a carefully planned policy is adopted, school officials can proceed with a clear sense of direction to establishing goals and the guidelines for teaching and program implementation.*

Such controversial topics as drugs, alcohol, tobacco, and sex education have often been the source of tension and conflict concerning the school's responsibility. The problem of adolescent risk-taking behaviors including drinking, drug abuse, teenage pregnancies, and sexually transmitted diseases has brought about a new awareness and concern as to the school's role in preventive education. Past difficulties with school programs point to limitations in the policy statements. Such weaknesses indicate that the policies have not been sufficiently representative of the community's views. School officials have been urged to include recommendations from all relevant school and community groups in the policy-making process.

Several of the controversial issues are examined in detail together with a consideration of their policy implications. Goals and recommendations for the instructional program are offered. The development of effective school policies requires a detailed and comprehensive review of all aspects of the issues. This, together with appropriate participation of school and community groups, provides the basis for effective programming. School policies that evolve from this process and are supported by educational research provide the basis for successful school programs.

OBJECTIVES   **After reading this chapter, the student should be able to:**

1. Explain the purposes that policies serve in the planning and conduct of programs.
2. Identify several steps that are involved in the policy development process.
3. Explain the effects of environmental tobacco smoke and the implications for school smoking policy.
4. Explain why determining the purposes of alcohol education is more difficult than determining the purposes of smoking education.
5. Explain why past efforts in drug education and sex education have been unsuccessful.

6. Explain the trends in drug use among adolescents.

7. Identify at least three issues that should be considered in developing a school drug education program.

8. Explain how the AIDS problem has affected the school sex education program.

9. Explain several guidelines for developing a school AIDS education program.

10. Identify several findings from research on teaching that are important to health education.

Policies are general statements often forming the guiding principles in relation to an adopted position. Policies determine the course of action to be taken by an organization, group, or an individual. In government, policies bear the same relationship to regulations as rules to law, except that, unlike regulations, policies do not have the force of law.

Porter (1982) stated that the process of formulating policy typically involves five steps: (1) identifying the problem or issue, (2) creating an awareness among relevant groups, (3) achieving a consensus position on the problem, (4) issuing a statement of the desired goal, and (5) developing a plan of action that is both prudent and consistent with the goal.

"The influence of volunteer health organizations on national health policies is both unique and necessary" (1982). The altruistic nature of organizations such as the American Heart Association, the American Lung Association, and the National Cancer Society adds not only to the importance of their statements and recommendations, but also to their influence upon American society.

The policy-making responsibilities for schools rest with the local school board. School policy reflects not only state education laws and regulations, but also state legislation pertaining to the health and safety of students and school personnel. In addition, the board seeks information from the community including parents, teachers, and business and professional leaders. On health issues, the local health department, medical and dental societies, as well as voluntary health agencies may each be called upon for information and technical advice.

The focus of this chapter is on school policies in regard to the controversial health issues including drug education, sex education, and the policy implications for AIDS education. A brief review of public education history indicates that these issues have been a source of continuing tension between the school and the community. In some instances school policies have failed to provide the scope and the direction needed for effective school health education.

School boards have frequently failed to establish a sufficiently broad base of community support to enable the school to implement its programs. If the school board has not established strong community support for its policies, small-program pressure groups can easily exploit the situation. Such confusion and disruption adversely affect the school's instructional program, which, in fact, may be supported by the community at large.

Good policy-making procedure is directly related to quality education. The Midwest Center for Drug-Free Schools and Communities (1988) has taken the initiative to develop a guidebook to assist schools in establishing sound school-community drug education policies. The staff of this center has recommended that an advisory council of representatives from the community, the school, and law enforcement agencies be created as a first step in developing a drug policy. This council, in addition to helping formulate policy, would also serve as an ongoing reviewer. Specific responsibilities of the council would include defining and redefining the drug problem, updating materials, distributing information, and advising on policy implementation issues.

SCHOOL POLICY ON SMOKING

All the elements for an effective school policy on smoking are in place. In the years since the surgeon general issued the landmark report *Smoking and Health* (1964) linking smoking and lung cancer, literally thousands of additional studies have been conducted reaffirming the finding that indeed smoking is a cause of disease. The voluntary health agencies together with the federal government have conducted massive informational and educational campaigns to alert the public to this health hazard. In recent efforts aimed at achieving a consensus approach to the smoking problem, the National School Board Association, the American Cancer Society, and the American Heart Association have joined forces on a project calling for a "Tobacco-Free Young America by the Year 2000."

Findings and conclusions drawn from the 1986 surgeon general's report on the Health Consequences of Involuntary Smoking have major implications for school smoking policies. The findings summarized in this report reveal that anyone who breathes environmental tobacco smoke is exposed to an increased risk of disease. The principal conclusions from the report are as follows:

1. Involuntary smoking is a cause of disease, including lung cancer in healthy nonsmokers.
2. Children of parents who smoke when compared to children of nonsmoking parents have more respiratory infections and lower lung function at maturity.
3. Although separating smokers from nonsmokers may reduce exposure, it does not eliminate the nonsmokers' exposure to environmental tobacco smoke and the increased risk of disease.
4. Laboratory research has now demonstrated that sidestream smoke, the aerosol from the burning tobacco between puffs, is much more toxic than is the exhaled mainstream tobacco smoke (USPHS, 1986).

Although the National School Board Association and the national voluntary health associations have called for a tobacco-free environment by the year 2000, can the educational community afford to wait this long to take steps that will protect the health of today's school children? Providing a special smoking room for school staff, teachers, and administrators is hardly doing the addicted smoker a favor. Being forced to smoke in an even smaller indoor space places the already-at-risk smoker and other inhabitants of the space at an even greater health risk because of the highly concentrated environmental tobacco smoke and its increased levels of toxicity. Separating the smokers from the nonsmokers indoors is not enough; the nonsmoker's right to breathe clean air should not be compromised. A policy that provides indoor restricted smoking areas is no longer defensible, at a time when schools are required to teach about the harmful effects of smoking and when an increasing number of schools are enacting expanded health and wellness programs for students and staff. An increasing number of states are passing legislation banning smoking in public places and work sites, and airlines are prohibiting smoking on planes. Now is the time for educators to assume leadership in the drive for a tobacco-free environment.

Results from a study of school smoking policies conducted for the National School Board Association (Rist, 1986) show that 87% of the responding schools have adopted policies regulating cigarette smoking. Many schools have adopted more restrictive policies since 1980. An important finding from this survey shows that once the school has adopted policies prohibiting smoking, students have been quite cooperative in supporting the policy. However, these results show a serious omission in schools' antismoking policies, since only 2% of the school systems prohibit smoking by school employees. The survey also shows that some 81% of the school systems provide designated smoking areas in school buildings for teachers and administrators. This points to a glaring inconsistency between the policies established for students and those established for adults at the school site. Although the motives of the National School Board Association and the national voluntary health agencies are laudable, their call for action is too delayed and insufficient given the results from recent research on the toxic effects of environmental tobacco smoke.

Such a policy need not pit youth against adults. As Sagor (1987) has warned, school officials must proceed with caution, lest their position be misunderstood. "The school community's war on drugs has the potential for pitting the two generations against each other."

ALCOHOL AND DRUGS POLICY

Research on adolescent involvement with tobacco and alcohol reveals a common pattern of use. Those teenagers who smoke or use alcohol are more likely to smoke marijuana and use other illicit drugs. Concentrating efforts on the development of a nonsmoking policy and the implementation of an effective ban on tobacco use at school has been shown to be an effective first step toward achieving a comprehensive drug policy. For example, one year after implementation of a "no-tobacco-use" policy in the Marietta, Georgia, schools (Phillips, 1984) the following positive results were noted:

1. There was a healthier, cleaner environment for all students.
2. There were fewer drug-related problems; there was no evidence of marijuana use at the school.
3. Fewer students were tardy to classes.
4. There were no reported incidents of students being under the influence of drugs.
5. Students performed better academically.

In general, the school drug education policy should address the issues of alcohol, tobacco, and marijuana use. Such a policy, carefully developed and implemented, would make unmistakably clear the school's role in establishing a drug-free environment. More importantly, it would create by precept and by example the essential environmental support and reinforcement so vital to the success of the school drug education program.

Policy statements issued by school officials, as in the following examples, range from one of strict punishment to a caring and advocacy role for the school.

> The schools especially must be unyielding. Students who drink alcohol, smoke marijuana, or use other drugs must understand that the consequences of their behavior are unalterable: expulsion from school and disqualification from all extra-curricular activities. (Strong, 1983.)

The second position is much more compassionate in tone.

> In our zeal to create policies and sanctions that will curb drug abuse, we must not lose sight of the fact that mentally healthy people become that way as a result of a series of caring, one-to-one relationships with parents, teachers, counselors and others." (Sagor, 1987.)

Obviously there are problems that must be recognized. A significant number of teenagers will start using psychoactive substances. As a rule, such experimentation is viewed as a natural curiosity, well within the range of normal behavior for the growing and developing young person. Often, after a brief period of experimentation with the drug, the person will refrain from further use. However, there is the risk that such experimentation will lead to the serious problem of habituation and chemical dependency. What may have begun out of a normal curiosity may unfortunately become an acquired habit that is extremely difficult to break. There is a consensus among the public at large that school officials must be unequivocal in their position regarding the use of alcohol, marijuana, and other drugs. Schools must teach abstinence, concentrate on the prevention of drug abuse, make young people accountable for their behavior whenever it deviates from this behavior norm and administer swift and firm discipline.

THE ALCOHOL PROBLEM AND ALCOHOL EDUCATION

Luce and Schweitzer (1984) calculated that approximately 25% of the total economic cost of illness to the nation is attributable to smoking and alcohol abuse. In addition, there are other costs of alcohol that are estimated to be as high as 6 billion dollars including property damage from accidents, fires, criminal justice costs, highway safety, and the social welfare system. Not only does alcohol impose a heavy burden of illness on adults, but also alcohol use places teenagers and young adults at great risk. Motor vehicle crashes are the leading cause of death for the age group 15 to 24 years. Young persons are 2½ times as likely to be involved in alcohol-related crashes. Data from a recent longitudinal study of a midwestern high school student's drinking pattern reveals that an increasing majority of teenagers are using alcohol during the high school years. Use of alcohol rises from 76% in the ninth grade to 95% at the twelfth grade level. In addition to this increasing prevalence of alcohol use during the high school period, an increasing number of students are drinking to excess. Social drinking in American society is part of the ritual of growing into adulthood (Adeyanju, 1987). Tables 15-1 and 15-2 show the average prevalences for alcohol use, smoking, and other drugs for all students in grades 7 through 12.

Investigators attempting to develop strategies dealing with the drinking problem cannot ignore the cultural and the social milieu that tolerates drinking and its consequences. The problems of drinking arise from many factors: economic, social, and cultural. These, plus cultural values and society norms, interact in this situation. No single intervention policy can solve society's problem with alcohol.

Instead of a single strategy designed for a single high-risk group, Stoudemire and colleagues (1987) have argued that many initiatives will have to be undertaken through a coordinated plan, for this society to move toward achieving a national goal—"the healthiest possible use of alcohol." Although social drinking is a well-established American custom, the achievement of a consensus position on the use of beverage alcohol has proved to be very

TABLE 15-1. Annual percentage drug use for youth 12 to 17 years of age

Drug	1972	1974	1976	1977	1979	1982	1985
Marijuana and hashish	—	18.5	18.4	22.3	24.1	20.6	20.0
Hallucinogens	3.6	4.3	2.8	3.1	4.7	3.6	2.8
Cocaine	1.5	2.7	2.3	2.6	4.2	4.1	4.4
Heroin	†	†	†	0.6	†	†	†
Nonmedical use of:							
Stimulants	—	3.0	2.2	3.7	2.9	5.6	4.4
Sedatives	—	2.0	1.2	2.0	2.2	3.7	3.1
Tranquilizers	—	2.0	1.8	2.9	2.7	3.3	3.7
Analgesics	—	—	—	—	2.2	3.7	4.4
Alcohol	—	51.5	49.3	47.5	53.6	47.3	52.0
Cigarettes	—	—	—	—	13.3*	24.8	26.0

National Household Survey on Drug Abuse, Rockville, Md., 1985, National Institute on Drug Abuse, Division of Epidemiology and Statistical Analysis.
— Not Available.
*For 1979, includes only persons who ever smoked at least five packs.
†Less than 0.5%.

TABLE 15-2. Onset of drug use by age

Age	Cigarette %	Alcohol %	Marijuana %
12-13	10	13	4
14-15	22	28	15
16-17	35	25	29
18-21	51	71	31

From Abelson, H.J., Fishburn, P.M., and Cisin, I.H.: National Survey of Drug Abuse, Rockville, Md., 1982, National Institute on Drug Abuse.

difficult. Aside from the religious objections to beverage alcohol, critics of the goal "responsible use of alcohol" argue that the human interaction to alcohol is so varied and unique that it is not possible to know who is likely to cross the line from a socially responsible drinker to a problem drinker.

Despite these difficulties, the nation has no workable alternative but to continue the effort to achieve this goal of responsible use. If such an ideal is to be achieved, it will require a coordinated school-community alcohol education program that is based upon the following societal norms:

1. Accepting a moderate consumption in *low-risk* situations
2. Actively discouraging moderate consumption in *high-risk* situations
3. Actively discouraging heavy consumption in any situation
4. Accepting abstinence
5. Establishing a high priority on safety and health protection in motor vehicle transportation

Policy initiatives for school also call for comprehensive educational approaches with careful attention given to the mobilization and coordination of all community resources. In addition to the school, this should include family, churches, voluntary associations, societies, professional organizations, and the local media.

GUIDELINES FOR THE SCHOOL

1. Alcohol education in the schools should begin not later than 12 years of age.
2. The curriculum should include information on the potential risks of alcohol and its misuse.
3. The myths and realities of drinking should include the effect of alcohol on the body, reasons for drinking and not drinking, and the social acceptance of drinking.
4. In addition to cognitive development, the program for preteens and early adolescents must focus on developing decision making, critical thinking, and social skills to help the student cope and resist the pressures to use alcohol and drugs.

TEACHING APPROACHES TO DRUG EDUCATION

As Botvin (1983) has observed, the traditional approach to teaching students about smoking, alcohol, and drugs has tended to focus on the factual data and the harmful effects of substances. This approach is based on the assumption that an increase of the students' knowledge will lead to wise choices and ultimately to the rejection of drug use.

This emphasis on the facts of hazardous substance use is a reminder of the past national drug education program of the 1970s and the war on drugs during President Nixon's administration. In its effort to solve this drug problem, the federal government set as a national goal providing every classroom teacher and school administrator with the facts about the nation's drug crisis. A timetable of 1 year was set to accomplish this goal. This plan was based on the assumption that once the administrators and the teachers were informed they in turn could inform the students, and in short order the drug crisis should be solved. However, it became apparent very early that this factual information program was falling short of its goal to reduce drug experimentation and drug abuse. In fact, some of the early studies conducted during this period revealed that not only were the programs not succeeding, but in some instances students who scored the highest on their knowledge of drugs were also the students who were most likely to be experimenting with drugs (Halpin and Thomas, 1977). Generally, an information-based approach to alcohol and drug abuse prevention has not been successful in changing attitudes and behavior.

Because of the concern that drug education was not effective, a national commission on marijuana and drug abuse was appointed in 1973 to evaluate the programs. After an extensive review the commission concluded that it could not find a drug education program anywhere in the country that it could recommend. The commission went on to state in its report

> that policy makers should also seriously consider declaring a moratorium on all drug education programs in the schools, at least until programs already in operation have been evaluated. . . . (National Commission on Marihuana and Drug Abuse, 1973, p. 357.)

The Midwest Regional Center for Drug Free Schools and Communities (1988) offers the following as guides for the development of effective drug education policies:

1. As a first step in the development of policies there should be a careful analysis of existing state and local laws along with an interpretation of these statutes especially

as they relate to school law. This may require consultation from the state department of education, law enforcement agencies, as well as the judicial system concerning questions that pertain to such topics as the individual rights of students, parents' consent, and the specific interpretation of "in loco parentis."

2. The school policy making body should not be confined to the school board and the school district administrator, but rather it should include all of those persons who, because of interest, knowledge, or job responsibility can make a contribution. In addition to school administrators, for example, teachers, counselors and coaches should be represented. Others who should be included are representatives of the court system, city officials, medical and health personnel, representatives of the business community, parents, students, and youth serving agencies.

Once the policy making body is organized, it should consider several issues such as:

1. The adoption of an appropriate and standardized procedure for reporting substance abuse and suspected illegal substance use activity.

2. A consideration of the appropriate roles of school personnel such as the role of administrators, teachers, and counselors in the implementation of drug policy.

3. Establishment of appropriate due process safeguards to protect the rights of the students as well as those of school personnel.

4. Establishment of consistent and reasonable policies relating to suspension and expulsion from school.

5. Establishment of policies concerning substance abuse which reflect a consistent standard of behavior to be applied in evaluating the actions of students and staff.

SEX EDUCATION POLICY

The first step in establishing a policy for sex education, as in all policy development, requires a careful definition and analysis of the subject. When the issue has been sufficiently delineated to secure a general understanding and agreed-upon goals, a plan of action can be undertaken.

Policies are the general guideline statements of principle that provide a frame of reference for school-community agreements. The specific rules or regulations derived from the general principles give direction to the standards of conduct derived from the policy statement. The over 1 million teenage pregnancies that occur each year serve as a reminder of the need for a more effective program of sex education.

Factors affecting the adolescent pregnancy rates include divorce, the increased number of single-parent families, working mothers, a mobile society, which has underminded the traditional role of the family, and changing cultural values. These forces, together with the influence of the mass media and the lack of supervision and parental involvement for many children, have contributed to the problems of alcohol abuse, drug use, and teenage pregnancy. Authorities point out that the first sex experience typically occurs when both adolescents are intoxicated.

The difficulties encountered in establishing an effective sex education program are somewhat similar to those encountered in establishing an effective program in drug education. In both instances past programs have tended to rely too much on narrowly based information programs without a recognition of important social forces contributing to drug use and sex behavior. Sex, alcohol, and drugs are associated for a variety of reasons. The adolescent boy may use psychoactive substances such as beer or marijuana to overcome his shyness and anxiety in social situations, especially those that include the opposite sex (MacDonald, 1987). The loss of inhibition and control under the influence of alcohol can easily lead the adolescent boy and his partner into sexual intercourse and the possibility of an unwanted or unexpected teenage pregnancy.

MacDonald (1987), a leading public health authority, has spoken out forcefully on the urgent need to upgrade the quality of the sex education program in schools. Gordon (1981) has also identified the ambivalence that characterizes American society's efforts to deal with sexuality in the educational setting. Despite the fact that surveys indicate that the great majority of parents support sex education in the public schools, studies show that very few comprehensive, high-quality sex education programs exist in American schools.

As a public health official concerned about the teenage pregnancy problem, MacDonald has proposed two models or approaches to more effective sex education: (1) an abstinence ("just say later") model and (2) broad-based school-community approach similar to that recommended for school-community drug education. Whatever approach is undertaken, it is essential that schools be quite clear about the objectives and goals for the sex education program. School officials have characteristically been hesitant to express a strong value preference for fear of being misunderstood and of offending certain persons or groups in the community. However, it has become increasingly evident that a neutral approach has not been effective for either sex education or drug education.

There is little doubt as to the information parents and the public want in the sex education course. A strong, clear message "abstinence for now" is the cultural imperative standard of behavior. Unfortunately, neither parents nor school officials have made the goal of sex education clear to students. Parents, in particular, have reflected an uncertainty and an ambivalence in communicating with their children about the desired standard of behavior.

Table 15-3 provides important data for analyzing the sex education needs of teenage girls 15 to 19 years of age. The rates of sexual activity given for 1971 and 1982 and the changes that have taken place over this period reveal at least three distinct groups whose needs should be recognized when one is planning the sex education program: (1) those girls who remain *sexually inactive*, (2) those who are *sexually active*, and (3) the 16%, labeled the

TABLE 15-3.   Rates of sexual activity of girls 15 to 19 years of age

Status	1971 (%)	1982 (%)
Active	27	43
Inactive	72	58
Swing group	16	

For 1971, Zeinick, M., and Kantner, J.F.: "Sexual and contraceptive experiences of young unmarried women in the U.S., 1976 and 1971," Fam. Plann. Perspect. **9**:55, 1977; for 1982, Pratt, W.F., et al.: "Understanding U.S. fertility: findings from the NSFG cycle III," Popul. Bull. **39**:Table 2, Dec. 1984.
NOTE: The disparity in the percentage differences is attributable to rounding of errors.

swing group, who are in the process of becoming sexually active. An examination of these data by year show that the shift to a large extent occurs among the older teens in this age group, an indication that these girls have delayed their decision about sexual activity until 18 and 19 years of age.

If a certain proportion of girls are delaying their decision to become sexually active until 18 or 19 years, sex education in high school provides an important opportunity to reinforce these students' decisions to remain sexually abstinent for now and to protect themselves and others against the threat of AIDS.

Obviously, school officials cannot ignore the needs of the sexually active students. However, this situation places both the parents and school officials in the ambivalent position of teaching abstinence on one hand while at the same time teaching about "safe sex" to the sexually active student. The school sex education program must stress the important responsibility these students have for protecting their own health and the health of their partners.

In view of the urgencies of the public health need, school officials must take the initiative to secure public understanding and the broad-based community support essential to the implementation of an effective sex education program. Emphasizing the "abstinence for now" approach is important because it provides the positive reinforcement for the majority of teenagers who have remained sexually abstinent. This message is particularly important to the 16% of the adolescent girls who are most likely to become sexually active. It is these students who are most likely to be responsive to a strong educational message, to peer groups, and to other forms of influence. Teaching students the benefits of delaying their sexual activity should stress the very considerable health risks that pregnancy poses for the teenage girl. In addition, there are the major social risks, such as interrupting educational plans to take on the heavy economic, social, and personal burdens of pregnancy, marriage, childbirth, and parenting. Teenagers, especially boys, must be helped to realize that sexual activity is not the teenage social norm. The reality is that the majority of teenagers are abstinent. In fact, the rates of sexual activity have leveled for white adolescent girls and have begun to decline for black adolescent girls. For the boys, the objectives are to develop an attitude of respect and caring for one's sexual partner and to appreciate the need to delay the relationship until both persons are prepared to accept the responsibilities that such a relationship entails.

What other topics should be stressed in the sex education curriculum? The concerns over AIDS and the resulting state and national legislation have had a major impact on school sex education. Traditionally, the local school has been given the option of whether to offer sex education and, if taught, what topics to include. However, with the advent of the AIDS legislation, Illinois and many other states now mandate the teaching of sex education. The law in Illinois requires that the specific topic AIDS shall be taught, beginning in grade 6.

IMPORTANCE OF COMMUNITY SUPPORT FOR SEX EDUCATION

One of the reasons for the lack of success in sex education during the 1960s and 1970s was the tendency to focus too much on the student to the exclusion of the parent. Also there was the tendency to assume that the schools could do the job of sex education more or less on their own. Moreover, parents were often neither comfortable nor sufficiently competent to provide the sex education of their own children and to teach children how to make goal decisions.

This experience has also revealed that certain errors were made in teaching approaches. The well-intended effort to teach children how to make responsible choices and decisions failed to realize that young, immature students may not be able to make decisions in their own best interests. Development of such a highly complex skill requires the support and guidance of parents, teachers, clergy, and others to help the child evaluate the competing options, to anticipate consequences, and to appreciate the full meaning of the consequences that may result from their choices.

AIDS AND PREVENTIVE EDUCATION

Major national policy making groups, after detailed and exhaustive studies of the acquired immunodeficiency syndrome (AIDS), have all issued statements emphasizing the importance of education in the prevention and control of this disease. The Centers for Disease Control, the National Academy of Sciences, the Surgeon General of the United States, and the U.S. Department of Education have recognized that until an effective vaccine and treatment for AIDS has been developed, education is the only effective means by which people can protect themselves.

In addition to these national governmental bodies, leading national professional organizations in the fields of education, public health, and medicine have also endorsed the Guidelines for Effective School Health Education to halt the spread of AIDS. These guidelines were developed through the leadership of the National Centers for Disease Control of the United States Public Health Service (USHHS, 1988).

The manner by which the disease AIDS is spread in children is quite different from the way it is transmitted among adults. In adults, AIDS is spread primarily by sexual intercourse. Surveys show that approximately two thirds of adult AIDS patients are homosexual or bisexual men who have a history of using intravenous drugs. Among children, nearly 80% of AIDS cases are contracted perinatally from infected mothers who are usually linked to intravenous drug usage. Transfusions with infected blood products is a much more significant cause of AIDS in children than in adults. Excluding hemophiliacs, only 2% of the adults have contracted AIDS from transfusions, in contrast to 13% of children. Most children who have contracted AIDS from transfusions were infected during their first year of life.

Nearly 90% of pediatric AIDS cases are under 5 years of age and about 50% are diagnosed in the first year of life (Dalton, 1987).

POLICY FOR AIDS EDUCATION

The AIDS epidemic is of such a magnitude that it threatens to overshadow all other experiences with disease in modern history. The fact that there is no likelihood of developing an effective vaccine or therapy for treating the disease in the near future makes preventive education the only option available to society. As a consequence, schools are faced with an unprecedented health education challenge.

This situation requires that all schools should have an advisory body to help develop the policies and plans needed to implement an effective AIDS education program. In addition to the preventive education effort, the advisory council must help the schools and the community keep abreast of current information and developments at the national and state level. Schools should be able to establish orderly procedures that are both appropriate and scientifically sound for the handling of children infected with AIDS. A host of other issues must be considered such as the problem of confidentiality, screening, the legal authority for protecting the infected child, as well as the rights and responsibilities of all parties concerned.

In addition to policy statements developed by governmental, professional, and commercial agencies, a wide range of curriculum materials on AIDS education is now available. Two such curriculum examples are (1) *Guidelines for Effective School Health Education*, developed by the Centers for Disease Control of the USPHS and (2) *AIDS Education: Curriculum and Health Policy*, prepared by Yarber (1987) at Indiana University for the Phi Delta Kappa Educational Foundation. This curriculum includes the following guidelines:

1. A team of representatives from the school board, PTA, school administrators, physicians, nurses and counselors should receive general training about AIDS.
2. Education about AIDS in the elementary school should be provided by a regular classroom teacher who has been given special in-service preparation on the scientific concepts and teaching strategies for AIDS education.
3. At the secondary level, the regular health education teacher should provide the instruction about AIDS. Special in-service preparation may be needed, depending on the circumstances and the teacher's background.
4. Schools should provide a curriculum that has adequate time and resources including a carefully planned sequence of concepts appropriate to each grade and developmental level of the students. Ideally AIDS education would be incorporated as a part of the school comprehensive health education.
5. A set of nine criteria are suggested for assessment of the extent to which the local school program is consistent with the CDC guidelines. Several of these criteria statements are embodied in the foregoing recommendations.

TEACHING STRATEGIES FOR PROMOTING HEALTH BEHAVIORS

The traditional approach utilizing informational dissemination and fear-arousal messages characteristic of many early drug education programs has not been effective in preventing drug use. Important as student knowledge and attitudes are in the health of the student, researchers have now concluded that the behaviors of smoking, drinking, and other drug uses are symptomatic of larger and more fundamental needs of students. Targeting a specific health behavior and a specific so-called high-risk group of students may not be the most productive approach. As Jessor (1984) has established, adolescence is a high-risk time for all youth, many of whom are experimenting with health-compromising behaviors such as alcohol and drugs.

Although there are youths with special needs and who are at special risk, Benard (1986) has recommended that the school instructional program be placed within a larger context, utilizing a comprehensive approach involving youth, families, schools, and community organizations. The causes of substance abuse are multiple, including personality, environmental, and behavioral factors.

Research concluded during the past decade has provided the basis for new teaching strategies emphasizing personal and social skills, which are proving to be effective in developing students' intellectual and social competencies and at the same time helping them to resist the pressure to become involved with drugs and other risk-taking behaviors.

The personality characteristic of student low self-esteem has taken on increasing significance in the designing of teaching strategies for preventing health-compromising behaviors. Studies have shown that virtually all maladaptive defense behavior patterns in childhood, adolescence, and adulthood are a product of the pain associated with low self-esteem (Mack, 1983). This lack of self-esteem has been hypothesized as an important element in many of today's social problems including child abuse, sexual abuse, domestic violence, delinquency, crime, teen-aged pregnancy, alcohol and drug abuse, and school failure. A direct concern of the school is those students who lack problem-solving skills. An important corollary to these findings is the research showing that children, adolescents, and adults who lack problem-solving skills also share the personality chacteristic of low self-esteem.

This research has brought about a new interest and emphasis on teaching skills for problem solving, decision making, and participation in social situations. Preventive education rests on the assumption that improving the students' problem-solving skills will have a positive effect on several important health behavior outcomes. For example, developing the students' social skills usually leads to improvement in their communication skills and a corresponding reduction of their anxiety in social situations. With these new skills students are able to face challenges with a sense of relaxed confidence that greatly enhances the chances for academic and social success. Achievement in these areas raises students' self-esteem and perception of self-efficacy, enabling them to participate more effectively in the problem-solving activities, which continue the cycle of positive outcomes. Problem solving and decision making involve critical thinking; the same skills that are applied to solving interpersonal problems can be applied to solving classroom intellectual problems (Bernard,

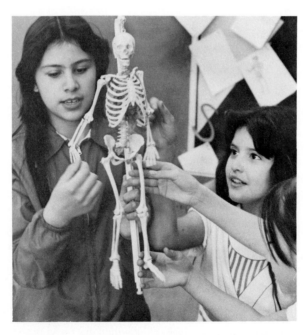

FIG. 15-1.   Girls examining skeleton illustrate students' active involvement in learning.
(From The School Health Curriculum Project. Pub. no. [CDC] 78-8359, Atlanta, 1977, Public Health Service, Center for Disease Control, U.S. Department of Health, Education and Welfare.)

1986 and 1988). Longitudinal research demonstrates the value of teaching social problem-solving skills. Observations from these studies show that persons with good problem-solving skills lead productive lives. Children who lack such skills have demonstrated problem behaviors. (See box below.)

ESTABLISHING AN EFFECTIVE TEACHING-LEARNING ENVIRONMENT

Once the general design of the curriculum has been adopted, it then becomes the responsibility of the teacher and the local school officials to translate the curriculum into workable learning experiences for the students. Until the curriculum is experienced by the student, it is nothing more than a plan. The process of implementation — moving from a teaching plan into active learning — requires special care in selecting teaching strategies, the content and

---

Drug education curriculum — personal and social skills

1. Cognitive skills
   a. Myths and realities of drugs
   b. Smoking
   c. Alcohol
   d. Marijuana and other drugs
2. Cognitive skills for personal control
   a. Self-image, self-improvement
   b. Goal setting
   c. Interpersonal influences
   d. Media influences
   e. Cognitive coping skills
3. Problem solving and decision making
   a. Steps in problem solving
   b. Analyzing solutions and consequences
4. Communication skills
   a. Verbal and nonverbal
   b. Avoiding misunderstanding
   c. Asking questions
   d. Communicating with parents
5. Social skills — interpersonal
   a. Overcoming shyness
   b. Conversational skills
   c. Conversing with opposite sex
   d. Social activities
6. Social skills — assertiveness
   a. Resisting peer pressure
   b. Reasons for being assertive
   c. Verbal assertiveness
   d. Nonverbal assertiveness
   e. Resisting peer pressure to drug use

Adapted from Botvin, G.J.: Life skills training: teachers manual, New York, 1983, Smithfield Press, Inc.

learning experiences, and the study materials and in assessing the effects of instruction on students.

Although there will always be some intangibles that make for effective teaching (i.e, personality factors and the "art of teaching"), nevertheless, there is also a growing body of research literature that is establishing the scientific basis of education. Given this research base, which generalizations can now be made that will help to ensure an effective learning environment for the student?

Research on learning

Walberg and associates (1983) have conducted an exhaustive review of the instructional research covering the period from 1969 to 1979. The following points summarize the key findings from the critical reviews of these authors.

1. *Instructional time* is positively correlated with learning achievement. In general, the more time devoted to instruction, the more students learn. Planning instruction for primary and intermediate level students must give priority consideration to helping students develop their fundamental skills in reading, writing, and mathematics and to the development of their skills for acquiring information. In this regard, health instruction that is carefully designed in terms of student reading and vocabulary levels has been shown to contribute significantly to the achievement of these fundamentals (Redican, Olson, and Stone, 1979).

2. *Students learn more when taught in small classes.* For example, elementary school students who are taught in class sizes of 20 or fewer will achieve as much as a 2-year advantage over children taught in larger classes (e.g., 40 students) during the course of their elementary school experience (K-6).

3. *Individualization,* sometimes referred to as a personalized system of instruction (PSI), is superior to all other forms of group instruction for cognitive learning. This form of instruction may be characterized as follows:

    a. Reliance on written words

    b. Specific instructional objective

    c. Small units of instruction

    d. Self-pacing of the student through instruction (students proceed through the material at their own rate)

    e. Mastery or near-perfect performance required before the student is allowed to proceed to the next unit

    f. Frequent assessment of the student by repeated testing with maximal credit for success and no penalty for failure

In this form of instruction, the amount of time for learning is flexible. Although the focus of instruction is on the individual student, providing alternative forms of instruction with opportunities for the student to participate in cooperative group learning with peers has also been found to improve learning.

4. *Direct instruction* has been shown to be particularly effective for student cognitive learning. The term *direct* refers to the fact that the teacher is in control of the teaching-learning situation including the selection of learning activities, sequencing the lessons, choosing instructional materials, and monitoring student performance. There is frequent

questioning of students with immediate feedback, emphasizing development of correct responses.

5. *Discussion* as a teaching method is more effective with the older, more mature student. Studies have shown that discussion is almost as effective for student achievement as the traditional lecture method. However, this research has revealed that the discussion method is more effective in helping students to retain information.

6. *Student-centered discussion* (compared with teacher-centered discussion) tends to produce superior results in the effective domain or in attitude changes. The same is true for student-led discussions, which are more effective than teacher-led discussions in achieving desired attitude changes.

7. *Teacher characteristics* are important. These include (a) being able to maintain class control — with gestures, eye contact, proximity control, and use of humor to release tension; (b) being able to restructure lessons that are not effective; and (c) providing clarity and firmness in communicating expectations regarding students' performance and behavior (Ornstein and Levine, 1981).

8. *Teacher skill in classroom management* has also been shown to be an important factor in student learning. Students' negative perceptions of the classroom tend to have a negative effect on their learning. For example, students may sense friction among classmates, the pressure of small-group cliques, or apathy toward the lesson, or they may perceive that the lesson is disorganized. On the other hand, if students have positive perceptions of the classroom environment, the effect on learning is also positive. For example, students may see the classroom as one of cohesion, in which lessons are difficult but challenging, in which democratic procedures are followed, and in which the physical setting and the materials used are necessary to learning.

Although the results from research on classroom management are less clear, there is the general conclusion that planning and preparation on the part of the teacher are the single most effective way to provide a suitable environment for individual and group learning (Ornstein and Levine, 1981).

Research on school health education

After conducting a comprehensive review of the research literature on school health education, Bartlett (1981) has offered the following perceptive assessment of school health education: "Evaluative studies of school health education curricula generally reveal that these programs are very successful in increasing knowledge, somewhat successful in improving attitudes, and infrequently successful in facilitating life-style changes."

As previously noted, Botvin and colleagues (1983) have begun to document the positive effects of the life-skills training program (cognitive and social skills) on the knowledge and attitudes of students with respect to cigarette smoking, drinking, and drug use. This research for the first time demonstrates consistent, positive, behavioral changes in addition to the traditional effects on knowledge and attitudes.

Moreover, teaching for health-behavior change, in addition to involving the student, must go beyond the traditional didactic or information-giving form of teaching. Instead, it is necessary to involve the student much more deeply in the self-management and self-concept development approach to behavior modification. Teaching for behavior change will also require the schools to reach out and involve parents and community agencies if the goal of improved health behavior is to be achieved.

Examples of specific health problem areas that have been found to have high potential for success in developing positive health behavior include the following: (1) the problem of dental care, especially when students perceive the severity of the problem and their susceptibility to dental disease; (2) the problem of unwanted teen-aged pregnancies, when there is a close working relationship with community agencies coupled with parental support; and (3) smoking prevention education, when there is the opportunity to involve older students in cross-age teaching and peer counseling or tutoring. Also, nutrition education has contributed to improved diet patterns by use of self-management behavior modification techniques with the social support of the family.

Regardless of whether schools will be able to secure the necessary material and human resources to undertake special health education programs aimed at specific health behavior changes, the responsibility to provide basic health information to the public still exists. This health information will form the basis of the public's health knowledge enabling the individual to exercise his or her full responsibilities of citizenship to make informed decisions affecting personal health, the health of one's family, and the health of the community.

SUMMARY

This chapter discusses policies and their importance in providing a mechanism that establishes a basis for communication and understanding as well as guidelines for program action. Policy discussion in this chapter is limited to schools and more specifically to several of the controversial issues in school health education: alcohol, marijuana, tobacco, and sex education including AIDS education. Several steps in the policy development process are reviewed.

School boards are charged with the responsibility for making school policy. An important step in this process is securing strong community support. Historically, schools have had difficulties with the teaching of controversial topics. Because of their sensitive nature, it is very important that the objectives, the teaching methods, and the curriculum materials be approved by the school administration, the school board, and the parents. School boards must involve all the community groups to assure that all views are properly represented in the policy development. Controversial issues relating to school health education are examined to help school officials clarify the goals and most appropriate teaching methods. The threat posed by the disease AIDS means that schools no longer have a choice as to whether to teach such a controversial issue. All schools are now required to teach sex education and AIDS education as a matter of national interest and public health.

Research has strongly supported the teaching of personal cognitive skills (e.g., problem solving, decision making, and critical thinking) and social skills to help students resist the pressure to engage in risk-taking behaviors. Each of these teaching strategies has been found effective in dealing with the controversial issues.

The chapter concludes with a review of the research on the effective teaching-learning environment. Conclusions are drawn from an exhaustive review of the research literature covering a 10-year period.

STUDY QUESTIONS

1. Why are policies important to the teaching of controversial topics in health education?
2. What is your position on a school policy that would ban all smoking from school facilities?
3. Explain why you would or would not favor a policy that expels students from school for a smoking violation.
4. From the standpoint of prevention, what is an ideal time for introducing drug education into the curriculum?
5. What is the rationale for using a social-skills approach in drug education?
6. What is meant by the statement "responsible use" in alcohol education and what might that imply from the standpoint of societal alcohol consumption?
7. Identify three points you believe should receive special emphasis in a teenager sex education program.
8. What are the principal conclusions to be drawn from the research on school health education?

REFERENCES

Adeyanju, M., et al.: The relationship among attitudes, behaviors and biomedical measures of adolescents "at risk" for cardivascular disease, J. Sch. Health **57**(8):326, 1987.

American Heart Association: The influence of voluntary health organizations on national health policies, Current Perspectives in Hypertension **4**:5, Sept.-Oct. 1982.

Barlett, E.E.: The contribution of school health education to community health promotion: what can we reasonably expect? Am. J. Pub. Health **71**(12):1384, 1981.

Bennett, W.J.: What works: schools without drugs, United States Department of Education, 1986, Washington, D.C.

Bernard, B.: The issue of self-esteem, Prevention Forum **6**(3):4, 1986.

Bernard, B.: Peer programs: the lodestone to prevention, Prevention Forum **8**(2):6, 1988.

Brion-Meisels, S., et al.: Decisions about drug use, Adolescent Decisions Curriculum, Adolescent Issues Project, United States Office of Education, Special Education Project Grant G008001910, Judge Baker Guidance Center, 1982, Boston, Mass.

Botvin, G.J.: Life skills training, a self-improvement approach to substance abuse prevention, New York, 1983, Smithfield Press, Inc.

Carr, T.F.: Drug abuse: Catholic schools are not immune, Momentum, pp. 11-14, May 1982.

Center for Population Options: AIDS and adolescents, Resources for Educators, Washington, D.C., 1987, the Center.

Crandall, D.P.: Planning issues that bear on the success of school improvement efforts, Educ. Admin. Q. **22**(3):21, 1986.

Dalton, H.L., and Burris, S., editors: AIDS and the law, New Haven, 1987, Yale University Press.

Dielman, T.E., et al.: Elementary school–based prevention of adolescent alcohol misuse, Pediatrician **14**:70, 1987.

Dielman, T.E., et al.: Susceptibility to peer pressure, self-esteem, and health locus of control as correlates of adolescent substance abuse, Health Educ. Q. **14**(2):207, 1987.

Ellickson, P.L.: Designing an effective prevention program: principles underlying the Rand Smoking and Drug Prevention Experiment, Santa Monica, Calif., 1984, Rand Corp.

Ellickson, P.L., and Abby, R.: A Rand note: toward more effective drug prevention programs, Santa Monica, Calif., 1987, Rand Corp.

Ellickson, P.L.: Project Alert: a smoking and drug prevention experiment, first year progress report, Santa Monica, Calif., 1984, Rand Corp.

Hansen, W.B., et al.: Evaluation of a tobacco and alcohol abuse prevention curriculum for adolescents, Health Educ. Q. **15**(1):93, 1988.

Halpin, G., and Thomas, W.: Drug education solution or problem? Psychol. Rep. **40**:372, 1977.

Health is basic: an introduction to the THTM program for teachers and students, Newton, Mass., 1983, Education Development Center, Inc.

Jessor, R., and Jessor, S.L.: Problem behavior and psychosocial development: a longitudinal study of youth, New York, 1977, Academic Press, Inc.

Kirby, D., et al.: Emerging approach to improving adolescent health and addressing teenage pregnancy, Washington, D.C., 1985, Center for Population Options.

Lovick, S.R., and Wesson, W.: School-based clinics: update, Houston, Texas, 1986, Center for Population Options.

Luce and Schweitzer in USDHSS, Fifth Spinal Report to the U.S. Congress on Alcohol and Health, Washington, D.C., 1984, DHHS Publ. no. (ADM) 84-1291.

MacDonald, D.I.: An approach to the problem of teenage pregnancy, Public Health Rep. **102**(4):377, 1987.

Mack, J., and Ablon, S., editors: The development and sustaining of self-esteem in childhood, New York, 1983, International University Press.

Midwest Regional Center For Drug-Free Schools and Communities, Chicago, 1988, Brass Foundation.

National Commission on Marihuana and Drug Abuse, Washington, D.C., 1973, USDHEW.

Phillips, J.A., Jr.: Abolishing tobacco use in secondary schools: a school-based management problem, NASSP Bull., pp. 121-123, Jan. 1984 (National Association of Secondary School Principals).

Ray, O.: Drugs, society, and human behavior, St. Louis, 1978, The C.V. Mosby Co.

Redican, K.J., Olsen, L.K., and Stone, D.B.: Health education: a positive force in increasing the reading skills of low socio-economic elementary students, Urban Rev. **2**(4):215, 1979.

Rist, M.C.: Antismoking policies are good for your school system's health, American School Boards Journal, pp. 25–28, Nov. 1986.

Sagor, R.: Seeking peace in the war on drugs, NASSP Bull., pp. 85-87, 1987 (National Association of Secondary School Principals).

Stoudemire, A., Wallack, L., and Hedemark, R.: Alcohol dependence and abuse. In Amler, R.W., and Dull, A.B., editors: Closing the gap: the burden of unnecessary illness, New York, 1987, Oxford University Press.

Strong, G.: It's time to get tough on alcohol and drug abuse in schools, American School Boards Journal, pp. 23-24, Feb. 1983.

Sex Education in the Public Schools, J. Sch. Health **51**:4, April 1981.

U.S. Department of Health and Human Services: Guidelines for effective school health education to prevent the spread of AIDS, MMWR **37**:S-2, Jan. 29, 1988, Centers for Disease Control, Center for Health Promotion and Education, Atlanta, Georgia.

Vincent, M.L., et al.: Reducing adolescent pregnancy through school and community-based education, JAMA **257**:24, June 1987.

Walberg, H.D., Schiller, D., and Haertel, G.D.: The quiet revolution in educational research. In Moore, G.W.: Developing and evaluating educational research, Boston, 1983, Little, Brown & Co.

Yarber, W.L.: AIDS education: curriculum and health policy, Bloomington, Indiana, 1987, Phi Delta Kappa Educational Foundation.

16

Healthful School Environment

OVERVIEW   *The principles of epidemiology indicate that the understanding of a health problem depends on three things: the host, or the person who has the illness; the causative agent, which brought on the illness; and the environment, which brings the causative agent and the host together.*

Traditionally school health practice focuses most resources on the host. Through education the school hopes to reduce the risk of illness caused by inappropriate behavior. Through health services the school strives to ensure optimal health, including the early detection of illness and initiation of subsequent treatment. The school environment cannot be overlooked although it is the least conspicuous element of school health practice.

OBJECTIVES   **After reading this chapter, the student should be able to:**

1. Describe the health risk posed by the school environment
2. Note significant questions to be asked about the location of a new school building
3. Identify responsibilities in monitoring a healthy school environment
4. List the basic requirements for adequate heating and ventilation in a classroom
5. Describe the effects of color, glare, and brightness difference and of desk placement on the learning process
6. Define footcandles, footlamberts, and decibels as important measures in meeting environmental standards
7. Describe lighting standards appropriate for different educational activities
8. Identify basic requirements for school toilet facilities
9. Describe basic requirements and suggest how teachers can establish a healthy social environment in the school
10. Suggest why water supply is a potentially dangerous source of infection in a school
11. Discuss basic standards for school food services
12. Specify special environmental concerns in special use areas such as gymnasiums, locker rooms, playground space, swimming pools, and shower rooms

For the student, school and home are the two environments where he or she spends the most time. The school environment is important to learning in that physically it must not create undue risk of accident or disease and socially it should encourage and support the teaching and learning process. The environment is one of the three elements of public health concern: the agent, the host, and the environment (see Chapter 3). A good environment contributes to the outcomes of health education and service programs, greatly improving society's investment in the total educational process.

Architectural, sanitary, esthetic and social aspects of the school environment must be considered (Fig. 16-1) though the health implications of school architecture may be over-emphasized. A very wholesome environment can be provided in a school of rather poor architectural design; yet a well-designed school has greater potential for healthful function than a less well-designed building. Whether esthetic, social and functional possibilities are developed is the responsibility of those who occupy the building.

Sanitation depends on adequate facilities, properly used through sound housekeeping (or school-keeping) practices. All people using the school should actively participate in school keeping. It is unjust to permit children to believe that the building is kept clean and orderly by someone hired solely for the task. To develop pride in this home away from home is a laudable educational objective. Each child should participate in the chore of keeping "our" school clean, orderly, and attractive.

RESPONSIBILITY FOR HEALTHFUL SCHOOL ENVIRONMENT

Theoretically responsibility for initiating and providing for school construction and maintenance rests with the board of education. As a matter of practice such action originates with the superintendent, a professionally qualified expert on such problems.

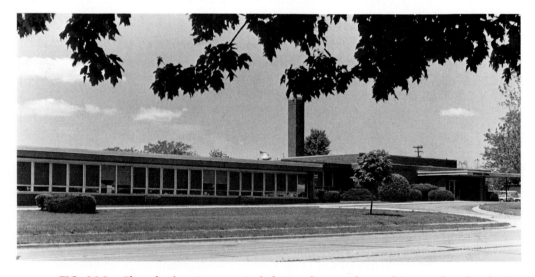

FIG. 16-1. The school environment includes much more than architecture, but the pleasing appearance of a school is important to students and community members alike. *(Copyright 1983 by David Riecks.)*

Frequently overlooked in discussions of the school environment is consideration of the ways the environment can promote health. The social and psychologic dimensions of the environment are as important as the temperature of the air or the light in a classroom.

Administrators

Full-time school administrators constantly appraise the school district's needs. Classroom enrollments, age-group populations, migrations, consolidations, real estate developments, industrial changes, and other factors that affect present and future school needs are used as bases for constructing new school buildings or remodeling old ones. Knowledge of the present plant — its shortcomings and possibilities — is necessary to the administrator. The economics of building anew or rebuilding are important.

Once administrators agree on plant expansion, they develop a tentative estimate and general plan. The superintendent submits these recommendations to the board for its consideration.

Maintaining the school plant is the responsibility of the superintendent and the administrators, especially the principals. General policies apply to the whole system, and each principal administers the policy to the best advantage for the building for which he or she is responsible. Although the superintendent does not intend to veto or even investigate problems or procedures of a particular school, he or she does need to know of unusual situations and circumstances.

In addition to the physical environment, administrators are also responsible for psychologic and social aspects of the environment.

Maintaining staff and student well-being is the responsibility of administrators and school boards. The development of personnel policies and discipline codes, the public image of the school, and relationships with parents represent important aspects of the school's responsibility to maintain an environment that encourages learning. Both physical and psychosocial aspects of the school environment are discussed in this chapter.

Board of education

Sovereignty, or ultimate authority, rests with the people, who delegate its exercise to the board of education. However, the board does not act on its own initiative in plant construction but judges the merits of recommendations made by the professional administrator. A wise board asks a representative community committee to review the plans and make suggestions. This ensures adequate study of the plan and community understanding of the proposal. When representative community leaders approve the plans, the board of education can proceed in the knowledge that the community understands and supports the project.

If the plan goes forward, an architect is engaged by the board to draw preliminary plans and to make preliminary estimates. The board then takes the necessary steps for financing — usually a bond issue for approval by the electors in a regular or special school district election. If the voters approve, final plans are drawn, bids are called for and opened, and a construction contract is awarded. Because of better school architects, better engineers, illuminating specialists, ventilation experts, and a host of other specialists, school buildings today are a vast improvement over those of a generation ago.

Regulations governing school maintenance are approved by the board. Often certain board members have an extensive background in the needs and procedures of plant maintenance.

Architect

In recent years school architecture has become a specialty in the architectural profession. As a result, school districts receive better plant designs. The most competent architect consults the school personnel who will "live" in the building. For effective school living the plan must be adapted to the needs of children. Who should know these needs better than the teachers? A wise architect solicits the composite judgment of all people who may have valuable suggestions in the planning of the building. In addition to drawing plans, the architect supervises construction.

Teachers

Once the structure is completed and furnished, the teacher's task is to make the building serve the needs of healthful school living.

A teacher's classroom becomes her or his domain and reflects his or her interests and personality. In this way each classroom assumes a different character and the school becomes a place of great diversity and considerable interest. The school environment itself should be included as an object of study. Class activities such as safety surveys, testing for light and noise intensity, learning to check water in swimming pools, and learning about sanitation standards in cafeterias are examples of ways teachers can maximize the use of the school as a learning environment.

Students

As much as possible, students should assume the primary responsibility for the order and cleanliness of their school. On a cooperative basis classes can supply additional furnishings for the building. Pictures, vases, bowls, flowerpots, stands, lecterns, and a host of other furnishings have been class contributions at various times. *School organizations* also contribute to building maintenance and obtain additional equipment.

Special projects such as *Don't Be a Litterbug Week,* pickup projects, locker cleanups, rake-up campaigns, and other activities add to the interest of the students, especially in elementary grades, in maintaining a healthful school environment.

Student pride in the school is not difficult to develop, but it does require some planning and promotion. Loyalties to the school and what it stands for create a desirable atmosphere for wholesome living. With stimulation and guidance, students usually develop appreciation. This can be solidified by having the students assume responsibility for preserving and extending the attractiveness of their common home. Monitors may be designated for specific tasks, but all children should feel they have a responsibility. Monitor selection procedures should be designed to award every youngster a regular assignment.

Custodians

The once nonskilled janitor has been replaced by the qualified custodian. Beside the mechanical skill needed for the assignment, the custodian should know sanitation, control of communicable diseases, and safety. Most states provide in-service preparation to assure the schools of well-qualified custodians. In addition to possessing job know-how, the custodian should be dependable and in good health. A competent custodian can care for 10 to 12 rooms properly. Some administrators supply the custodian with a printed list of duties and instructions.

A custodian has many miscellaneous duties, but some are of specific health significance. These include heating and ventilating, dusting, gathering trash, cleaning plumbing fixtures, filling soap dispensers, sweeping floors, mopping, cleaning steps, walls, and windows, cleaning chalkboards and erasers, taking care of the school grounds, checking playground apparatus, inspecting for safety, and eliminating hazards.

Custodian-staff cooperation is a two-way street. Insofar as is possible the custodian's schedule should avoid interfering with the school routine. Time after school and on Saturday is used for cleaning and minor maintenance. When students, teachers, and custodians cooperate, everyone's task is lighter and the school's atmosphere is healthier.

Although the custodian should be friendly with the children, the custodian's role is *not* the role of a teacher or counselor. The custodian should not be regarded as a personal servant for any one teacher. A custodian has specified duties to carry out, but a healthful school environment is not solely the responsibility of the custodian.

The principal should make periodic inspections of the custodian's work. Understanding on the part of the whole staff, plus tact on the part of the principal, results in maximal service from the custodial force. An incompetent custodian, like an incompetent teacher, should be dismissed.

Lunchroom personnel

Sanitation is more important in the lunchroom than anywhere else in the school. A situation where sanitation prevents the spread of disease also provides an opportunity for children to observe and understand proper food-handling conditions and procedures. Lunchroom experiences integrate health practices and instruction.

The facilities and practices in school lunchrooms are those prescribed by public health departments for sanitation regulation in public food establishments. Observance of these regulations is doubly important in the school.

Lunchroom personnel should feel a special obligation to the children, which can be demonstrated by pride in lunchroom work. Personal health habits should be exemplary. If the lunchroom workers suffer from a communicable disease, they should isolate themselves voluntarily. The worker who strives for perfection in sanitary measures is a valuable member of the health instruction team.

LOCATION AND PLAN OF SCHOOL BUILDING

Certain factors in the location and plan of a school building are of direct health significance. To these factors the elementary classroom teacher and the secondary school health instructor should direct their attention. It is not suggested that other things about the building are unimportant, but for present purposes health factors alone will be considered.

Site

School sites should be considered from the standpoint of accessibility, safety, quietness, air cleanliness, adequate drainage, and recreation space. Distance is not so important today as formerly because of improved transportation. Railroad areas, main highways, and through streets are physical hazards to be avoided. City ordinances and state laws usually specify what distance from the school alcoholic beverage dealerships must be located. For clear air and a quiet neighborhood, residential and rural areas are preferable to industrial or other congested areas. Adequate play and recreation space can be provided by setting a minimum of 5 acres for an elementary school, 12 acres for a junior high school, and 20 acres for a senior high school. A standard of 100 square feet (26 sq m) of play space per child will be adequate for any situation.

For esthetic reasons the surrounding area should be attractive, and the school site itself properly landscaped.

Standards of physical comfort

For the usual school situation, standards for physical comfort have been determined by scientific investigation and practical experience. These standards are expressed in terms of temperature, humidity, and movement of air. Properly all three should be discussed together, but practical consideration dictates that they be dealt with individually.

Temperature in the schoolroom should be held between 66° and 70° F (19° to 21° C). In the winter the lower half of this temperature range will feel comfortable as will a room temperature of 70° F (21° C) in the hotter seasons.

Humidity, or air moisture, should be between 30% and 70% of the maximal amount of moisture the air will hold. A humidity of 50% and a temperature of 70° F (21° C) are ideal. Several instruments, such as hygrometers and psychrometers, precisely determine humidity. Without an air-conditioning unit it is difficult to affect the humidity of a classroom.

Air movement carries away body heat and moisture. To be effective, a current of air should be perceptible. The least perceptible current is called the threshold velocity. Under ordinary room conditions air movement should at least be of threshold velocity. A current perceptible at one moment may not be felt a few minutes later. As room temperature declines, the perceptible velocity rises. Since temperature and air movement vary, window ventilation is highly effective because it permits these variations to operate in producing comfortable sensations of the skin. Modern mechanical ventilating systems now do an adequate job but are more expensive to maintain than window-gravity methods of ventilation, which depended on a draft caused by open or partially open windows.

Heating and ventilation

In heating and ventilating schoolrooms, emphasis must be on physical comfort. Body heat and moisture must be removed. When the elimination of heat and moisture is retarded, students experience drowsiness, lassitude, depression, headache, and loss of vigor. For an alert and stimulating class the room must have proper temperature, humidity, and movement of air.

Heat for each room should be controlled individually by a thermostat placed 5 feet (1.5 m) above the floor. Ordinary window-gravity ventilation can be highly satisfactory if a glass deflector in the window starts the air current upward and an outlet high on the opposite wall permits circulation. Glass deflectors are recommended because they do not reduce the light from outdoors.

Mechanical ventilating systems are usually designed to provide 15 cubic feet (3.8 cu m) of air per occupant per minute. Ventilation in one room does not depend on ventilation in another room. Zoned ventilation is necessary in large school buildings. The gymnasium, auditorium, shop, and cafeteria usually have independent ventilating units. Cloakrooms have separate ventilation. Toilet rooms have ventilating ducts and fans independent of the rest of the system. To remove objectionable fumes or odors, laboratories are provided with special means of ventilation. Chemistry laboratories are provided with fume hoods of acid-resisting construction. Technical standards for special ventilation needs are usually available through engineering and public health organizations.

Vent grills are placed in the walls as far removed from windows as possible. Fireproof exhaust ducts carry the air outside the building. Ventilator hoods protect the exhaust openings against back drafts and inclement weather.

Air conditioning

Air conditioning controls the temperature, humidity, movement, and purity of air. The air is filtered to remove dust, smoke, obnoxious gases, and pollen. Temperature is maintained at 68° F (20° C). Humidity is maintained from 40% to 45% during winter and from 45% to 50% during hot weather. Air conditioning is used more widely in warmer climates than in colder climates.

ILLUMINATION

No one has ever become blind or had eye damage from poor schoolroom lighting, but proper lighting contributes to the effectiveness of students' work and helps prevent fatigue (Fig. 16-2). Efficiency and comfort of vision are the major considerations of illumination.

A distinction should be made between the terms *light, illumination,* and *brightness*. Light

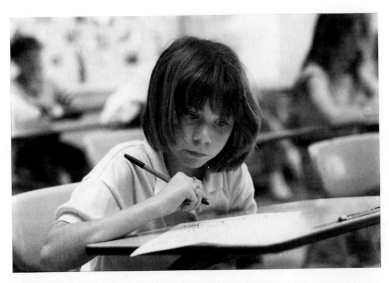

FIG. 16-2. Good illumination is essential for learning.

is the source, illumination is the effect, and brightness is the amount of light returned from a surface.

Intensity of visible light is measured in footcandles. A *footcandle* is the amount of light received at a point 1 foot removed from a source of standard candle power. The universal standard unit of light is at the Bureau of Standards, Washington, D.C. Footcandle meters, adjusted to the standard unit, measure the intensity of illumination.

A *footlambert* is the brightness of any surface produced from the illumination in footcandles and the surface's reflection factor. Thus, if the light units on a task are recorded as 50 footcandles and the reflection factor of the task is 70%, the units reflected to the eye would be 35 footlamberts. The equation is $FC \times RF = FL$. Footlamberts must be considered when the environment is conditioned for visual efficiency and comfort.

Three factors in lighting are important—sufficient light, proper distribution of light, and absence of glare. The amount of needed light depends on a person's activity. A corridor requires less light than a reading area. Distinctness of vision (visual acuity) attains its maximal effectiveness at about 5 footcandles. Speed of vision attains its maximal effectiveness at about 20 footcandles. On a sunny day outdoor illumination may be up to 10,000 footcandles. In a schoolroom the illumination near a window may be above 200 footcandles.

Proper distribution of light demands that all areas of the visual field have the same approximate intensity. Recognition of brightness difference has led to the use of lighter-colored chalkboards, woodwork, floors, furniture, and equipment in schoolrooms. *Brightness difference* expresses the brightness of the task as compared with brightness of the surrounding area.

Brightness balance is essential to visual efficiency and comfort. This can be attained when low brightness differences between the task and the surrounding area are maintained. Absolute brightness balance in the classroom is not possible; however, the footlambert brightness of the best-lighted area in the room should not be more than 10 times the footlambert brightness of the poorest-lighted area where tasks are being performed.

Glare is light that causes discomfort, annoyance, or distress to the eyes. It is annoying to face a window or an uncovered light bulb. Reflected light from a tabletop produces glare. Contrast in light disturbs vision. All these conditions produce glare and are much too common in schoolrooms.

Classroom factors

Satisfactory illumination in a classroom depends on more than just the necessary window space and light units. All surfaces should be dull or semiglossy to reduce glare. This means that the furniture must be a light color and have a dull finish. A highly reflective semiglossy paint should be used for the walls and ceiling. Reflective values indicate the colors that should be used in schoolrooms.

The ceiling and the first 3 feet (0.9 m) down on the wall should be painted white, ivory, or a light cream color. Tasteful pastel tints on the walls provide both attractiveness and good reflective value. Some architects recommend a buff color for the lowest portion of the wall.

Chalkboards should be dull and light colored but should never be located between windows. When placed in front of the room or on the wall opposite the windows, chalkboards may cause glare. Such glare can be prevented if the lower edge of the chalkboard is pulled out about 2 inches (5 cm). If the board is tilted, reflected rays are thrown above the children's heads.

Seats should be placed so that no child faces the window light. By the same token, the teacher should not face the light or stand in front of the windows so that the children must face the windows to see the teacher.

Standards of light

Minimal intensity of light for different purposes has been determined by scientific study and practical experience (Table 16-1). Other standards have been set up in terms of footlamberts (Table 16-2).

Although sufficient light is important, contrasts should be avoided. The peripheral field and background should be nearly as intensely illuminated as the work field.

Natural light

Both for psychologic effect and for good visual conditions, natural light should be used to the fullest and most effective extent possible. Ideally, window space should be one fifth of the floor area in rooms not more than 24 feet (7.2 m) wide. Unilateral lighting or lighting from one side is recommended. The left side is preferred, but the right side is acceptable.

NOISE

Noise is unwanted sound. Noise distracts students and teachers from the business of learning and also causes undue fatigue (Fig. 16-3). Noise can be reduced at its source or in its

TABLE 16-1. Recommended lighting levels in schools

Location	Recommended footcandles on task
Classrooms—on desks and chalkboards	70
Study halls, lecture rooms, art rooms, offices, libraries, shops, laboratories	70
Drafting rooms, typing rooms, sewing rooms	100
Auditoriums (not for study), cafeterias, washrooms	50
Open corridors, storerooms	20

TABLE 16-2. Recommended footlamberts

Area	Footcandles		Reflection factor		Footlamberts
Average task	30	×	70%	=	21
Desk top	30	×	50%	=	15
Floor	20	×	30%	=	6
Chalkboard	50	×	30%	=	15
Tack board	50	×	50%	=	25
Walls	30	×	75%	=	22.5

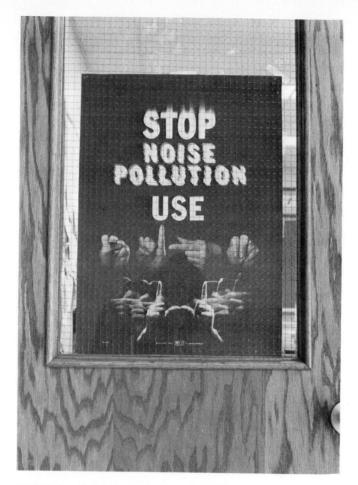

FIG. 16-3. Noise is unwanted sound. Simple reminders to reduce noise level are an effective part of any noise control program.
(Mary E. Allen.)

transmission by special modification of the environment. Carpeting and acoustic tiles are two obvious ways to reduce noise transmission.

The original decision of school placement should consider possible noise problems. Traffic and industrial noise can be reduced by the judicious placement of buildings and careful planting of trees.

Students and teachers should not be subjected to average noise levels over an 8-hour period that exceed 85 decibels on scale A. Sound can be measured on many frequencies. Scale A measures sound in the frequency range most closely resembling human speech. Recognizing that noise levels above 65 decibels interfere with speech communication gives meaning to decibel measures.

For students who may be in an especially noisy area such as a shop, swimming pool, or gymnasium, high noise levels for short periods of time are acceptable, but for the teacher who stays in these areas for long periods noise presents a significant health hazard. Such areas should be carefully surveyed to make maximal use of noise-reducing materials, and teaching schedules should be arranged to allow adequate time away from excessive noise. An alternative, but not a particularly satisfactory one except when certain equipment is used in shop classes, is the use of ear plugs. Teachers working in noisy areas should conduct regular noise surveys of these areas, seek ways to reduce noise at its source, and regularly have their hearing checked.

VERMIN CONTROL

Flies, rats, mice, cockroaches, and other vermin should be controlled by securing doors and windows, eliminating breeding places, and depriving them of food and water sources. These pests are most common in kitchens and lunchrooms. Flies, rats, and mice are easier to control than cockroaches. Because these insects inhabit warm, dark areas and survive on limited amounts of food and water, even scrupulous cleanliness usually cannot eliminate them once an infestation is established. Insecticide sprays should only be used by licensed exterminators and should be used with great care in food preparation areas. Special care should be taken if insecticides and pesticides are stored in school buildings. Containers should be clearly labeled and stored completely separate from any food-related materials.

WATER SUPPLY

School authorities are responsible for providing a safe and adequate water supply for school use. When a municipal water supply is used, primary responsibility for its source and purity rests with the municipality and the public health department. Yet the school district is responsible for proper installation and maintenance of water facilities in the school. In addition to being free from contamination, water should be palatable and sufficiently abundant for normal school needs.

Source

Most schools obtain their water from an established public water system. These supplies are under the surveillance of the health department, and the school can accept this supervision as adequate. Some schools provide their own water supply, usually by drilling wells. Some school, may use shallow wells less than 30 feet (9 m) deep. Deep wells more than 30 feet (9 m) are the recommended water source for a school when no public supply is available. Regardless of source, school officials should work cooperatively with local public health officials to ensure safe water and an adequate program of surveillance.

Bacteriologic examination should be taken at least once a month. This test is for the Enterobacteriaceae (usually *Escherichia coli*) group of bacteria. Their presence indicates that the water has been exposed to human or livestock contamination and may be dangerous for drinking purposes. A positive test does not reveal the presence of disease organisms, but the possibility that they may now or later get into the water.

Fountains

Fountains are the most sanitary school drinking facility. One fountain per 75 pupils is an acceptable standard. Recesses in corridor walls provide a safety factor (Fig. 16-4). The height of the nozzle should be adapted to the age of the students.

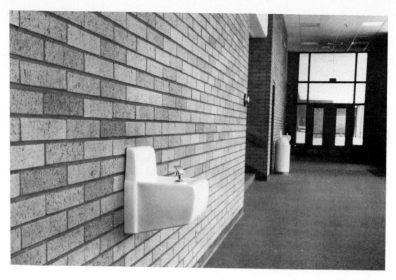

FIG. 16-4. Hazardous location for a fountain. To avoid possible injuries to students, a fountain should be set into the wall so that no part of the fountain protrudes and those using the fountain are not likely to be accidentally bumped while drinking.

Grade level	Height of nozzle
Kindergarten	23 in (59 cm)
Primary grades	25 in (64 cm)
Intermediate grades	29 in (74 cm)
Junior and senior high	35 in (90 cm)

GENERAL TOILET ROOMS

One washbasin or lavatory for each 40 pupils is recommended. Wash fountains can be substituted for washbasins. Height of the washbasins is important.

Grade level	Height to rim
Kindergarten	20 in (52 cm)
Primary grades	22 in (57 cm)
Intermediate grades	25 in (64 cm)
Junior and senior high	28-30 in (72-77 cm)

Washbasins should have no stoppers so that students wash their hands in running water. Each basin should have potable water that flows through one spigot with hot and cold water valves.

Liquid soap dispensers are preferred. Powdered soap is satisfactory. Bar soap is acceptable. No one has demonstrated that disease is spread by bar soap. *Paper towels* should be available. *Wastepaper receptacles* large enough to hold waste towels for a half day are necessary for an orderly toilet room.

Toilets and urinals

The number of fixtures will vary for different age levels. Any suggested standard may be unsatisfactory for a specific situation.

Elementary school	**Junior and senior high school**
1 toilet to 30 girls	1 toilet to 45 girls
1 toilet to 60 boys	1 toilet to 90 boys
1 urinal to 30 boys	1 urinal to 30 boys

Toilets for elementary schools should be 13 inches (33 cm) to the rim, or junior size. Standard size is proper for both junior and senior high schools. Construction should be of porcelain or vitreous china, with flush rim, siphon jet, extended lip or elongated bowl, and open-front seat without a cover. Flush valves and vacuum breakers are preferable to flush tanks. Individual compartments with doors should be provided for each toilet.

SPECIAL TOILET ROOMS

Kindergartens, locker rooms, faculty lounges, health service facilities, office suites, and other locations in a school building may have special toilet rooms. The number of fixtures in the kindergarten toilet room can follow elementary school standards. In locker rooms the number of fixtures should be adequate for the largest physical education class. Toilet rooms should be equipped to meet all needs of those enrolled, including easy access for handicapped students.

FOOD SERVICE

A food service unit is properly located on the ground floor, conveniently accessible from the outside. It should be planned to facilitate the most direct route from corridor to serving line, water cooler, tables, soiled-dish counter, and finally corridor again. A large school has a serving room, kitchen, and dining room. In smaller schools a serving counter between the kitchen and dining room replaces the serving room. Some schools use the dining room for a classroom, for a study hall, and for student activities such as student council meetings. The dining room should be pleasant and well lighted and have smooth, washable walls in attractive pastel shades.

Storage rooms should be cool (50° to 60° F [10° to 16° C]), well lighted, adequately ventilated, and vermin free. There should be adequate shelves and clean barrels, boxes, and bins for vegetable and fruit storage.

Refrigeration units should be spacious enough to allow ample room for all foods requiring refrigeration. Temperatures must be below 50° F (10° C). Dairy products should be separated from meats or other foods from which they may absorb odors.

Manual dish-washing facilities must include an adequate supply of hot water, a wash sink with detergent and warm water (100° F [38° C]), a rinse sink, and a sanitizing sink containing decontaminant or water above 170° F (77° C). Use of dish baskets allows dipping, speeds up handling, and eliminates wiping.

Dish-washing machines should be checked regularly to assure unblocked nozzles and adequate water pressure. Temperature of wash water should be between 140° and 160° F (60° and 71° C), and rinse water should be at least 170° F (77° C). Detergent dispensers should regularly be checked. Dishes removed from the machine should dry without toweling in 45 seconds.

Dishes and *trays* should be of smooth nonporous materials for easy cleaning. Discard rusted utensils and cracked or chipped dishes.

Hand-washing facilities should be available in the kitchen, with hot and cold water, soap, and paper towels. Lockers for storing outdoor clothing and uniforms should be provided for the lunchroom workers.

Practices

The best facilities available are of little value if the food service personnel do not follow sound practices. These are simple but important requirements:

1. Food service personnel should meet the same health standards as teachers.
2. Symptoms of communicable disease or open sores should be sufficient cause to remove a worker from duty.
3. A susceptible worker who has been exposed to a communicable disease should have clearance from a physician before reporting to duty.
4. Workers should wear light-colored, washable uniforms while serving and aprons while preparing food.
5. Caps, bands, or hair nets should be worn.
6. Workers should wash their hands *before* beginning work, handling food, and serving food and *after* coughing and sneezing, using a handkerchief, returning from the toilet, fixing the hair, and using objects handled by others; paper towels should be used for drying hands.
7. Dishes and utensils should be scraped and prerinsed.
8. Tightly covered garbage receptables should be emptied daily.
9. Forks, tongs, or spoons should be used for serving.

Inspections

Administrators are responsible for food service sanitation, and although health department sanitarians may periodically inspect and make recommendations, school administrators should require in-school inspections. A common administrative practice is to delegate the task to the school health program director. In the absence of a health director the health instructor may be assigned. A constructive inspection will improve conditions and encourage lunchroom personnel in the performance of their duties.

PLAY AREAS

The school environment where most accidents and injuries occur is the outside play area. Frequently teachers and administrators overlook this area as an important element of the school environment. Unprotected posts, gravel-covered playing surfaces, poor drainage allowing ice or mud to accumulate, slippery concrete surfaces, hedges and trees that scratch, uneven surfaces, and poorly constructed or supervised play equipment constitute significant environmental hazards. Although the play area cannot and should not contain challenges, the environment should be suited to those who use it. Secondary school students can tolerate a greater variety of circumstances in their recreation space than kindergarten students can. Common sense, simple rules, and caution reduce play area hazards to a minimum.

GYMNASIUM AND ACTIVITY ROOM

The gymnasium in junior and senior high schools and the activity room in elementary schools should be clean, well lighted, adequately ventilated, and free from hazards. A hard-

Sanitation report

School and institution food-handling facilities

S Milk, cream _____   Name _____
O Ice cream _____   Location _____
U Cream-filled   No. served daily _____
R   pastry _____   Water supply _____
C Meats _____   Sewage system _____
E Shellfish _____
S Ice _____

All items are satisfactory unless otherwise indicated.

Superintendent's name _____ Mailing address _____

Physical plant	Items	Remarks

1. Floors _____
   Clean and good repair

2. Walls and ceilings _____
   Washable, clean, good repair

3. Doors and windows _____
   Clean screens if needed

4. Lighting _____
   Clean fixtures; adequate light

5. Ventilation _____
   Free from cooking odors (hoods or fans or forced ventilation)

6. Toilet facilities _____
   Clean, good repair; proper vestibules and signs; convenient

7. Lavatory _____
   Located in kitchen or toilet room or both; hot-cold water; soap; paper towels

8. Water supply _____
   Bacteriologically safe

9. Sewage disposal _____
   Adequate

10. Plumbing approved _____

11. Rodent, insect control _____
    Building free of rodent harborage

12. Employee's locker space _____
    Clean, adequate

Equipment

13. Cooking utensils _____
    Good construction; satisfactory condition

Continued.

Sanitation report — cont'd

14. Worktables _____
Durable; easy to clean

15. Plates, silverware _____
Good condition; sufficient for size of operation

16. Refrigeration _____
Adequate; proper temperature

17. Protected display for exposed foods _____

18. Dish-washing equipment _____
Approved construction for hand or machine dish washing; sufficient hot water

19. Storage room _____
Clean; dry; well ventilated; vermin-free shelves; racks

20. Garbage cans _____
Cover; sufficient supply

Operation

21. Dish washing _____
Proper washing and sanitizing

22. Food preparation _____
Proper refrigeration (cream products, etc.); clean and minimal handling

23. Wholesomeness of food _____
Free from spoilage and contamination; canned foods properly processed
from inspected sources

24. Equipment _____
Power equipment; stoves, utensils, etc. kept clean

25. Storage _____
Kept clean; food off floor; bulk food in tight containers

26. Employees _____
Clean uniforms or aprons; hair confined; free from infectious disease; no
open or inflamed skin lesions

27. Garbage and refuse handling _____
Cans kept covered and washed; proper disposal of garbage;
no trash accumulation

28. Premises _____
Kept clean; free from rodents and insects

29. Storage of cleaning supplies _____
Separate from food storage

30. Cloths _____
Kept clean

Date of inspection _____ Sanitarian _____

wood floor with a nonslip finish cleaned daily keeps dust at a minimum. Windows are often more of a detriment than an asset in a gymnasium. Glass bricks should fill window space when masonry is used in construction. Screens over the windows reduce illumination but may be necessary. "Artificial lighting as the sole form of illumination is entirely satisfactory. Forced ventilation is necessary when large crowds occupy the gymnasium, though for classes of 30 to 40 students window-gravity ventilation can be adequate. Regular inspections of conditions and practices promote safety in the gymnasium.

LOCKER ROOMS

A well-lighted locker room is usually attractive and sanitary. Located adjacent to the gymnasium, the locker room should provide at least 12 square feet (3.3 sq m) of floor space per student, based on the class with the largest number of students. Floors and walls constructed of nonporous material promote sanitation. Floors should have excellent drainage and be cleaned daily. Adequate heat and mechanical ventilation complete the requirements for excellent sanitation.

SHOWER ROOMS

Nonslip tile flooring is necessary in the shower room. At least 10 square feet (2.7 sq m) of floor space should be allowed for each shower head. The recognized standard is one shower head for every four students, based on the class with the largest enrollment. Shower heads should be at chin height (Fig. 16-5). Whether individual or gang showers are used, water-mixing chambers with wheel-control valves are recommended. The control of water temperature is quicker and easier with this type of equipment. Drying rooms between shower and locker rooms are important.

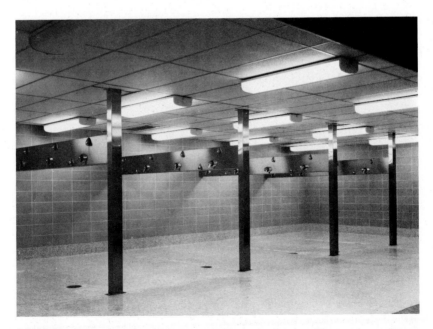

FIG. 16-5. Adequate and careful use of light limits fungi and bacterial growth.

SWIMMING POOL

Sanitation of the swimming pool is the physical education staff's responsibility. Two factors maintain a sanitary swimming pool — construction and regulation. A properly constructed pool provides for water filtration, chlorination, recirculation, and straining. A chlorine content of 0.2 to 0.5 parts per million inactivates all pathogenic organisms in the water. Daily samples are taken to determine bacteriologic and chlorine contents.

Essential to swimming pool regulation is a qualified person to supervise pool use. Standard regulations to govern pool use are personal cleanliness, freedom from communicable disease, and proper conduct and personal habits. It is essential that everyone who uses the pool take a cleansing shower, wear a clean suit, and use clean towels. Water temperatures between 72° and 78° F (22° and 26° C) and room temperatures between 75° and 82° F (24° and 28° C) should be maintained.

FIRE PREVENTION

Eliminating all risk of fire is impossible, but fire risk can be reduced to a minimum. Construction techniques now make maximal use of fire-resistant building materials, but a great deal of education material, namely books and paper, is flammable. Important considerations for fire safety include a building design for easy escape, posted directions for emergency exits, and careful preparation of students and teachers to leave the building quickly and orderly in case of fire.

Areas such as home economics rooms, shops, and laboratories present high fire risk and are usually equipped with special fire-fighting equipment. Students and teachers should be familiar with the use of this equipment and be able to operate it in an emergency. However, the first responsibility of all is evacuation. Containing the fire is a secondary concern better left to fire department personnel.

PSYCHOSOCIAL ENVIRONMENT

Important as the physical environment is, the psychosocial environment must not be neglected because it is less tangible and thus more difficult to control than the physical one. A healthy social environment must be maintained by recognition of factors that affect each child's adjustment.

Characteristics

There are certain characteristics of a healthy psychosocial environment in the schoolroom, as follows:

1. The children are relaxed and at ease.
2. They feel that the teacher and their classmates regard them well. Their age mates become their peer group, and approval of their peer group becomes progressively more important to such a degree that many high school students will rate peer approval to be more important than parental approval.
3. They have high levels of self-esteem.
4. They are challenged by the situation.
5. They are confident they can succeed.
6. They experience success.

7. They receive adequate personal gratification from their success.

To attain this atmosphere in the classroom, the school has certain responsibilities:

1. Recognize and identify any children who have special educational needs.
2. Provide all children with experiences that will stimulate the progressive development of desirable patterns of emotional behavior.
3. Provide students with esthetic experiences that will develop an awareness of beauty in life and help them identify with cultural groups.
4. Provide opportunities for the development of concepts of values and for practice in conduct arising from these concepts.

To create a psychosocially healthy environment, a teacher can make many contributions:

1. Adjust the curriculum's difficulty to the student's mental capacity.
2. Adjust the curriculum to the students' educational maturity.
3. Make special provisions for specific deficiencies.
4. Develop high expectations and good conduct habits through reading, discussion, visual aids, and other procedures.
5. Utilize the social influence of the group to aid in the child's development and to enhance learning.
6. Give students opportunities to make decisions.
7. Develop responsibility and leadership.
8. Develop a wholesome interest in law and order within the classroom, the school, and the community.
9. Provide desirable social experiences (Fig. 16-6).
10. Create a desire in each child to participate in extracurricular activities.
11. Instruct pupils in extracurricular activities.
12. Restrict or extend extracurricular functions in keeping with the needs of each student.
13. Give due encouragement and credit to each child for each accomplishment.
14. Be an understanding listener.
15. Make assistance as real as possible by helping pupils to help themselves.
16. For the poorly adjusted child, find the groups and teacher to which he or she will best respond.
17. Help parents know their child better.
18. Help parents develop a wholesome attitude toward a child's ability.
19. Help parents acquire a sensible attitude toward success in school and recognize the school's expectations.

Building a healthy psychosocial environment

Assuming that the physical environment is without undue hazards and is designed to encourage health, attention should be directed at creation of a healthy psychosocial environment. Here the stress is on relationships and the management of human resources. In this section we discuss the management of time, the school's relationship with the community in general and parents in particular, the relationship between school boards, administrators, and teachers, and the relationship of teachers to students and males to females.

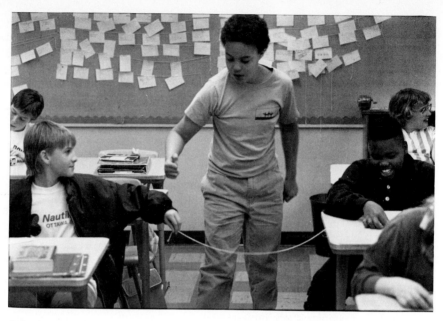

FIG. 16-6. Teachers can provide desirable social experiences to create a wholesome environment.

Time.   Misjudging time can create havoc with health. Time management is difficult, but good time management can reduce stress and prevent tensions in the school environment. Time affects the school program in many ways.

The starting time of the school year was originally based on the need for young people to work in the fields. Today early school openings may conflict with family vacation time, work opportunities for the students, or unseasonably hot weather. For example, in parts of the United States unusually hot weather in the fall frequently leads to the closings of un–air conditioned schools.

More important are issues relating to daily time. How long do students spend on school buses? What time in the morning do they leave for school? What time do they arrive home from school? How much time is left to study and do homework after school athletic teams, debate teams, cultural clubs, and music groups have completed their practice? Is there sufficient time between classes to move safely throughout the building? Is the lunch recess sufficient to eat comfortably? Do all student tests occur on Friday rather than spread throughout the week to reduce anxiety and stress? Do some students, especially athletes, miss excessive class time at the expense of learning? Are parent-teacher conferences scheduled at convenient times, and do they allow a flexible enough schedule to meet the needs of parents and teachers? Do buildings open early enough before school to allow for all needed activities?

Do teacher contracts allow sufficient time for their various responsibilities to be carried out? Is sick-leave time for all staff adequate to allow full recovery and to encourage absence for even mild conditions that may be contagious?

Is classroom time spent well or is it wasted? Do administrative matters interfere with learning time? Are teaching and learning resources adequate to maximize learning? Is it time to consider extending the school day or the school year?

Do we teach young people to manage time in the same way we teach them to manage money, responsibilities, and natural resources, or do we leave it up to them to learn from our example?

Everyone agrees that time is money, but few plan ahead for managing time. Recognizing the importance of time management in creating a healthy environment, one can use the preceding questions to form a time and health inventory to suggest possible modifications in school operations that may increase the likelihood of encouraging psychosocial health.

Community relations.   The school in general needs to maintain an equitable relationship with its community. In terms of health and health promotion this is especially important. The greatest potential for gaining consistent support for the school health program and increasing its effectiveness is to recognize and organize a school-community health council or team. Representatives of parents, administrators, students, physicians, dentists, school nurses, counselors, and teachers form the school health team. In this way the value of each member's contribution increases when she or he combines efforts with the others.

School-community health councils, because members have both a common interest in health and different backgrounds, are more likely to see health implications of school policies not always visible to any one individual policy maker. Encouraging the promotion of health throughout the school and the community and coordinating these activities greatly increases the quality of the environment.

Parents.   If parents know what the school is attempting to do, they are likely to be supportive. Active schools and supportive parents make for an environment that promotes health and learning. In addition to communication with parents by newsletters and conferences, such things as homework activities can be used to help parents become more aware of the school's health programs. Many health curriculums encourage students to ask parents or other adults about health matters, such as reasons for not smoking. Other curriculums encourage health promotion activities for the whole family, such as family blood pressure screenings. Of course not all parents cooperate, and sometimes students who need the most parental assistance get the least. However, this doesn't decrease the need to gain parents' support. The key is to encourage consistency within the environment. Consistency and clear expectations at school and at home make for a good psychosocial environment.

School boards.   Consistency in policies developed by school boards also enhances the psychosocial environment and encourages health. Policy making reaches into the classroom. When teachers' contracts are being negotiated, there is often a degree of tension that affects the teaching and learning process. Changes in relationships caused by difficult personnel issues like terminations are also felt by students directly or indirectly.

Even more direct in their effect are policies on tobacco use, seat-belt use, and drug abuse. The school board that prohibits student smoking, encourages tobacco and drug education, and yet does nothing to curtail smoking by teachers, staff, administrators, or visitors, creates an obvious contradiction. The hypocrisy of such actions is likely to disturb students and to undermine the health teacher's efforts. This is not a healthy situation.

More and more schools are reviewing their board-directed operating policies to remove such inconsistencies and clarify standards to create physically and psychologically health-enhancing environments.

Administrators and teachers.　Even closer to students is the relationship between school administrators and their staff. A spirit of cooperation between all staff members is essential for learning. An atmosphere of congeniality depends on clear job descriptions, clearly assigned responsibilities, hiring policies that ensure staff competence in areas of responsibility, and supportive administrative procedures. In this regard school personnel should not accept tasks that are pushed on them by others in the interest of "education." Teachers, for example, should not allow themselves to be drawn into time-consuming counselor roles when a competent counseling staff exists. Likewise, they should not be compelled to accept coaching responsibilities that interfere with teaching responsibilities.

Teachers.　Teachers must be realistic and deal objectively with student adjustment. All school activities directly or indirectly contribute to a student's personality growth. Because each student is unique, teachers should provide for all types and degrees of participation. The classroom environment established by the teacher is, for most students, second only to the home in terms of exposure.

Males and females.　Psychosocial health can also be advanced by sensitivity in the way teachers deal with male and female students. There is, for example, a documented tendency for teachers to ask male students tough analytical questions but to ask female students simple factual questions. Female students are less likely to be called on in class, and females are more likely to be interrupted. Students report that teachers are often more abrupt and impatient with female students than they are with male students.

Such behaviors are unacceptable. In some cases they are not recognized, but in others they may be a conscious reflection of prejudice. Often these behaviors result from bias that exists in the larger community and goes unrecognized. It is important, however, for teachers to be conscious of these behaviors and to guard against their occurrence.

The Chancellor's Commission on the Status of Women at the University of Nebraska–Lincoln has produced a document containing a series of suggestions that are particularly helpful:

1. At the beginning of the semester, teachers should inform students that they are all expected to participate in class discussions.
2. Give women students a fair opportunity to express themselves.
3. Be attentive when women students ask or answer questions.
4. Verbally reinforce contributions by women students as well as those by men.
5. Monitor discussions to prevent women from being interrupted.
6. Encourage women, as well as men, to speak out.
7. Avoid sexist grammar.
8. Avoid stereotypes that portray women as helpless or less competent than men.

9. Choose course materials that do not use sexist language and that recognize contributions by women.
10. Mention contributions by females as well as males in the discussions of course materials.
11. Entertain the same expectations for males as for female students.
12. Ask a knowledgeable student or colleague to monitor your class.
13. Include a question on classroom equity in course evaluations.
14. Avoid telling sexist jokes.
15. Avoid commenting on a female student's appearance.
16. Avoid using sexist diction, such as the generic "he."
17. Avoid presenting women in traditional or subservient roles.

SUMMARY

Changing the environment is the fundamental principle of primary prevention. We change the environment to reduce the likelihood that disease conditions can occur. Sometimes, however, we overlook this principle in the day-to-day conduct of education. For schools, not only is there a responsibility to provide an environment that is safe from undue hazards, but there is also a responsibility to provide an environment that facilitates learning. Such an environment includes the physical characteristics that encourage good teacher and student interaction and also the psychosocial characteristics that create an atmosphere of calm and confidence that enhances learning.

It is not adequate to expect that an ideal environment be presented to teachers and students for their daily tasks. The environment is the responsibility of all who work and learn in a school and also reflects the values of the total community. The ideal environment enables all to work together to maintain optimal standards.

STUDY QUESTIONS

1. Identify the areas of a school most likely to create a risk to health.
2. Who has the responsibility for monitoring a healthy school environment? What are the actual responsibilities of the people you have just listed?
3. What are the important environmental considerations in planning the location of a school?
4. List the variables important to a healthy environment inside the school.
5. For what purpose do we use footcandles and footlamberts, and why are these concepts important?
6. In what ways are brightness balance and glare important to the students' learning?
7. What would dictate practical standards for noise in the school building?
8. Outline basic standards for school toilet facilities.
9. How can the psychologic environment of a school be improved?
10. Why are public health officials greatly concerned about the possible spread of infection via the school lunchroom?
11. What is the primary purpose of school ventilation?
12. Why do some school authorities prefer all artificial lighting in schools?
13. Rate the illumination in the room in which your health class is held.
14. What would you rate as the most important requirements in school sanitation?
15. What can each teacher do to promote more healthful school living?

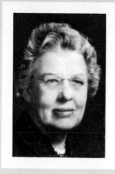

Mabel E. Rugen

BORN   May 13, 1902, Glenview, Illinois

EDUCATION   B.S., University of Wisconsin, 1925; M.A., New York University, 1929; Ph.D., New York University, 1931; postdoctorate work, University of Michigan School of Public Health

Dr. Rugen's career reveals a broad and varied spectrum of professional activities in both education and public health. It is evident that her first commitment was to education and teaching. Her teaching experience ranged from public elementary and secondary schools through undergraduate and graduate education. Her public school experience included positions in the states of Illinois, Kansas, New Jersey, and New York, where she taught physical education and health education. Her long and productive career at the University of Michigan began in 1930, as a junior faculty member, and covered a span of 40 years. She became a full professor, holding appointments in both the School of Education and School of Public Health. Her work in higher education encompassed teacher education, public health, medicine, and her special interest — health education.

Through the experience, contributions, and professional leadership of Dr. Rugen and other leaders, the field of health education emerged as an independent field of study and professional work. In a true sense, she can be called the "great interpreter." She was truly a multidisciplinary person, who devoted much of her professional career to developing understanding and to strengthening relationships among professional disciplines such as education, nursing, public health, and medicine. Her overriding objective was to promote health and well-being through education.

One of her early, important appointments occurred during World War II, when she became the director of the Community Health Service Project for the Michigan Department of Education. It was funded by the W.K. Kellogg Foundation and was later known as the Kellogg project. Initially the purpose of the project was to teach high school girls to serve as nurses' aides. The popularity of the project spread throughout the United States and evolved into a strong school-community cooperative effort to promote child health through health education.

Dr. Rugen was a prodigious worker, who carried a major leadership role as chairperson or project director of important committees and commissions throughout her academic and professional career. In addition to this very active leadership role, she was a prolific writer, contributing well over 120 publications as editor, writer, and researcher. The emphasis of much of this work is on the interpretation of health education — its contribution to general education and its function as a profession.

Among her significant publications is *History of Public Health Education,* which was written for the American Public Health Association; it is a series of books and monographs on school health published by the Joint Committee of the National Education Association and the American Medical Association, during the period when she served as chairperson of this committee. She was a frequent contributor to yearbooks, commission reports, and special editions of the *Reviews of Educational Research.*

She received many honors and awards — an honor award from the American Alliance for Health, Physical Education, and Dance, the Elizabeth Prentiss Award for Health Education, and an honorary doctorate of laws from Central MIchigan University. She was elected to the American Academy of Physical Education and was given the American School Health Association's highest honor, the William A. Howe Award.

REFERENCES

Basic concepts of environmental health, Pub no. 80-1254, Washington, D.C., 1980, National Institutes of Environmental Health Sciences, Public Health Service/National Institutes of Health, U.S. Department of Health, Education and Welfare.

Castaldi, B.: Educational facilities: planning, remodeling, and management, Newton, Mass., 1977, Allyn & Bacon, Inc.

Chancellor's Commission on the Status of Women: Chilly classrooms: equity for female and male students, Lincoln, Neb., May 1986, University of Nebraska–Lincoln.

Christensen, J.F.: IES lighting handbook: the standard lighting guide, ed. 5, New York, 1972, Illuminating Engineering Society.

Franklin, P.: Sexual and gender harassment in the academy: a guide for faculty, students and administrators, New York, 1981, Commission on the Status of Women in the Professions, Modern Language Association of America.

Hall, R.M., and Sandler, B.R.: The classroom climate: a chilly one for women? Washington, D.C., 1982, Association of American Colleges, Project on the Status and Education of Women, Association of American Colleges.

Hall, R.M., and Sandler, B.R.: Out of the classroom: a chilly campus climate for women? Washington, D.C., 1984, Project on the Status and Education of Women, Association of American Colleges.

Olds, R.S., and Eddy, J.M.: Negative health messages in schools, J. Sch. Health **56**:334, 1986.

Purdom, W.P.: Environmental health, New York, 1979, Academic Press, Inc.

Reid, C.R.: Environment and learning, Rutherford, N.J., 1977, Farleigh Dickinson University Press.

Rowe, D.E.: Healthful school living: environmental health in the school, J. Sch. Health **57**:426, 1987.

Sadker, M.P., and Sadker, D.M.: Sex equity handbook for schools, New York, 1982, Longman, Inc.

Schultz, E.W., Glass, R.M., and Kamholtz, J.D.: School climate: psychological health and well-being in school, J. Sch. Health **57**:432, 1987.

Wagner, R.H.: Environment and man, New York, 1978, W.W. Norton & Co., Inc.

Wiatrowski, M.D., Gottfredson, G., and Roberts, M.: Understanding school behavior disruption, Environment and Behavior **15**:53, Jan. 1983.

Willgoose, C.E.: Environmental health: commitment for survival, Philadelphia, 1979, W.B. Saunders Co.

Zeisell, J.: Stopping school property damage, Arlington, Va., 1976, American Association of School Administrators.

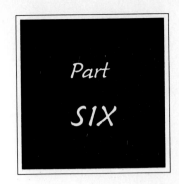

Part

SIX

APPRAISALS IN SCHOOL HEALTH PRACTICE

17

Evaluation

Evaluation is both enthusiastically recommended by most people and enthusiastically resisted by those whose programs are about to be evaluated. It is a mistake, however, to believe that the purpose of an evaluation is to prove programs a success or a failure; the purpose of an evaluation is to improve.

Evaluation data provide the basis for decision making. Frequently persons are unaware that they are carrying out evaluation activities. A simple action such as crossing the street requires an evaluation of existing conditions compared to the recollections of what happened the last time similar conditions occurred. If evaluation is considered an ongoing process, an integral part of living, it becomes less ominous than when viewed as an action to tell whether a program was good or bad.

In school health practice, evaluation continues on many levels. Each day the teacher, nurse, principal, and aide evaluate aspects of their programs. As a result of these ongoing evaluations they also change and improve programs. Ongoing evaluation of this type, when more formalized, is referred to as process, or formative, evaluation. The second principal type of evaluation is product, or summative, evaluation and is carried out after a program is completed. Both types are equally important.

Evaluation activities begin when project objectives are established. And today, more than ever before, evaluation activities are seen as important considerations in program planning. Well-conducted evaluations provide the single greatest opportunity to improve school health practice.

OBJECTIVES

After reading this chapter, the student should be able to:

1. Define evaluation
2. Differentiate between formative and summative evaluations
3. Outline basic procedures in any evaluation activity
4. Describe a variety of evaluation devices and techniques
5. Define and differentiate between the concepts of objectivity and reliability
6. Suggest ways that the health status of children can be evaluated and how these evaluations would be significant in the planning of health services and health education
7. List important program elements that would be examined in an examination of health practice administrative policies and practices
8. Describe important criteria in evaluating the school environment
9. Describe, develop, and use a variety of measurement techniques to assess the outcomes of health education programs

How much has the school health program improved children's health status? How effective is the school health program? Does it measure up to recognized standards? Is health instruction effective? Does the school meet healthful living standards? All these are inevitable and logical questions for those concerned with the school health program. To what extent school health activities meet the general and specific objectives of the health program is of concern to students, parents, the community, school administration, and, particularly, health teachers and school health service personnel.

Ideally, evaluation includes both objective measurements and the subjective judgments of experts. In school health, evaluation determines the effectiveness of the program by measuring the degree to which the school's health objectives are achieved. It encompasses the purely subjective, transient judgments as well as highly objective, scientific measurement of factors affecting health. Thus evaluation is inherent not only in the teacher's observation of a child's attitude but also in the dental examination.

PURPOSE OF EVALUATION

The purpose of evaluation is not to prove or disprove but to improve. Evaluation has as its single most important purpose program improvement. Program improvement occurs in two general ways: through better organized programs and through improved program outcomes. Evaluating the conduct of a program is called *formative* evaluation, and evaluating program effectiveness is called *summative* evaluation.

Evaluation audience

The actual conduct of any evaluation follows some generally accepted steps. However, the most important decision is determining why the evaluation is being conducted. Who wants the evaluation? Who will use the results of the evaluation? Why is the evaluation being carried out? If the school board wants an evaluation of a health education program, they will be interested in such things as the evaluation of teachers, the curriculum materials used, parents' satisfaction with the program, and student interest in elective health courses. Teachers, on the other hand, are likely to be interested in students' knowledge gains, satisfaction, and unmet needs.

Why an evaluation is needed is also necessary information to understand evaluation results. If the evaluation is requested because of public complaints about a program, it will differ significantly from one conducted as a part of a self-study in preparation for an accreditation review.

When an evaluation is planned, knowing clearly why it is conducted and who will use the results are equally critical to the planning process. Formal evaluations should be conducted for a specific cause, which focuses the evaluation efforts. Informal evaluations are ongoing. Anyone involved in educational programs will, consciously or unconsciously, evaluate the program constantly. At the same time minor program changes result from these informal evaluations. Most of what is discussed in this chapter refers to the more formal and structured evaluation activities carried out to meet a specific purpose.

Reasons for planning and carrying out evaluation activities include but are not limited to the following:

1. To determine the present status of the school health program

2. To assess progress toward achievement of program objectives
3. To provide information about program strengths and weaknesses
4. To provide data that will justify additional support and funds for the program
5. To provide information about program activities such as health services and health instruction to modify the program and improve it

Important purposes of pupil health evaluations are as follows:

1. To determine pupil health status as well as individual health education status
2. To provide information that will enable students to adjust their study programs in order to improve progress
3. To inform parents of their children's health status
4. To provide data on students' learning achievement that can serve as a basis for grading students
5. To enable teachers and school officials to adapt school programs to meet the health and educational needs of children

EVALUATION PROCEDURES

Because of the number of factors in the school health program that must be evaluated and the variety of conditions and situations under which evaluation must be done, it is not possible to set up a step-by-step procedure that will serve all purposes. Yet certain principles apply, some of which are as follows:

1. The general program objectives must be clearly stated.
2. Specific objectives must be stated precisely in order to serve as measurable outcomes.
3. All products, records, and instruments of an evaluation should be preserved, since they can be of value in assessment of the effects of the program on participants.
4. Methods and instruments used to collect program information must meet the standards of objectivity, reliability, and validity.
5. Information about the program should be collected early enough to be useful in revising or modifying the program.
6. In health education evaluation, efforts should be made to determine whether students apply what they learned or exhibit skills they learned from the health instruction program.
7. Evaluation of the total school health program may require that information be collected from many different sources, including the school, the home, the neighborhood, and the larger community.
8. The value of any school health program will depend on the collection of valid data followed by expert judgment to arrive at decisions and program recommendations.
9. The results of the evaluation must be presented in a usable and easily readable form for application to future situations.

EVALUATION DEVICES

There are few things that can be proved without qualification. The best that can be done is to present evidence one way or another. One should keep this in mind in selecting and using any evaluation instrument, which is merely a device for obtaining evidence. A human being must interpret and weigh the evidence. Some devices provide fairly precise data, whereas others yield only general tendencies or relative differences. Many evaluation devices that have recognized mechanical faults and qualitative shortcomings may, nevertheless, serve worthwhile purposes in certain situations. A critical analysis should be made of every measure used, but the device should also be appraised in terms of the service it performs and the purpose for which it is used.

This section will present a wide range of devices and techniques useful in program evaluation. It is important to keep in mind that the school health program includes services, education, and the provision of a healthy environment. Some of the techniques described will be especially useful in evaluating one aspect of the school health program but of little value in evaluating others. No single instrument or technique is equally effective in evaluating all areas of the school health practice.

Observation.   Observation, the most frequently used instrument in school appraisal, can be both meaningful and valuable in health evaluation. To be most effective, observation must be critical and precise. By using carefully prepared observation protocols and monitoring clear standards of objectivity a teacher can develop a highly accurate level of discrimination.

Interviews and conferences.   Interviews and conferences reveal information that other techniques cannot elicit. Conferences involving parents and friends who know a child are highly productive in providing health-related information.

Self-appraisal.   Student analysis of their own health provides information and stimulates interest. A checklist is a useful tool to guide self-appraisals. Original comments will add to the data gathered.

Questionnaires.   A series of specific questions can be used to obtain information on health practices and problems. A variety of standard health questionnaires are available.

Checklist.   Checklists are composed of objective items that usually consist of yes-or-no answers or descriptive lists. They are frequently used for studies of such things as sanitary conditions or health practices.

Surveys.   Surveys relate to people, including sociologic facts and psychologic data, such as knowledge, attitudes, and practices, as well as health status.

Records.   Family and personal health records can be rewarding sources of data. School health records should be sufficiently complete to be a dependable source of information.

Reports.   Accounts, descriptions, or statements, either incidental or developed for a special purpose, have value, especially when correlated with other data.

Achievement tests.   The most commonly used form of measurement in the school is the written or oral test. Both are adaptable to health instruction and are particularly effective in revealing the nature and extent of student learning.

Simulations.   To assess how students may behave, the conditions of an actual situation are simulated. Sometimes simulations are called situation tests. Role playing can be used to simulate real health-related situations.

•   •   •

From each of these techniques two types of information can be obtained. One type of information is the numeric data that come from counting, such as test scores, screening results, or the number of times a behavior was observed. This type of information, amenable to statistical analysis, has long been an important part of evaluation. From statistical data, the establishment of norms provides a standard for comparison. Numeric scores are precise, objective, and definite. Averages, variations, and consistencies can be determined with a high degree of accuracy. Health knowledge tests are particularly amenable to statistical treatment. Raw scores can be made more meaningful if specific sections of the test and of the types of errors are analyzed. Statistical methods, when applicable in the measurement of health outcomes such as knowledge and attitudes, should be given preference. However, care should be taken in the interpretation of statistical results as well as other data. A high correlation does not establish a cause-and-effect relationship.

The second type of information is less objective and less amenable to statistical analysis but no less valuable. These are data from observations and interpretations, often described as clinical appraisals or clinical evaluations. Clinical evaluations, less precise and standardized than statistical evaluations, are the only means available for appraising some activities in health. The determination of a child's health status does not lend itself readily to statistical treatment. The findings of the physician and dentist, the observations of the nurse and teacher, the personal history of the child, and the report of the parents may be adequate for clinical evaluation of the child's health. Although lacking statistical precision, the purpose of health evaluation may be well served. Up to now, no completely satisfactory standardized test of health attitudes has been developed. Nevertheless, teachers can devise techniques for attitude appraisal by systematically observing children in situations that reflect their choices and attitudes toward health. Norms cannot be determined and perhaps are unnecessary. Many health activities and objectives involve too many intangible values to be gauged with objective test instruments. Until such measures are available, clinical appraisals will have to be utilized to obtain a general evaluation of various health factors.

ESTABLISHMENT OF EVALUATION CRITERIA

The processes of evaluation, including procedures and instruments, should meet the criteria of objectivity, reliability, validity, and the practical considerations of use.

Objectivity

Objectivity implies the elimination of personal bias and self-interest. It is the opposite of subjectivity, where personal interest colors the decision or choice. Certain laboratory tests used in health examinations may be totally objective. An electrocardiograph gives an objective measure of the frequency and rhythm of the heartbeat and the action of the heart. Perhaps the recording of blood pressure is considered objective, though human judgment is involved. However, whenever human judgment is involved, the evaluation cannot properly be totally objective.

No test a teacher uses to measure learning is totally objective. Although the test may be written in an objective form, such as a multiple-choice test, the selection of the item and judgment as to its quality constitute a subjective process. The practical approach in evaluation is to reduce subjectivity to a minimum. Understanding validity is a way to increase the objectivity of any testing procedure.

Validity

Validity is the extent to which a test measures what it is designed to measure. In testing terms, validity can be assessed in four ways: content validity, concurrent validity, predictive validity, and construct validity.

Content validity indicates how well a test or evaluation instrument actually samples the unit being measured. In some cases this is obvious. If a teacher wants to test students' knowledge of the bones in the arm and leg, he or she can ask them to list all the bones in the arm and leg. If, however, the educational task is more complex, for example, learning all the major bones in the body, it would be impractical to ask students to list them all. However, questions asking students to name a sample of the entire list of bones would be adequate to estimate students' knowledge.

Concurrent validity indicates how well a test score relates to an accepted performance criterion. Knowing the names of all the major bones in the body, for example, probably has little relationship to knowing how to lift heavy weights without risking injury. However, knowledge about levers, muscle origins and insertions, and kinesiology relates to knowing how to lift heavy weights.

Concurrent validity is a control issue in evaluation of health education programs. The question is how well knowledge, attitude, and practice measures on a test actually relate to behavior. Since teachers are teaching the most healthful way to behave and have healthy student behavior as an objective, the question arises of how to evaluate outcomes. High concurrent validity indicates that there is a good correlation between test scores and actual health practice.

Predictive validity is concerned with present test scores and future measures of performance. If students who score well on a written test of skills to resist social and peer pressure to smoke are actually less likely to be cigarette smokers, this test has good predictive validity for future smoking behavior.

Construct validity, the last of the four types of validity, is the least specific and is based on logical inferences drawn from various evidence to indicate that the test actually measures what it was designed to. If one hypothesizes that knowledge about advantages of a particular behavior relates to the likelihood that the behavior will be carried out, a degree of construct validity exists.

Validity is not a simple generalized concept but should be viewed four different ways as an indicator of an evaluation tool or a technique's usefulness.

Reliability

Reliability is the consistency of measurement and can be assessed three ways: internal consistency, equivalence, and stability.

Reliability is usually expressed as a correlation coefficient. Measures of *internal consistency* show the consistency of performance of two parts of a single test. The coefficient is computed by comparison of one part of the test with another part ("split half") using a Spearman-Brown formula or by an item analysis using the Kuder-Richardson formula.

A *coefficient of equivalence* measures the relationship between two forms of the same test administered at close to the same time.

The relationship of two measures taken at two different times using the same test represents a *coefficient of stability*.

High reliability coefficients indicate that what is being measured has a degree of constancy and is therefore probably a stable construct, not affected by transient pressures but can be affected over time by focused programs.

EVALUATION OF CHANGE IN THE HEALTH STATUS OF CHILDREN

Because the school health program emphasizes building up and maintaining the highest possible health level in every child, a reliable means for measuring health status change would be extremely valuable. No single scale or measure has been devised, but combining several tests and methods can obtain a workable profile of a student's health status.

A recent thorough health examination obviously gives the best indication of the child's health. Comparison with previous examinations will be relatively simple for children who have had defects corrected during the interim. However, for many youngsters no such corrections will have been necessary, and evaluating any change in health status commands the skills and expert judgment of the physician.

In the absence of a health examination the teacher's own assessment of a child's health level will be of value. Although highly subjective, the appraisal considers attitude, pleasure in activity, vigor, endurance, ability to relax, absence of defects, and adequate social adjustment. The appraisal can be supplemented by data from the child's school health record, such as dental corrections, vision tests and corrections, hearing tests, weight and height changes, and records of illnesses. The physical growth charts in Chapter 4 can be used to chart the child's developmental status.

Supplementing the teacher's appraisal with the judgment of other teachers who have had ample opportunity to observe the child and obtaining the parents' assessment will reduce the subjective factor.

More objective measures can also be used to assess health status, for example, the number of days absent for illness, the number of visits to the school nurse, and the need for medication. Certain measures of fitness and strength taken in physical education classes and grades received for regular classwork also add perspective to health status. Taken together several of these measures would give a useful evaluation of changes in health.

EVALUATION OF ADMINISTRATIVE PRACTICES AND POLICIES

School health work is advanced or retarded in terms of administrative policies and practices related to it. An insight into the success or failure of the health program may be gained by a survey of administrative practices and policies that relate to the health program. The usual survey is made by means of a checklist of widely accepted school health responsibilities of the administrator. Such a list should include the following:

1. Recognize health as a basic objective of education and reflect this priority in the school's written administrative practices and policies
2. Secure and budget adequate funds for health programs
3. Regularly keep parents informed of the health program
4. Establish an appropriate cooperative relationship with community health agencies
5. Maintain communication with community organizations
6. Employ qualified school health service personnel
7. Become informed about health problems of the school-aged group
8. Arrange the school day in accord with sound health practice
9. Establish an effective system for keeping health records
10. Establish a policy on school health examinations
11. Provide for health observations by the teachers
12. Establish a systematic referral program
13. Promote measures to ensure services for every child in need of such services
14. Establish program policies aimed at control of injuries and communicable diseases
15. Procure necessary materials, facilities, and equipment for health instruction
16. Provide time and facilities for health instruction in the secondary school
17. Appoint only qualified teachers for health instruction
18. Provide a healthful and safe physical environment
19. Establish a school safety program
20. Provide facilities, personnel, and an established plan to meet emergencies
21. Provide health services for professional personnel
22. Provide in-service health education for teachers
23. Provide adequate faculty sick leave

This checklist does not include all the health responsibilities of the administrator but specifies essential minimal practices to serve as a practical, realistic measure of the administration's contribution to the school health program.

EVALUATION OF THE SCHOOL HEALTH PROGRAM

Appraisal of the overall school health program is necessary to measure the completeness of the program, its function, and its effectiveness. A valid program evaluation points up its strengths and weaknesses. Despite the recognized need for such an evaluation instrument, very few such appraisal forms are available. In consequence, most program assessments are either general surveys or evaluations of specific phases of the program, notably the health instruction phase.

Available standard forms differ in purpose, scope, and composition. They can be used to advantage, particularly if supplemented by other evaluative devices to serve specific situations and needs.

An example of a comprehensive instrument is included in Appendix B. This self-

appraisal checklist was originally developed through a cooperative effort among representatives from state agencies and professional groups in the fields of education and health.
Published by the Ohio State Department of Education, the checklist contains an excellent set
of standards pertaining to administration, health instruction, health services, and school
health environment. Although the standards have been written specifically for the state of
Ohio, school officials will find this checklist useful in evaluating their own programs.

EVALUATION OF HEALTH SERVICES

Circumstances may make it desirable to evaluate health services independently of other
phases of the health program. Such an evaluation includes the nature and frequency of
health examinations; dental examinations; screening of vision, hearing, weight, and height;
and the teacher's appraisal of the child's health. The follow-up program and correction of
defects must be included. Prevention and control of diseases, emergency care, and first-aid
provisions are also appraised.

Teachers and administrators can make effective use of two types of resources in evaluating school health services: (1) the evaluative checklist type of instrument, such as Part II
of the checklist included in Appendix B, and (2) the published formal statements of standards from authoritative bodies such as the American Academy of Pediatrics. The academy's
book *School Health: a Guide for Physicians* presents a useful set of standards and supplementary information.

EVALUATION OF HEALTHFUL SCHOOL LIVING

Any assessment of the school environment must extend beyond the mere static physical
environment. It should encompass the activities and practices in the school that affect health
promotion, disease prevention, safety, social adjustment, and esthetic appreciation. Evaluation should include factors affecting physical and mental health. The construction of the
school plant and sanitation facilities is important, but an evaluation of healthful school living
must extend to the total school program and the people who are part of the child's environment.

No phase of the school health program is as easy to appraise as the physical environment. Sanitary facilities are tangible, can be counted or tabulated, and involve relatively little
analysis or subjective judgment. Even the safety elements of the school environment are easy
to identify and tabulate. Perhaps for these reasons sanitary surveys of schools have long been
routine in school practice. Certainly these surveys should continue, but they should be
expanded into an evaluation of total healthful school living. Part III of Appendix B provides a
useful checklist for this purpose.

A functional evaluation of healthful school living can be made by use of Part III in
Appendix B. In this section the school is visualized as a dynamic community of students and
school personnel. The various forces and factors that affect the child's well-being are included and evaluated in terms of their influence on the student's total health. In addition to
appraising school life in action, this scale can serve as a stimulating instructional instrument.
Students can participate in the evaluation when this type of scale is used.

EVALUATION AND HEALTH INSTRUCTION

Two aspects of evaluation can be applied to health instruction. One aspect is evaluation of the health instruction program based on the quality and appropriateness of instructional activities. The second aspect can be based on the learning achieved by students.

What should be included in a health instruction program? What objectives should be recognized? What time allotment is made? What facilities, equipment, and materials are available? What methods are being used? To what extent do integration and correlation take place? What preparation should teachers have in health education? These are questions that must be answered in an evaluation of the school health instruction program.

Because schools vary greatly in their perception of health instruction aims, developing a universally applicable scale is difficult. Any form broad enough to encompass all purposes and situations would be so all-inclusive as to be impractical. The problem is to determine essentials of health instruction and to construct a scale to evaluate such a program. Each school can rate itself in terms of these basics and then supplement the rating with an evaluation of the special features of its own program.

An evaluation of a specific health course can be done with a checklist or inventory that includes the important criteria of classroom practice applied to health education.

Inventory of the health course

1. Objectives of health instruction
   a. Are there both general and specific objectives?
   b. Are the objectives stated in terms of student behaviors?
   c. Do the statements of objectives specify the type of behavior and the content or subject matter to be learned?
   d. Are the objectives related to the health needs and interests of both students and society?
   e. Are objectives stated in terms of attitudes, skills, and practices as well as knowledge?
2. Course organization and content
   a. Is there use of conceptual statements or generalizations to facilitate organization and understanding of health content?
   b. Is there a logical order of health content?
   c. Is there a logical sequence of topics to be covered?
   d. Is the content or subject matter scientifically accurate?
   e. Are health topics correlated or integrated with other school subjects?
3. Learning activities and materials of instruction
   a. Do class activities relate to student interests?
   b. Are a variety of methods used in teaching?
   c. Are there a variety of materials and instructional aids used in teaching?
   d. Are provisions made for individual differences and for individualized instruction?
   e. Are materials current and scientifically accurate?
   f. Are students given frequent reviews of instruction?
4. Evaluation of instruction
   a. Is the classroom atmosphere conducive to learning?
   b. Do students appear alert and interested in the health instruction?
   c. Are students given ample opportunity for class participation?
   d. Are student objectives, content, learning activities, and materials effectively related?
   e. Is student progress effectively measured in terms of course objectives?
   f. Is the course of curriculum regularly evaluated and revised?

Developing instruments to evaluate health instruction effectiveness requires an understanding of the subject, a grasp of outcomes toward which health instruction is directed, competency in test construction, and a willingness to put forth creative effort. Whether a teacher needs a simple survey of health practices or a complex objective test to measure students' understanding and appreciation of health values, demands on time, patience, ingenuity, and energy are involved.

Test construction and testing are competencies that every classroom teacher should strive to master. Standard tests have their place and value, but constant reliance on such tests indicates a limited classroom testing program. Standard tests cannot replace teacher-made tests. A rich, meaningful evaluation program means that tests and testing are integrated with the objectives, procedures, activities, experiences, techniques, concomitant learning, skills, and values developed in the class. Testing can be mastered by study and practice. A teacher need not attain the competence of a specialist to do an acceptable job of testing. In addition to its contribution to the instructional program, testing competency personally and professionally gratifies the teacher.

Tests are used for diagnostic purposes, to determine progress and to measure final achievement. In all cases, tests should reveal the nature and extent of learning. They can be tailored to fit each situation and can be both enjoyable and stimulating. Tests should be considered a means to facilitate learning. Students should be encouraged to view tests as an opportunity to demonstrate knowledge and skill. Students' fear of tests can be overcome by using tests frequently as another method of teaching. Instead of using test results only for the purpose of grading, tests can be used as a means of review and of stimulating learning. By developing high quality tests and using them properly, teachers help students develop positive attitudes toward testing. In all testing, teachers should make an effort to put students in a proper frame of mind before the test.

The steps in test construction should follow a fairly well-developed set of procedures such as the following:

1. Prepare a list of major objectives
2. Develop a content outline of topics to be covered
3. Develop a comprehensive list of specific objectives
4. Classify the objectives into categories such as the following:
    a. Cognitive or knowledge facts, terminology, application, analysis, interpretation, synthesis, and evaluation
    b. Affective interests, attitudes, appreciations, and values
    c. Psychomotor skills, practices, and technical performances
5. Devise test situations to reveal what students have learned in relation to the specific objectives
6. Prepare test items appropriate to the different types (domains) of objectives and different levels of learning
7. Try out the test to determine the following:
    a. The degree of difficulty of items
    b. The discrimination index of items
    c. General utility of the test
8. Revise the test to overcome weaknesses revealed in pretesting.

Health practices tests should do more than measure the pupils' knowledge of health practices. Such tests have decidedly limited value, for the pertinent question is whether this knowledge is being applied.

Since health practices are stressed at all grades, adequate evaluation of the health instruction program at this level must examine the extent to which health practices are established. Daily observation by the teacher is an acceptable, though not completely satisfactory, means of determining student health practices.

Some teachers have developed a short *health practices questionnaire* for parents of younger students that asks them to indicate their child's health practices. Group discussions can identify behaviors.

A *health practices inventory* is a good way to call the teacher's attention to the progress of the program in general and specific practices in particular.

However, in the higher grades many important health practices are considered either personal or in some cases illegal. It is reasonable to expect a student to report food choices in a food diary but not to report alcohol, marijuana, or tobacco use, at least not very accurately. Therefore health practices inventories are limited by the validity and reliability of the data obtained and will vary greatly from one area of health behavior to another.

For research and special evaluation efforts there are sophisticated ways to obtain reasonably accurate information on health behavior. Such procedures often require persons other than the teacher to gather the data, with assurances of anonymity and the fact that school personnel will see only the data in aggregated form. Sometimes these inventories include the gathering of physiologic measures to assure more accurate self-reporting of behaviors. For example, gathering saliva samples for chemical analysis to detect chemical indicators of nicotine in the body usually increases the number of students who indicate on a health behavior inventory that they smoke cigarettes.

Health attitude tests

A great deal of attention has been paid to attitude as an evaluation measure in health education. Despite this attention there is much yet to be learned about attitudes and their measurement. The relationships between knowledge, attitudes, and behaviors are unclear. Although it is logical to assume that these relationships exist, it has not been shown, for example, that change in knowledge will result in a change in attitude or that a change in attitude necessarily predicts a change in behavior. Attitudes can exist in the absence of supporting knowledge, and behaviors can exist in the absence of attitudes and knowledge as to why the behavior is carried out.

Frequently attitudes are simply considered a response on a scale to a statement of fact:

	Strongly agree	Mildly agree	Neither agree nor disagree	Mildly disagree	Strongly disagree
Smoking is a dirty habit.	_____	_____	_____	_____	_____
Jogging is boring.	_____	_____	_____	_____	_____

Carefully conceived, this type of measuring technique provides some useful data, but frequently it is difficult to tell whether attitude or knowledge is being measured.

The construct of attitudes has great utility. Teachers and others readily admit that youngsters who smoke cigarettes have a different general attitude from those who do not. Counselors indicate that some youngsters have a poor attitude toward authority figures and others do not. Everyone acknowledges that attitudes are associated with behaviors, but the precise meaning of attitude escapes consensual definition. The psychologic and educational literature over the years has included a large number of definitions of attitude. Allport (1935) defined attitude as "a mental and neural state of readiness, organized through experience, exerting a directive or dynamic influence upon the individual's response to all objects and situations with which it is related." Thurstone (1932), on the other hand, defined an attitude as "the effect for or against a psychological object." In general, an attitude is often seen as an emotionally toned idea.

More recently Fishbein (1973) has described an attitude in a way useful to health educators and has suggested some effective ways of measurement. Fishbein has defined an attitude as a "learned predisposition to respond in a consistently favorable or unfavorable manner with respect to a given object." Although Fishbein's work with behavior acknowledges the influence of social norms, his means of measuring an attitude has clarified the value of attitude measurement in health education.

Fishbein suggests that an attitude can be derived from an assessment of *beliefs* about a behavior and an *evaluation* of the *consequences* of these beliefs. Beliefs are an assessment of the subjective probability that performing a behavior may lead to a particular consequence. For example, the belief that smoking cigarettes can be habit forming may be assessed by some to be very likely whereas others may judge it to be very unlikely. The second component of attitudes, according to Fishbein, is the evaluation of the consequences of this particular behavior. In this example the second component of attitude measure is an assessment of whether respondents consider the forming of habits to be good or bad. An attitude then is a representation of the beliefs concerning the consequences of a particular behavior and an evaluation of the consequences.

A series of scales could be developed to measure both beliefs about cigarette smoking and beliefs about the consequences of smoking, as follows.

BELIEF ABOUT THE BEHAVIOR

1. Smoking cigarettes in the company of others is upsetting to them.
   Likely _____:_____:_____:_____:_____:_____:_____Unlikely
2. Smoking cigarettes is an unnecessary expense.
   Likely _____:_____:_____:_____:_____:_____:_____Unlikely

EVALUATION OF THE CONSEQUENCES

1. Upsetting others is
   Good _____:_____:_____:_____:_____:_____:_____Bad
2. Unnecessary expenses are
   Good _____:_____:_____:_____:_____:_____:_____Bad

This is not the only way to measure attitude, but it is an especially interesting one because it measures two important components. These components of attitude can be summarized as follows:

Attitude = Beliefs × Evaluations

Using the types of scales illustrated above and scoring each response +3 to -3 provides a standardized way to compare attitude scores. Each belief score is multiplied by its corresponding evaluation score, and the resulting scores are summed to provide an attitude score.

It is clear that this technique for measuring attitude has clear advantages over the single-dimension scales frequently used for attitude evaluation.

Health knowledge and understanding tests constitute the health teacher's principal evaluation instruments. Knowledge as a recognized objective of health is amenable to fairly precise measurement, and many test forms can serve this purpose. Understanding is equally important as an objective and, though more difficult to measure than knowledge, can be evaluated by means of tests built on recognized principles of test construction.

Certain forms and criteria are recognized in test item construction. They are helpful in aiding the health teacher to develop classroom tests that both are challenging to the students and truly evaluate aspects of health education.

Essay tests

The essay examination has considerable merit. It can reveal the students' general grasp of a subject and their ability to organize and express understanding. These are skills or attitudes that the whole school program seeks to develop. The essay test is especially valuable for diagnostic purposes. An essay question should call for a sequence of ideas, for the development of logical thinking, or for support for an idea.

Some suggestions for the construction, use, and scoring of essay tests can be channeled into the health teacher's needs. Questions might be structured as follows:

1. Elicit reactions to a situation, not merely a description of it.
2. Base items on how, why, or the significance of a particular piece of information rather than merely restating facts.
3. Call for definite, precise points and ask that the most important points in the answers be underlined.
4. Work out several model answers for use in grading and set up certain pertinent points.
5. Read the first question on all papers, then the second on all papers, and on through the last in order to give uniformity to grading; subjectivity can be reduced when you take the average score of several qualified graders, but there is not likely to be such a luxury as several graders in the usual school situation.
6. Use either the positive approach in scoring by adding points for each contributing statement or the negative approach of starting the reading by giving the question an arbitrary value (e.g., 20) and then deducting from the maximal score as the answer is deficient in meeting the model or standard answer.
7. Read selected answers in class to help students evaluate their own performance and understand what a high-quality answer is.

True-false tests

To many people an objective test means only one thing—a true-false test. Most widely used, most abused, and most maligned, the true-false test can be a useful testing technique. It is easy to construct, is useful in testing for misconceptions, is especially suitable for situations involving just two alternatives (such as infectious or noninfectious), provides for wide sampling, and is easy to score.

Testing as well as teaching should discourage rote learning without understanding. For this reason, subtracting the number of wrong answers from the number of right ones (R − W = S) to obtain the score discourages both rote memorizing and guessing. For a single test, correction for guessing (R − W = S) quite likely will produce a distribution of letter grades different from that when no penalty is received for an incorrect answer.

R   equals number of right answers
W   equals number of wrong answers, not counting omissions
S   equals score corrected for guessing

The most acceptable scoring procedure for objective tests is to give the same credit for each correct answer and to provide a correction for questions omitted. Correcting for omissions is in effect a correction-for-chance, as shown by the following example. On a 100-item true-false test, student A had 60 correct answers and 40 incorrect answers. Thus he received a score of 20. Student B, on the same test, also had 60 correct answers but he had only 20 incorrect answers with 20 items omitted. Therefore student B received a higher score of 40 (60 − 20 = 40). However, over a period of time (e.g., a semester) that involves several tests the final distribution of letter grades will be much the same under either plan.

A good test uses new terms and phrases, cast in a new mold, and avoids common word associations and textbook statements. A good test favors the student whose preparation has been thorough and who understands the material. It penalizes and confuses the student whose preparation has been superficial and who tries to get by through cleverness and outguessing the tester. A few suggestions may be helpful.

1. Use true and false statements approximately in equal proportions.
2. Make the important factor in the statement apparent to the student.
3. Use straightforward statements, not confusing or trick statements.
4. State exactly what is meant and avoid ambiguity.
5. Use quantitative rather than qualitative terms.
6. Do not depend on recalling a precise figure or word to determine whether the statement is true or false.
7. Exercise caution in the use of the following:
   a. Absolute words, such as *only, never, always,* and *all* are usually found in false statements.
   b. Qualifying words, such as *usually, frequently,* and *almost* are more often employed in true statements.
   c. The longer the statement, the more likely it is to be true.

A modified true-false test has items in which one or more key words are underlined. If the statement is correct, it is marked true. If the statement is incorrect, the underlined term is crossed out and a correct term substituted in the blank space.

Other variations of the true-false test include the alternate response test, which permits only two possible responses such as yes-no, correct-incorrect, and same-opposite. Still other forms of this test include the use of S and U for satisfactory and unsatisfactory or the use of A, D, and U to designate agree, disagree, and undecided.

The following sample true-false items illustrate the enumerated suggestions. Some common errors in item construction have been purposely included. Can you identify these? The last item shows a different way to construct true-false questions.

Items 1 to 5 are true-false questions. If the statement is true, circle the T; if false, circle the F.

T F 1. There is no single index of the quality of a child's health.
T F 2. Large persons always have good health.
T F 3. A mentally healthy person never gets angry.
T F 4. A balanced diet is one having the same number of calories each meal of the day.
T F 5. Alcohol is always a *stimulant* to the human body.

Material that lends itself to modified true-false items can usually be converted to simple true-false or short-answer items.

Multiple-choice tests

Superficially all multiple-choice questions appear to be similar, but a wide variety of items are included. In general, multiple-choice items should contain at least four responses, and five responses are preferred if all the options appear plausible.

The first type is a direct question followed by five possible responses, one of which is correct or the best answer. For example:

_____6. The statement "In solving one problem we often create a new problem" is best illustrated by which of the following?
   A. The discovery of penicillin put the producers of tincture of iodine out of business.
   B. Controlling infectious diseases has made new immunization methods necessary.
   C. Prolonging the length of life has resulted in new economic and social needs.
   D. The decline of infectious disease has created the problem of an oversupply of physicians.
   E. The discovery of the electron microscope has added new diseases to be conquered.

In the second type of multiple-choice test, the items are stated as incomplete sentences; there are five proposed completions, one of which is the best:

_____7. The expression "Nature grants biologic function without social favor" means
   A. Reproduction is solely a function of socially well-adjusted people.
   B. Only responsible people should have children.
   C. Some people, capable of being fathers and mothers, are incapable of being proper parents.
   D. The ability to reproduce is independent of economic or educational level.
   E. Sterility does not occur among the more socially fortunate.

In the third type of multiple-choice test, one key with five responses for a series of statements is used:

Key for items 8 to 12
A. Favorable for prevention of respiratory infection
B. Unfavorable for prevention of respiratory infection
C. Not related to prevention of respiratory infection
D. Favorable for prevention of respiratory infection only when a person is under 10 years of age

_____ 8. Vigorous exercise

_____ 9. Avoiding crowds

_____ 10. Avoiding night air

_____ 11. Fatigue

_____ 12. Taking a laxative

Another example of the same type of multiple-choice test that has some characteristics of a matching test is as follows:

Key for items 13 to 19
A. *An A level of mental health*
B. *A B level of mental health*
C. *A C level of mental health*
D. *All of the above levels*
E. *None of the first three*

_____ 13. Improvement in mental health possible

_____ 14. Alcoholism

_____ 15. Never gets angry

_____ 16. Minimum of friction; maximum of enjoyment

_____ 17. Uninspired, everyday boredom

_____ 18. Perfect mental health

_____ 19. Constructive, effective adjustment

Another design of multiple-choice test may stimulate analytic thinking:

Key for items 20 to 24
A. *Statement is correct; reason is correct.*
B. *Statement is correct; reason is incorrect.*
C. *Statement is incorrect; reason is correct.*
D. *Statement is incorrect; reason is incorrect.*

_____ 20. All overweight people should exercise vigorously because exercise increases metabolism.

_____ 21. Drinking fluids before or during a meal will stop digestion because water will dilute stomach acid.

_____ 22. Regularity is favorable to good digestion because it permits a cycle or rhythm in the function of the digestive system.

_____ 23. Dentifrices should be used in brushing teeth because dentifrices are antiseptics.

_____ 24. Fluoride prevents decay for adults because it destroys bacteria.

Another variaton in multiple-choice tests is a chart on which designations are used as the key and the items refer to the designations on the chart.

In the construction, use, and scoring of multiple-choice items, certain safeguards are suggested:

1. There should be only one correct or best answer.
2. The position of the correct response should be changed from item to item. There is a tendency to make the second response the correct one most frequently.
3. Skill in constructing foils is the key to good multiple-choice test construction.
4. Foils should be attractive and vary in degree of plausibility.
5. One item may ask the student to select the exception to the other four items.
6. Direct statements are preferable to incomplete sentences.
7. If incomplete sentences are used, the responses should come at the end of the sentence.
8. All responses to incomplete sentences should be grammatical completions.
9. Responses should be as homogeneous as possible.
10. When multiple-choice items are placed in a block, the student is aided and scoring is more simple.

11. Avoid words in the response that repeat words in the sentence, except when inserted as foils to counter attempts to outguess the test.
12. Correct responses should not be conspicuous by being long or short.
13. Avoid the use of direct phrases from the text.
14. If the five response items are well constructed, deducting ¼ point for each error $(R - \frac{1}{4}W = S)$ will spread the scores and reduce guessing.
15. The multiple-choice test lends itself to the effective measurement of understanding.

Matching tests

Matching tests are a modification of the multiple-choice test. Two columns are used; one is either incomplete statements or a list of questions, and the other column is a list of responses. Another form of matching test consists of parallel columns.

From the key at the right, select the best response to each statement in the column to the left. Place the letter of that response in front of the number of the statement.

_____25. Health of the gums	A. Vitamin A
_____26. Important for thyroxin production	B. Vitamin B
_____27. Elevates a schoolchild's intelligence	C. Vitamin C
_____28. Necessary mineral for red corpuscles	D. Vitamin D
_____29. Helps prevent infection	E. Fat
_____30. Bone growth and development	F. Iodine
_____31. Growth and repair of tissues	G. Iron
_____32. Citrus fruits	H. Protein
	I. None of the above

Statements in items 33 to 36 are to be compared quantitatively.

Key for items 33 to 36
A. Statement M is greater than statement N.
B. Statement M is less than statement N.
C. Statement M is the same as statement N.

Statement M	**Statement N**
_____33. Number of chromosomes in a sperm	Number of chromosomes in a mature ovum
_____34. Number of ova in newborn girl	Number of sperms in newborn boy
_____35. Rate of maturation in the male	Rate of maturation in the female
_____36. Action of progesterone before ovulation	Action of estrone before ovulation

Matching tests are quickly constructed and require little space. For broad subject areas they are satisfactory but are not readily adaptable to limited ones. Matching tests are excellent for testing knowledge and association but have limited value for testing analysis and interpretation.

In the construction, use, and scoring of matching tests, certain suggestions are helpful:

1. Using the same number of terms in each column should be avoided.
2. Statements should be in the left column and responses in the right column.
3. The same response may be used more than once.
4. Each statement should have at least two plausible answers that serve as foils in addition to the correct response.
5. A single block should contain only homogeneous material from a single area.
6. Sentence structure and the form of the responses should be consistent.
7. The students should understand the mechanics of the test.

Deduction for errors presents a problem. If a deduction is to be made, the number of possible choices must be considered. An arbitrary formula of $R - \frac{1}{4}W = S$ serves in most instances, since usually no more than four foils would likely apply to the statement.

Completion tests

Incomplete statements are given, and the student either selects the correct responses from a list or writes in the appropriate terms. This test is not satisfactory for grading purposes but has diagnostic value. It is used almost excessively because it is easy to construct. Convenient for small areas of subject matter, it can be objective if terminology is not a major consideration. Completion tests are used frequently to test student recall of sheer factual material. Care should be taken in sentence structure in order to prevent confusion.

For items 37 to 48 in each blank space place the letter of the term that best completes the statement.
Key for items 37 to 59

A. *Age*	G. *Organic*
B. *Building*	H. *Protein*
C. *Carbohydrate*	I. *Regulation*
D. *Energy*	J. *Sex*
E. *Fat*	K. *Upkeep*
F. *Height*	L. *Weight*

A food is any substance that provides cells with (37)_____, materials for (38)_____ and (39)_____, or that provides for the (40)_____ of functions. Only (41)_____ foods are digested and these are of three classes, (42)_____, the sugars and starches, (43)_____, which contains nitrogen, and (44)_____. Placed in alphabetic order four factors are important in determining a person's basal metabolic rate: (45)_____, (46)_____, (47)_____, and (48)_____.

There is merit in using more responses than blanks. This type of test can be challenging and even takes on some of the aspects of a puzzle. Deduction for errors is difficult to determine.

A simple type of completion test is one in which a short key applies throughout:

Key for items 49 to 53
A. *Increase (increased)*
B. *Decrease (decreased)*
C. *Not change (not changed)*

Regular exercise may (49)_____ one's resistance to disease and (50)_____ one's immunity to infection. Regular exercise will (51)_____ one's predisposition to a particular disease. Regular exercise will (52)_____ the output of the thyroid. According to present studies, an athlete's life expectancy will (53)_____ as a result of athletics.

Short-answer tests

In short-answer tests the student completes the statement by writing a short answer in the space provided. Credit should be given for reasonably correct responses. Textbook sentences should not be used, and care should be taken to avoid revealing the correct response. Sentence structure is highly important. The shorter the answer required, the less the grader's subjective judgment enters into the scoring. A few examples of short-answer items, shown in the following, illustrate this type of test.

Items 54 to 59 are short-answer questions.
In your words complete the following sentences with a brief statement:

54. A food is any substance that _____
55. The most nearly perfect food is _____
56. The best way for a person to lose weight is _____
57. Infection is _____
58. As a cause of death in the United States, communicable diseases are _____
59. Three of the five leading causes of death in the United States are _____

Although limitations inherent in the short-answer tests are obvious, they can be used to some advantage. They can be constructed quickly, which is especially helpful when a limited area of material is to be tested.

GRADING

No matter how you grade, some students will be unhappy. Grades are designed to communicate educational status rather than to guarantee happiness, and so it is important that grading schemes do indeed reflect educational status. Some schools have replaced grades with anecdotal records. Some use anecdotal records to supplement grades. However, the demand for a single indicator of grade equivalency means that grades will be with us for a long time.

Teacher-generated grades require the establishment of a standard against which to compare student performance. Standards for comparison are either absolute or relevant.

Absolute values

The absolute system of grading uses a preestablished standard for course or examination expectations. Subjectivity occurs in determining what the standard is. Three examples of absolute grading systems follow.

Percentage grading.   Percentage grading implies that 100% represents all possible learning and 0% represents no learning at all. Some arbitrary standard usually is established to represent the passing grade, for example, 70%. A 70% implies that 70% of the materials was learned or mastered. Percentage scores can be converted to letter grades by the establishment of a range, i.e., *A* equals 93% to 100%; *B* equals 85% to 92%.

The teacher's goal is to prepare a test that truly reflects course content and to write test items that allow the assessment of acceptable learning to fall in a relatively small range of scores such as 70% to 100%.

Adjusted percentage scores.   In recognition of the difficulty in test making, the "adjusted" approach usually allows the highest score achieved to be adjusted to equal 100%. If the highest grade is 85, then 85 is defined to equal 100%, and all the other scores are adjusted accordingly. In this way student performance anchors the scale. Comparison of scores between different groups of students becomes impossible, however, because members of each group are compared only with each other.

Competency-based grades.   The level of acceptable competency is determined *a priori*, and students are judged as passing or not passing a certain "benchmark" of competency. With this approach, students are given multiple chances to pass or master a defined area of competency.

Relative values

Grading on a curve.   This system implies that grade distribution reflects a normal curve and establishes quotas for each grade. For example, this system may dictate that only the highest 8% can get an *A*, even if many students cluster close to this cut-off point. This approach presupposes that even at the end of the course students will still be distributed across a normal curve, which implies that a significant number of students did not learn much.

Distribution gap grading.   Distribution gap grading involves ranking all grades achieved in the class and recording their frequency. Natural clusters are then assigned a letter grade. The highest grades may cluster anywhere on the scale, and they represent a common grade, i.e., the highest grade. The next cluster of grades represents the next highest grade, and so on. If grades do not cluster clearly, the teacher is still faced with the subjective task of

TABLE 17-1.   Comparison of absolute and relative grading systems

Relative grading system (comparison with other students)	Absolute grading system (comparison with an established standard)
Advantages	
1. Individuals with exceptional ability will be recognized.	1. Course expectations must be communicated clearly to students.
2. This is the common and accepted system in many schools, and so results can be interpreted easily.	2. Most or all students can obtain high grades if they work well.
	3. Course grades represent the degree of achievement of course objectives.
	4. Students do not influence their grades if they help each other in preparing for exams and tests.
Disadvantages	
1. No matter how good or bad the reference group is, some students will always get high grades and some will always get low grades. Accordingly these grades are difficult to interpret without additional information.	1. It is difficult to establish ahead of time what the course standards will be for each grade.
2. Grades are influenced as much by the quality of students in the class as by real differences in performance.	2. Reasonable student achievement levels need to be identified and measured by teacher-made tests.
3. Grades tend to fluctuate from one class to another depending on the quality of students.	

Adapted from Fisbie, D.A., et al.: Assigning course grades, Office of Instructional Resources, University of Illinois at Champaign-Urbana, 1979.

deciding the point where one grade ends and another begins.

A summary of the advantages and disadvantages of these two approaches is laid out in Table 17-1.

Grading tends to create a difficult situation for students and teachers. However, grades are inevitable, and in one form or another are experienced throughout life. The important point for teachers is to ensure that students know exactly what they are expected to learn, how their achievement will be measured, the consequences of not meeting certain standards, and where they can go for help and special assistance.

SUMMARY

Individual instructors find certain types of tests preferable to others. Doubtless the instructor's particular skill is reflected in the preference. Practical considerations of a busy teacher frequently determine the type of test developed. Ideally, test results should be analyzed statistically, but the health teacher has neither the time nor the inclination for such an analysis. For that reason the occasional use of a standard health knowledge test may be advisable. Several standard health knowledge tests are available.

To ask for perfection in a health test is to ask for the impossible. These tests depend on words, and although words are our best tools for conveying ideas, they are also the biggest obstacle to understanding. Different connotations and shades of meaning are an ever-present difficulty. Health tests need not be perfect to be valuable. A precise measure to the most minute increment is unnecessary in the practical affairs of life.

A health test is not the end of health education; it is a record of the past and a barometer for the future. Evaluation is a continuous and never-ending process, an integral part of learning.

The objective of evaluation is not to approve or disapprove but to improve. Evaluation outcomes should always be expressed in ways that are comprehensible and encourage improvement. Evaluation should always be presented as a positive and constructive process.

STUDY QUESTIONS

1. In the final analysis, what is the true measure of the effectiveness of a school health program?
2. Distinguish between subjective and objective evaluation.
3. What are the advantages of using a standardized test instrument in evaluation in the school health program?
4. How can a health evaluation be an inventory?
5. Why are objectives of a program necessary as a guide in developing evaluation instruments?
6. When subjective judgments are necessary, how can subjectivity be reduced?
7. To what extent is testing a specialty?
8. A youngster's health status may decline so little each day that it will be imperceptible to the teacher. How then can teachers identify the youngster whose health is declining?
9. Distinguish between the different types of validity and the different types of reliability of a test.
10. How valid are health attitude tests with which you are familiar?
11. "Essay tests are not outmoded and can be highly valuable for certain evaluation purposes." Explain.
12. Make an appraisal of true-false tests.
13. What is an attitude, and how can it be measured?
14. What is the relationship between attitudes, knowledge, and practice?
15. In multiple-choice tests why is the construction of foils the critical skill demanded?
16. Interpret the statement "A student who does well on one type of test usually does well on any other type of test."
17. What are the basic requirements of a good multiple-choice question?
18. What is the purpose of evaluation in school health practice?

REFERENCES

Allport, G.W.: Attitudes. In Murchison, C., editor: A handbook of social psychology, Worcester, Mass., 1935, Clark University Press.

Anderson, L.W.: Assessing affective characteristics in the school, Boston, 1981, Allyn & Bacon, Inc.

Berk, R.A., editor: Educational evaluation methodology: the state of the art, Baltimore, 1981, Johns Hopkins University Press.

Diederich, P.B.: Short-cut statistics for teacher-made tests. 1983-1984 test and measurement kit, Princeton, N.J., Educational Testing Service.

Fishbein, M.: The prediction of behaviors from attitudinal variables. In Mortensen, C.D., and Sereno, K.K., editors: Advances in communication research, New York, 1973, Harper & Row, Publishers, Inc.

Gay, L.R.: Educational evaluation and measurement, Columbus, Ohio, 1980, Charles E. Merrill Publishing Co.

Guide for planning educational facilities, Columbus, Ohio, 1976, Council of Educational Facility Planners International.

Hills, J.R.: Measurement and evaluation in the classroom, Columbus, Ohio, 1981, Charles E. Merrill Publishing Co.

Katz, M.: Selecting an achievement test: principles and procedures. 1983-1984 test and measurement kit, Princeton, N.J., Educational Testing Service.

Knapp, J., and Sharon, A.: A compendium of assessment techniques, Princeton, N.J., 1975, Educational Testing Service — CAEL.

Lidz, C.S.: Improving assessment of school children, San Francisco, 1981, Jossey-Bass, Inc., Publishers.

Making the classroom test: a guide for teachers. 1983-1984 test and measurement kit, Princeton, N.J., Educational Testing Service.

Nader, P.R., editor: Options for school health, Germantown, Md., 1978, Aspen Systems Corp.

Popham, J.W.: Educational evaluation, Englewood Cliffs, N.J., 1975, Prentice-Hall, Inc.

Proctor, S.E.: Evaluation of nursing practice in schools, J. Sch. Health **56**:272, 1986.

Rowe, D.E.: Healthful school living: environmental health in the school, J. Sch. Health **57**(10):426, 1987.

Siegel, L.P., and Krieble, T.A.: Evaluation of school-based, high school health services, J. Sch. Health **57**(8):323, 1987.

Swezey, R.W.: Individual performance assessment: an approach to criterion referenced test development, Reston, Va., 1981, Reston Publishing Co.

Thurstone, L.L.: The measurement of social attitudes, Abnormal Soc. Psychol. **26**:449, 1932.

Trotter, C.E.: Guide for evaluation of school facilities, Knoxville, Tenn., 1977, School Planning Laboratory, University of Tennessee.

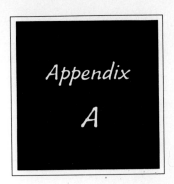

Appendix

A

General Criteria for Evaluating Instructional Materials

The following criteria are to help you evaluate instructional materials. Indicate your judgment by circling the appropriate number. Each item must be rated. A separate evaluating sheet is necessary for each set of materials considered for recommendation.

NOTE: Comments that would add to this evaluation would be appreciated. Please use last page.

Evaluated by _____ Date _____

Committee _____ School _____

DATA FOR EVALUATED MATERIALS

Author _____

Title _____

Publisher   or   producer _____

Copyright date _____ Type of materials _____

Grade level of material being evaluated _____

Is this material part of a series? Yes ☐   Series grade level _____
                                   No ☐

Title of series _____

Cost per item _____

SUMMARY OF EVALUATION

	High				Low	M*	NA†
I. Text format	5	4	3	2	1	0	0
II. Audiovisual format and considerations	5	4	3	2	1	0	0
III. Organization and overall content	5	4	3	2	1	0	0
IV. Bias content	5	4	3	2	1	0	0
V. Teacher's guide for texts or audiovisual materials	5	4	3	2	1	0	0
VI. Additional support materials	5	4	3	2	1	0	0

*Missing: material should have had item but does not.
†Not applicable.

1. TEXT FORMAT

	High				Low	M	NA
1. General appearance	5	4	3	2	1	0	0
2. Size and color practical for classroom use	5	4	3	2	1	0	0
3. Binding: durability and flexibility	5	4	3	2	1	0	0
4. Quality of paper	5	4	3	2	1	0	0
5. Readability to type	5	4	3	2	1	0	0
6. Appeal of page layouts	5	4	3	2	1	0	0
7. Usefulness of chapter headings	5	4	3	2	1	0	0
8. Appropriateness of illustrations	5	4	3	2	1	0	0
9. Usefulness of references, index, bibliography, appendix	5	4	3	2	1	0	0
10. Consistency of format	5	4	3	2	1	0	0

II. AUDIOVISUAL FORMAT AND CONSIDERATIONS

	High				Low	M	NA
1. Sound quality	5	4	3	2	1	0	0
2. Picture quality	5	4	3	2	1	0	0
3. Emotional impact	5	4	3	2	1	0	0
4. Other qualities: vitality, style, imagination	5	4	3	2	1	0	0
5. Authoritative and well-researched, free of propaganda	5	4	3	2	1	0	0
6. Length suitable to audience and content	5	4	3	2	1	0	0
7. Durability	5	4	3	2	1	0	0

8. Usefulness in more than one subject area: write areas here _____

_____

_____

III. ORGANIZATION AND OVERALL CONTENT

Use the specific criteria developed for the subject area if available. Otherwise, use the following guidelines.

Guidelines for organization and overall content	High	----	----	----	Low	M	NA
1. Currency of content	5	4	3	2	1	0	0
2. Consistency of organization	5	4	3	2	1	0	0
3. Clarity and conciseness of the explanation	5	4	3	2	1	0	0
4. Unit organization: follows logical sequence	5	4	3	2	1	0	0
5. Usefulness of illustrations in enhancing the content	5	4	3	2	1	0	0
6. Consistency of point of view with basic principles of subject area	5	4	3	2	1	0	0
7. Usefulness in furthering the systematic and sequential program of the course of study	5	4	3	2	1	0	0
8. Interest appeal: provisions for student differences and backgrounds	5	4	3	2	1	0	0
9. Usefulness in stimulating critical thinking (i.e., problem solving situations, etc.)	5	4	3	2	1	0	0
10. Usefulness in stimulating students toward self-evaluation and formulation of their own goals	5	4	3	2	1	0	0
11. Usefulness in facilitating lesson planning by the way the material is organized	5	4	3	2	1	0	0
12. Adaptability of content to varied instructional methods	5	4	3	2	1	0	0
13. Adaptability of content to varying abilities of individual students (i.e., vocabulary and reading levels)							
Above average							
Average	5	4	3	2	1	0	0
Below average	5	4	3	2	1	0	0
14. Adequacy of learning activities							
Quality	5	4	3	2	1	0	0
Quantity	5	4	3	2	1	0	0
15. Provision for review and maintenance of previously acquired skills	5	4	3	2	1	0	0
16. Provision for measuring student achievement	5	4	3	2	1	0	0

IV. BIAS CONTENT

	High --------------------------- Low					M	NA
1. Presents more than one viewpoint of controversial issues	5	4	3	2	1	0	0
2. Presents accurate facts when generalizations are made	5	4	3	2	1	0	0
3. Includes all socioeconomic levels and settings and all ethnic groups	5	4	3	2	1	0	0
4. Gives balanced treatment of the past and present	5	4	3	2	1	0	0
5. Promotes the diverse character of our nation by:	5	4	3	2	1	0	0

   a. Presenting the positive nature of cultural differences
   b. Using languages and models that treat all human beings with respect, dignity, and seriousness
   c. Including characters that help students identify positively with their heritage and culture
   d. Portraying families realistically (one-parent, two-parent, several generations)
   e. Portraying the handicapped realistically

	High					M	NA
6. Includes minorities and women by:	5	4	3	2	1	0	0

   a. Presenting their roles positively but realistically
   b. Having their contributions, inventions, or discoveries appear alongside men
   c. Depicting them in a variety of occupations and at all levels in a profession
   d. Having their work included in materials
   e. Presenting information from their perspective
   f. Having appropriate illustrations

V. TEACHER'S GUIDE FOR TEXTS OR AUDIOVISUAL MATERIALS

	High --------------------------- Low					M	NA
1. Easy to use	5	4	3	2	1	0	0
2. Answers provided	5	4	3	2	1	0	0
3. Background information	5	4	3	2	1	0	0
4. Teaching strategies	5	4	3	2	1	0	0
5. Ideas for motivation, follow-up, extension	5	4	3	2	1	0	0
6. Guidelines for evaluation	5	4	3	2	1	0	0
7. Inclusion of script	5	4	3	2	1	0	0
8. Bibliography	5	4	3	2	1	0	0

VI. ADDITIONAL SUPPORT MATERIALS THAT ACCOMPANY TEXT

Please list the materials (e.g., workbooks, tests) and use separate form for each one listed

USE THIS SPACE FOR COMMENTS:

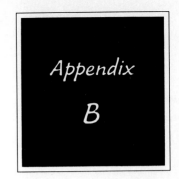

Self-appraisal Checklist
for School Health Programs

The Ohio Association for Health, Physical Education and Recreation, in cooperation with the State Department of Education, the State Department of Health, and the State Planning Committee for Health Education in Ohio, developed and distributed this self-appraisal checklist for evaluating all aspects of a school's health program.

This instrument is useful in surveying and comparing actual practice with ideal practice in three major areas:

1. School health services
2. Healthful school environment
3. Health instruction

The school health program is designed to maintain and enhance the health of students, school personnel, and the community. It should be a foundation for action programs in the community by providing a health-oriented school population. Students will be equipped to deal wisely with their own and their families' health problems and should provide a potential source of adult leadership for future community health problems. The program supplements and reinforces home and community programs. It utilizes the resources of official agencies, professional associations, voluntary organizations, and other community groups, including civic clubs.

Four interrelated parts make up the school health program:

I. *Administration of the school health program*
II. *School health services,* which strive to determine the total health status of the student and seek remedial action for health problems
III. *Healthful school living,* which designates the plans, procedures, and activities that provide a school environment conducive to optimal physical, mental, and social health and safety
IV. *Health education,* which provides formal classroom experiences for favorably influencing knowledge, attitudes, habits, values, skills, and behaviors pertaining to individual and group health

This guide can be useful in surveying what a school is doing in terms of health and comparing this to what is considered good practice. As a result, desirable changes can be undertaken to improve the school health program as the needs are indicated.

From Ohio Department of Education, Health, Physical Education and Recreation Section, Columbus, Ohio 43215.

HOW TO USE THIS GUIDE

It is recommended that an evaluation team be organized to include representatives from school administration, teaching staff, medical and dental professions, nursing, health departments, parents, and community groups.

The team should review and discuss the guide before its utilization and formulate a plan of action to help ensure that techniques and resources are available to complete the study. The team can then proceed to evaluate its health program by answering the questions and comparing the existing program with the recommended practices.

Shortcomings should be ranked by priority based on needs and the resources to correct them. A thorough plan of action will include deficiencies subject to immediate and easy correction as well as a timetable and methodology for the correction of problems requiring larger amounts of resources and time. Follow-up observation is encouraged to see that corrections are being made according to the specified plan of action.

The study group should not hesitate to request help from specialists or consultants from agencies listed, in addition to local community resources.

Also, this checklist should serve as a valuable tool for school personnel to point out strengths and weaknesses of their respective areas or responsibilities.

PART I. ADMINISTRATION OF THE SCHOOL HEALTH PROGRAM

A successful school health program involves understanding and leadership by the school administrator in the role of top-ranking coordinator and liaison with the board of education, staff members, and community. The administrator must be able to present school health needs to the board and utilize all resources and facilities in the community for fostering the health of schoolchildren. The administrator is responsible for the enforcement of the state laws regarding school health, including immunizations. The school experiences of students in our school health programs will largely determine their knowledge and their attitudes about health, and it is the responsibility of every school to offer a comprehensive and effective health education program taught by adequately prepared instructors. This effort should be supported by all groups in the community. The administrator sets the keynote for effective working relationships with school personnel, students, and the community. A school should be responsive to and involve the community in planning, developing, implementing, and evaluating programs in a variety of ways, including the establishment of school-community health committees.

Standards and recommended practices	What we are doing

Program organization and administration

A. 1. A well organized school health program should be planned jointly by the schools, the health department, educational and health professional associations and other responsible community groups.
   2. Both the Board of Health and Board of Education may be charged with specific responsibilities. If this is so, the administration of the duties should be the result of joint planning, and roles and responsibilities of personnel clearly defined.
   3. A school health program is best integrated when a well qualified school person is appointed to coordinate it.

A. 1. What are we doing with respect to joint planning of the school health program?
   a. on a community-wide basis?
   b. on an individual school basis?
   2. What are the responsibilities of the:
   a. School?
   b. Department of health?

   3. Who is responsible for the coordination and administration of the school health program?
   a. Superintendent ☐
   b. Health coordinator ☐
   c. Principal ☐
   d. School medical advisor ☐
   e. School dental advisor ☐
   f. School nurse ☐
   g. Other (list): ☐
   4. Who is responsible for the development of the health curriculum?
   a. Superintendent ☐
   b. Curriculum director ☐
   c. Health coordinator ☐
   d. Principal ☐
   e. Nurse ☐
   f. Supervisor, Health, physical education and recreation ☐
   g. Other (list): ☐
   5. Who is responsible for health services?
   a. Superintendent ☐
   b. Health coordinator ☐
   c. Nurse ☐
   d. Supervisor, Health, physical education and recreation ☐

B. Administrative objectives are:
   1. To develop sound school health practices and to facilitate and make more effective the work of teachers, school health service personnel, and other related nonteaching staff (cafeteria workers, bus drivers, custodians).
   2. To provide for special in-service education programs to be conducted for the personnel directly involved in the school health program.

B. 1. Does the school have written policies that:
   a. Clearly define agency responsibility including legal?   Yes ☐ No ☐
   b. Clearly define roles of personnel, e.g., nurses, administrators, teachers, etc.?   Yes ☐ No ☐
   c. When were the policies last reviewed?
   2. Special in-service education programs are conducted for these personnel?
   Yes ☐ No ☐
   How often?
   These in-service education programs are evaluated to determine their effectiveness?   Yes ☐ No ☐

Standards and recommended practices	What we are doing
3. To provide for periodic evaluation and improvement to help keep the program in step with changing needs and trends.	3. Periodic evaluations and improvements are provided in the program? In what ways? How often?
4. To define and develop sound and effective working relationships among agencies directly concerned with the school health program and to communicate school health concerns to the community at large.	4. There are sound and effective working relationships between those involved in the school health program and agencies? Yes ☐ No ☐ If not, what plans are being made to improve these relationships? Check ways the school health concerns are communicated to the community: PTA or PTO ☐ School health committee ☐ School communications ☐ Official agencies ☐ Voluntary health agencies ☐ The person responsible for helping to ensure sound and effective working relationships is: a. Superintendent ☐ b. Principal ☐ c. Health coordinator ☐ d. School nurse ☐ e. Supervisor, Health, physical education and recreation ☐ f. Other (list): ☐
C. Well prepared personnel, in all phases of the school health program, are essential for its effective and successful implementation.	C. Qualifications of school health personnel. 1. Check the qualifications and experience of the school health coordinator: a. Certificated ☐ b. 3 to 5 years experience in health education or school health programs ☐ c. Recent courses of workshops related to school health ☐ d. Other (list): ☐ 2. What percent of the school nurses are: a. Registered in the state of Ohio? ☐ b. Certificated? ☐ c. Have had postbaccalaureate courses in school health? ☐ 3. How many elementary teachers have background (a minimum of three semester hours) in health education, or health science? ☐ 4. Are the secondary teachers assigned to teach health certificated in health education? Yes ☐ No ☐

Standards and recommended practices	What we are doing

Program organization and administration — cont'd

5. The school provides an in-service education program for:
   a. Teachers?   Yes ☐ No ☐
      Date:
         One-half day or less ☐
         One day or more ☐
         College credit ☐
   b. Nurses?   Yes ☐ No ☐
      Date:
         One-half day or less ☐
         One day or more ☐
         College credit ☐
   c. Administrative personnel?
      Guidance counselors, social workers, etc.
      Yes ☐ No ☐
      Date:
         One-half day or less ☐
         One day or more ☐
         College credit ☐
   d. Nonteaching (noncertified) personnel?
      Yes ☐ No ☐
      Date:
         One-half day or less ☐
         One day or more ☐
         College credit ☐

D. The school administration promotes the integration of health and safety in all curricular and extracurricular activities of the school.

D. The school administration promotes the integration of health and safety in all curricular and extracurricular activities of the school by:
Leaving to individual teachers ☐
Combined efforts of teachers/coordinators ☐
Suggestions in teachers guides ☐
Written policies and procedures ☐

E. If available, schools utilize their community directory of health services.

F. Schools should know what health resources are available in the community and how they can be utilized effectively.

E. The director is readily available to all school personnel?   Yes ☐ No ☐

F. The school utilizes the following community resources:
Health department ☐
Other official agencies ☐
Medical society/auxiliary ☐
Dental society/auxiliary ☐
Voluntary agencies ☐
Civic groups ☐
Other (list): ☐

Standards and recommended practices	What we are doing

First aid for sudden illness and accidents:

A. State law (Sec. 3313.712) requires that an emergency medical treatment authorization form be annually filled out on each student by his parent or legal guardian before October of each year. This form is to be kept on file in the school.

A. Emergency medical treatment authorization forms for all students are filled out annually and are on file in each school?
Yes ☐ No ☐

B. First aid and sudden illness procedures agreed upon by administrator and staff are written and disseminated to all staff.

B. 1. Are policies agreed upon by administrators and staff? Yes ☐ No ☐
2. Are written copies of first aid and sudden illness policies made available to all staff?
Yes ☐ No ☐

C. Persons (other than nurses) trained in first aid procedures should be available for administering first aid or providing direction in cases of sudden illness.

C. 1. How many persons with current first aid preparation are available?_____
2. Are all teachers working in high risk areas qualified in first aid, such as:
Science labs ☐
Shops ☐
Home economics ☐
Physical education ☐

D. First aid procedures should be briefly written for quick reference and posted in special areas, such as science labs, shops, home economics rooms, school health clinic, and physical education areas.

D. Check areas posted:
Science labs ☐
Shops ☐
Home economics room ☐
Health clinic ☐
Physical education ☐

E. First aid equipment/supplies should be kept in stock and readily accessible. All medicines, compounds, bandaging materials should be clearly labeled for use. A designated person should be responsible for ordering supplies.

E. 1. In what locations are first aid supplies stored?
2. All supplies clearly labeled?
Yes ☐ No ☐
3. Check the person responsible for ordering and restocking supplies?
Superintendent ☐
Principal ☐
Nurse ☐
Supervisor, Health, physical education and recreation ☐
Health coordinator ☐

Accident reporting system

A. Written policies and procedures (developed by administration and faculty, outlining a system for reporting school accidents) should be available to all school personnel.

A. Policies are written and made available to all staff?
Yes ☐ No ☐

B. The Ohio Department of Health has an Accident Reporting Form, No. 4966.32. They may be utilized if the schools will report the statistical data to the accident prevention program at the end of the year.

B. Does your school use the Ohio Department of Health Accident Reporting Form?
Yes ☐ No ☐

Standards and recommended practices	What we are doing

Accident reporting system — cont'd

C. The reporting system should:
  1. define a "reportable accident."
  2. indicate the time lapse in reporting the accident.
  3. record information to include: who, what, where, when, why.
  4. include follow-through on treatment or referral.
  5. indicate who is responsible for recording and reporting accidents.

C. Does the reporting system include:
  1. definition of a reportable accident ☐
  2. time lapse in reporting accident ☐
  3. who-what-where-when-why ☐
  4. follow-up —
    a. number of days lost from school ☐
    b. possible action in future to avoid or eliminate future occurrences ☐
  5. who is responsible for recording accidents?

D. School personnel should be familiar with school accident forms and should complete or use them uniformly.

D. School personnel are informed regarding the use of accident forms by:
  1. Staff conferences ☐
  2. News bulletin ☐
  3. Teacher handbooks ☐
  4. Other (list):

E. At the end of each school year, all accident data should be reviewed, analyzed, and compared with last year's records to determine the needs for next year's program.

E. List recommendations as a result of reviewing this year's records.

F. A safety committee is recommended to provide leadership for planning a comprehensive safety education program. It should include such people as administrator, safety specialist, teacher, driver education teacher, physician, school nurse, sanitarian, custodian, student, parent, etc.

F. 1. Do you have a safety committee?
    Yes ☐ No ☐
  2. Who is on the committee?
  3. List the name of the Specialist in Safety.

PART II. SCHOOL HEALTH SERVICES

To meet the educational and health needs of students, it is essential to secure data concerning their physical, mental, and emotional condition. Thus school health services are an important part of the school health programs. These services are planned to protect the health of the students and to help each pupil reach and maintain good health. Also, the school health service program serves as a learning experience for students, teachers, and parents, thereby helping to ensure positive health practices.

The school health program is influenced by local customs, the types of professional manpower, the resources available, and the understanding and cooperation of the community.

Standards and recommended practices	What we are doing

Teacher observation

A. To teach effectively it is important that the teacher keep informed of the health needs of all his/her pupils.
   1. Teachers should receive in-service education in the health observation of school children so that they may refer children who they suspect as having a health problem to appropriate health service personnel. This should be a year round program.
   2. A "Teacher Worksheet for Student Health Observation" would be useful to familiarize teachers with signs and symptoms of health and emotional problems. This may be ordered from the Ohio Department of Health. (No. 3611.13)

A. What type of in-service education is provided teachers to improve their skills of observation and referral procedures?
   1. Teacher/nurse conferences
      Yes ☐ No ☐
      Health education workshops
      Yes ☐ No ☐
      College/university credit courses
      Yes ☐ No ☐
      Other (list):
   2. Do teachers use "A Teacher Worksheet for Student Health Observation"?
      Yes ☐ No ☐

Health screening

Hearing

A. The following should be screened annually:
   (1) all children in grades K through 3
   (2) all teacher referrals
   (3) all children new to the school system
   (4) all children in grades 6 and 9
These tests should be administered with the individual pure tone audiometer.

A. Check grades you are screening with the pure tone audiometer:

	No. screened	No. failed 1st screening	No. failed 2nd screening	Failed threshold test and referred
K				
1st				
2nd				
3rd Other grades				
Referrals New students				
Total				

Standards and recommended practices	**What we are doing**

Health screening — cont'd

Hearing — cont'd

B. All students failing the first screening should be re-screened within two weeks.

B. The number of children who failed to pass threshold screening tests represents _____ percent of all children screened.

C. Refer all children who fail to pass the threshold screening test to appropriate resources as: medical or audiological.

C. What percentage of the children referred for follow-up care are known to have received it?

_____

D. Assure that follow-up care has been obtained for each person referred for care.

D. Procedures used to secure follow-up care
 ☐ Visit to home
 ☐ Telephone call (by teacher or nurse)
 ☐ Note sent home
 ☐ Other (list):

Vision

E. Ideally, all children (kindergarten through grade 12 and all teacher referrals) should be screened annually with a Snellen chart. Minimum: K and grades 1, 3, 5, 7, 9.

E. Check grades you are screening with the Snellen eye chart:

	No. screened	*No. failed 1st screening*	*No. failed 2nd screening and referred*
K			
1			
2			
3			
4			
5			
6			
7			
8			
9			
10			
11			
12			

F. Screen all children for ocular muscle imbalance, excessive farsightedness, and near acuity in grades 1 or 3, and screen for color deficiency in either elementary or junior high grade.

F. Are you screening all children in grades 1 or 3 for:

Ocular muscle imbalance	Yes ☐ No ☐
Excessive farsightedness	Yes ☐ No ☐
Near acuity	Yes ☐ No ☐
Color deficiency	Yes ☐ No ☐

(elementary or jr. high grade. Please indicate which grade _____).

Standards and recommended practices	What we are doing

Health screening — cont'd

Hearing — cont'd

G. Refer all children who fail a screening test to a vision specialist.

G. How many children were referred for eye care after last screening? This represents _____ percent of the children screened.

H. Determine that follow-up care has been obtained for each child referred for eye care.

H. What percentage of the children referred are known to have received follow-up care? _____%

Health room (clinic)

A. A health room or clinic should be provided and adequately equipped to carry on essential school health services: examinations, tests for vision, hearing, speech, psychological, and private conferences.

A. Does your school have a room where the school physician, school nurse and other specialists can perform:

Examination	Yes ☐ No ☐
Vision testing	Yes ☐ No ☐
Hearing testing	Yes ☐ No ☐
Psychological testing	Yes ☐ No ☐
Speech therapy	Yes ☐ No ☐
Private conferences	Yes ☐ No ☐

1. Does it have a place where pupils who are injured or who become suddenly ill can wait until someone can transport them home? Yes ☐ No ☐
2. Does it have space for use by health services personnel for individual or small group conferences? Yes ☐ No ☐
3. Is there adequate space for storing first aid supplies, school health records, etc.? Yes ☐ No ☐

Medical examinations

A. "School Health: A Guide for Physicians," American Academy of Pediatrics, suggests that the priority of medical appraisal should be:
(1) children identified as having problems
(2) children entering school
(3) children in midschool (6-7 grades)
(4) children before leaving school (11-12 grades)
Medical examinations should be done by a physician in his/her office or in a clinic. Parents of elementary children should be present. These examinations should be comprehensive and any abnormal findings of the school screening tests should be provided to the physician. The results of the physician's examination should be reported to school personnel.

A. Do pupils receive a medical examination upon entrance to school? Yes ☐ No ☐
1. Are they examined at midschool? Yes ☐ No ☐
2. Are referrals with special problems examined? Yes ☐ No ☐
3. Are they examined at senior high school? Yes ☐ No ☐

Standards and recommended practices	What we are doing

Medical examinations — cont'd

B. Arrangements should be made for children of low income families to receive examinations. Plans should be formulated whereby school and physicians share necessary information.

B. Is this examination done by:
Health department   Yes ☐ No ☐
School health service   Yes ☐ No ☐
Other (list):
If there are no arrangements for this examination, give reason:

C. Medical examinations should be given to students enrolled in athletic programs. Consideration should be given to students enrolled in other groups, such as marching bands, intramural and interscholastic sports, etc.

C. Are boys and girls in the athletic program provided medical examinations?
Boys   Yes ☐ No ☐
Girls   Yes ☐ No ☐
By whom? _____
When? _____
Other groups such as:
Marching band members   Yes ☐ No ☐
Drill teams   Yes ☐ No ☐
Intramural sports   Yes ☐ No ☐
Interscholastic sports   Yes ☐ No ☐

D. All families receiving ADC should be enrolled in the Early Periodic Screening Diagnosis and Treatment (EPSDT) Program.

D. How many children are enrolled in EPSDT Programs in:
Elementary _____
Secondary _____

E. Plans should be developed with Department of Welfare to share this information as needed by professional personnel planning health services for the child.

E. Check the method the Welfare Department utilizes to share EPSDT screening information on students:
Phone   Yes ☐ No ☐
Written form   Yes ☐ No ☐
Other (list):

Health records

A. A health record should be started when the child enters school and should follow the student as he moves from grade to grade and from school to school. Confidentiality of all health and mental health records should be respected. All personnel should be very careful of sharing any information that might prove speculative or damaging to any student.

A. Does each pupil have a health record on file?
Yes ☐ No ☐
Does your school use School Health Records, form 3613.13 Rev. 1974, from the Ohio Department of Health?
Yes ☐ No ☐
If not, what form is used:
Is the permanent health record transferred when a child changes schools?
Yes ☐ No ☐

Health counseling

A. A definite plan of continuous follow-up should be established. The school nurse should be a liaison with school, parents and community resources.

A. Has your school established a plan of referral and follow-up?   Yes ☐ No ☐

B. Health counseling is one of the main functions of the school nurse, and important information should be shared with and utilized by school counselors, psychologists, teachers, etc.

B. Is the nurse given time for counseling?
Yes ☐ No ☐

Standards and recommended practices	What we are doing
C. The school nurse follows through to help the parent with remedial action. Upon discovering a health defect in a student, the school nurse should follow-up by assisting parents with a plan of remedial action. This could involve a team, such as: physician, psychologist, public health nurse, visiting teacher, speech therapist, school counselor, etc.	C. Does the nurse communicate with parents regarding child health defects and remedial action by: Written note Yes ☐ No ☐ Telephone Yes ☐ No ☐ Home visit Yes ☐ No ☐ Conference at school Yes ☐ No ☐
D. The school nurse should have some training in mental health counseling. The school nurse and counseling psychologist should have agreed-upon procedures for mutual referral and collaboration on students with significantly overlapping physical (somatic) and mental health problems.	D. Has the school nurse had any courses in mental health? Yes ☐ No ☐ Are there mutually agreed procedures for referral by school nurse and by psychologist? Yes ☐ No ☐

Teacher-nurse conferences

A. A teacher-nurse conference should be held at least once a year or as often as needed.	A. Is time provided for the nurse to schedule conferences with teachers? 1. Once a year Yes ☐ No ☐ 2. As often as necessary Yes ☐ No ☐

Children with special problems

A. Identification of and special provision for handicapped children; deaf and hard of hearing, crippled, visually impaired, neurologically and emotionally, educable mentally retarded, etc., is an important aspect of school health services. The school should make special provisions for handicapped pupils in regular classes when this is the most appropriate placement.	A. Number of children with special problems in: Elementary _____ Secondary _____ List types of handicaps:

Special facilities or programs should be made available to the children with any handicapping conditions.	What provisions is made for children with special problems? Check:
	1. Special facilities: ☐
	   Ramps ☐
	   Special toilets ☐
	   Rest areas ☐
	2. Special services:
	   Occupational therapy ☐
	   Physical therapy ☐
	   Speech therapy ☐
	   Psychological ☐
	3. In-service education for teachers ☐
	4. In-service education for auxiliary personnel
	   Types: ☐
	5. Transportation provided ☐
	6. Other (list):

Standards and recommended practices	What we are doing
Dental examinations	

Dental examinations

A. Examination by a dentist for school purposes should be given to all pupils entering the system and at the beginning of the secondary school level.

A. Do pupils receive a dental examination upon entrance to school? Yes ☐ No ☐
If yes, what percent? _____%
1. Do pupils receive a dental examination at the secondary level? Yes ☐ No ☐
If yes, what percent? _____%

B. These examinations should be done by a dentist in his/her office or clinic with the parents of elementary children accompanying them.

B. Outline your plan for making a concentrated effort to have all students visit their dentist regularly
1. Check reasons why students are not receiving dental care:
Lack of dental manpower ☐
Lack of funds ☐
Lack of transportation ☐
Other (list):

C. The school or the community should provide for the dental examinations of indigent pupils. The local dental society working with the school and community should formulate a program to provide services for indigent students.

C. What dental services are provided for children whose parents cannot afford such services?
1. What arrangements are made for the examination of indigent children?

D. All students involved in interscholastic contact athletics should be provided with mouth protectors. The local dental society should be contacted for assistance.

D. What arrangements are made for mouth protectors for students involved in interscholastic contact athletics?
Provided by student   Yes ☐ No ☐
Provided by schools   Yes ☐ No ☐
Provided by local dental society Yes ☐ No ☐
Provided by other (list):

E. The community water supply should be fluoridated.

E. Is your community water supply fluoridated?
Yes ☐ No ☐
1. If not, why?

F. In a good school health program, oral hygiene should be observed by the teacher, school nurse, and other personnel involved in the health of the student. Pertinent information should be recorded on the cumulative health record. Evidence of dental neglect should be reported by the school nurse or teacher to parents. Follow-up of this referral should be done by the responsible person.

F. Pertinent dental health information is filed in the cumulative health folder? Yes ☐ No ☐
Referrals from dentists   Yes ☐ No ☐
Recorded by nurse   Yes ☐ No ☐
Other (list):

Standards and recommended practices	What we are doing
G. Dentists, dental auxiliaries or affiliated groups are resources that can be utilized in a dental health education program.	G. Check the resources listed below which have been utilized in your dental program in the past. Dentists — Yes ☐ No ☐ Dental hygienists — Yes ☐ No ☐ Dental auxiliaries — Yes ☐ No ☐ PTA or PTO — Yes ☐ No ☐ Others (list): Future plans:

Health of school personnel

A. Pre-employment health examinations should be required of all school personnel.

B. Periodic medical examinations of school personnel are recommended.

A. Pre-employment examinations are required for all school personnel?　　　Yes ☐ No ☐

B. If periodic medical examinations are required, state the time intervals:

Communicable disease control

A. There should be well defined school health policies developed in cooperation with local health departments or with School Health Services and approved by the Board of Education.

B. School personnel and parents should be informed regarding these policies.

A. Does your school have written school health policies?　Yes ☐ No ☐

B. Parents and teachers are informed regarding these policies by:
Meetings — Yes ☐ No ☐
Newsletters — Yes ☐ No ☐
Other (list):

C. School nurses should report cases of communicable diseases, including pediculosis and scabies, to local health department.

C. Check the method the school nurses use in reporting communicable diseases to the local health department:
Phone ☐
Written form ☐

D. All students should comply with the law of Ohio regarding immunizations as stated in Section 3313.671 of the Ohio Revised Code. This law requires a pupil to be or in the process of being immunized against polio, rubeola, diphtheria, rubella, pertussis and tetanus. This is the responsibility of the administrator.

D. Does your school have a formal plan for enforcement of this law?
Yes ☐ No ☐

PART III. HEALTHFUL SCHOOL LIVING

The health of the students and school personnel is affected by the environment in which they work and play. Environment influences the health, habits, attitudes, comfort, safety, and working efficiency of school personnel. The environment is the responsibility of the school administration; helping to maintain it is the responsibility of all school personnel, and inspecting for environmental deficiencies is the statutory responsibility of the local department of health.

Standards and recommended practices	What we are doing
A. Semi-annual inspections of the school facilities are made by the local health department sanitarians and school health personnel (custodial staff—school administrators).	A. Date of school inspection: School official Name and title: _____ 1. Progress of inspection recommendations:
B. Semi-annual inspections of the school food service operation (if provided) are made by the local health department's sanitarian and school personnel (cafeteria supervisor—school administrators).	B. Date of food service inspection: School official Name and title: _____ 1. Progress in correcting (remedying) inspection violations:
C. Procedure has been established to ensure that inspection reports are properly interpreted to school authorities.	C. The inspection results are reviewed and explained with recommendations to the school officials at the time of the inspection. School officials consulted: 1. Superintendent or principal ☐ 2. School administrator ☐ 3. Custodial supervisor ☐ 4. Cafeteria supervisor ☐ 5. Others ☐
D. Copies of the inspection reports are sent to the appropriate persons.	D. Copies of the inspection reports are sent to: 1. Board of Education ☐ 2. School administrator ☐ 3. Health supervisor/coordinator ☐ 4. Custodial supervisor ☐ 5. Cafeteria supervisor ☐ 6. Others ☐
E. Plans for any new physical structure, (including all major improvements) are submitted to the appropriate agencies prior to construction.	E. Plans are submitted to: 1. State Department of Industrial Relations ☐ 2. State Plumbing Unit, Ohio Department of Health ☐ 3. Local health department ☐ 4. Others as required ☐
F. Periodic in-service education programs sponsored jointly by the health department and the school system for custodial and food service employees are recommended.	F. Check in-service education programs for custodial and food service employees during the last 12 months. 1. A program conducted by the Health Department for custodial and food service employees. Yes ☐ No ☐

Standards and recommended practices	What we are doing
	2. Personnel attended workshop in Columbus conducted by the Department of Education. Yes ☐ No ☐ List future plans for in-service education programs for the next 12 months.
G. The school environment should stimulate learning and the development of good sanitation practices such as: 1. Food handling instructions for students assisting in the lunch room. 2. Students to learn and appreciate good food handling practices. 3. Maintaining a more attractive lunch room. 4. Proper storage of food.	G. Check any activities initiated by school officials which serve to motivate environmental sanitation practices. 1. Enlists the help of student patrols to make inspections of the environment to check for good sanitation and safety practices. Yes ☐ No ☐ 2. Food handling class conducted for students assisting in the lunch room. Yes ☐ No ☐ 3. Group of students works with lunch room personnel in improving attractiveness of lunch room. Yes ☐ No ☐ 4. Invites local sanitarian to discuss sanitation and safety practices to school personnel or health classes. Yes ☐ No ☐ 5. Others (list):

Safe school environment

Accident prevention is a vital part of semiannual inspections conducted by local health sanitarians and school health personnel. These inspections place considerable emphasis on maintaining, planning and developing safety practices within the school environment and especially at specific locations.

A. the sanitarian's inspection of safety of the environment should include the following major areas: School grounds Parking area Playground and equipment Athletic field and equipment Floor areas, stairs, ramps Classrooms Dressing/shower rooms Gymnasium Vocational areas/chem labs/home economics rooms School cafeteria/kitchens Restrooms Fire fighting equipment/exits First aid emergency rooms	A. 1. Parking kept away from playground equipment? Yes ☐ No ☐ 2. Playground equipment maintained in good repairs? Yes ☐ No ☐ 3. Has soft, absorbent surface been provided around playground equipment? Yes ☐ No ☐ 4. Are floor surfaces kept clean, free of tripping, slipping hazards? Yes ☐ No ☐ 5. Classrooms arranged for best traffic pattern, least amount of congestion? Yes ☐ No ☐ 6. Classroom furniture kept in good repair, adequate lighting provided? Yes ☐ No ☐ 7. Adequate supervision provided for organized/unorganized activity on the school grounds and in the gymnasium? Yes ☐ No ☐

Standards and recommended practices	What we are doing
Safe school environment — cont'd	

8. Necessary safety precautions taken in vocational shop, chem labs, home economics areas, i.e.:
   Protective eyeware provided
   Yes ☐ No ☐
   Faucet for eye lavage if chemically burned
   Yes ☐ No ☐
   Fire extinguisher close to heating elements
   Yes ☐ No ☐
9. In-service safety programs presented for food service personnel in school kitchen?
   Yes ☐ No ☐
   Date of last in-service workshop?
   Projected date for next food safety program?
10. Restroom floors kept dry, free of debris?
    Yes ☐ No ☐
11. Fire extinguishers checked monthly to determine operability? Yes ☐ No ☐
    Date of last fire extinguisher check?
12. Proper class of extinguishers provided according to type of fire hazard, i.e., electrical, paper, chemical, etc.?
    Yes ☐ No ☐
13. Health department sanitarian meets with school personnel or safety committee to discuss findings of the school inspection and needed or recommended corrections?
    Yes ☐ No ☐
    Comments:

B. An effective school safety program encompasses many areas within the school system:
   1. Constant awareness to potential hazards of new products being introduced into the school environment.
   2. Special training, and drills of school bus drivers and children in school bus safety practices along with regular school vehicle inspections.
   3. School safety concerns integrated into appropriate curriculum designs.
   4. Fire drills
   5. Safety education

B. Check any special safety in-service education programs during the past school year for:
   Bus drivers   Yes ☐ No ☐
   Lunch room personnel   Yes ☐ No ☐
   Teachers   Yes ☐ No ☐
   Custodians   Yes ☐ No ☐
   Safety patrol   Yes ☐ No ☐

Standards and recommended practices	What we are doing
C. Safety concerns should be integrated into the health education curriculum.	C. Check safety concerns that have been integrated into the curriculum this past year, such as:

    1. Accident etiology   Yes ☐ No ☐
    2. Bicycle   Yes ☐ No ☐
    3. Home (urban/suburban)   Yes ☐ No ☐
    4. Home (rural)   Yes ☐ No ☐
    5. Toy safety   Yes ☐ No ☐
    6. Pedestrian safety   Yes ☐ No ☐
    7. Vacation   Yes ☐ No ☐
    8. Poisons   Yes ☐ No ☐
    9. Firearms and hunting   Yes ☐ No ☐
   10. Automobile and seat belt   Yes ☐ No ☐
   11. Pets   Yes ☐ No ☐
   12. Fires   Yes ☐ No ☐
   13. Athletic and playground   Yes ☐ No ☐
   14. Water and boating   Yes ☐ No ☐

School nutrition program

A. there is a food service provided in the school and all pupils are encouraged to participate.

A. Is there a food service program in your school?
Yes ☐ No ☐

B. The lunch served meets the national "type A" standard.

B. Does it meet national "type A" standard?
Yes ☐ No ☐

C. Even though it is legal to sell candy and sweetened beverages in the school, it is recommended that this practice not be permitted during school or lunch hours. Sale of such items is in direct competition with a good lunch program.

C. Does your school sell:
    1. Candy   Yes ☐ No ☐
    2. Soft drinks   Yes ☐ No ☐
    3. Chocolate milk or drink   Yes ☐ No ☐
    4. Other snack items   Yes ☐ No ☐

D. The school lunch program should be utilized as a learning laboratory for good nutrition in a child's life.

D. Check any of these activities related to lunch room and nutrition that are utilized in the health education program.
    1. Classroom units   Yes ☐ No ☐
    2. Pupils given an opportunity to evaluate menus to determine if they meet "type A" school lunch requirements   Yes ☐ No ☐
    3. Pupils or art classes make posters for the lunch room.   Yes ☐ No ☐
    4. Classes plan menus and solicit the assistance of head cook in serving it to students.
       Yes ☐ No ☐
    5. A class makes a survey of eating habits of students in lunch room to see foods rejected or wasted.   Yes ☐ No ☐
    6. Class tours the kitchen to observe dish washing, storage of food, etc. and to discuss why certain practices are necessary.
       Yes ☐ No ☐

Standards and recommended practices	What we are doing
E. School food service personnel should be required (expenses to be paid by the Board of Education) to attend workshops and conferences sponsored by the State Department of Education for the lunch room workers.	E. In this school year, how many school lunch personnel attended the workshops and conferences sponsored by the State Department of Education? _____ 1. How many attended local workshops?

PART IV. HEALTH EDUCATION

Schools are the official community agencies for the education of children. They have the major responsibility for the health instruction of children, grades K through 12. Health education instruction should be organized to provide learning experiences that favorably influence understanding, attitudes, and behavior with respect to individual and community health. In addition, the program should be designed to teach the individual to assume an ever-increasing responsibility for his or her own health status.

Careful and continuous planning on the part of the school is necessary for an effective health instruction program. Objectives must be established; a sequential curriculum (K-12) must be developed or adopted; content should be appropriate to the needs, interests, and intellectual ability of the pupils; adequate time and credit must be allotted; and, most important, well-qualified, certified, and enthusiastic teachers must be assigned to teach the health classes.

Standards and recommended practices	What we are doing
Administration A. Authorities recommend that health be taught 15-30 minutes daily at the elementary level; a full year course taught daily at the 7th, 8th, or 9th grade; and a full year course on a daily basis at the 10, 11th, or 12th grade. In the elementary schools, the Ohio State Department of Education requires a minimum of two 40 minute periods per week in grades 3 through 6, and two 45 minute periods per week in grades 7 and 8. The Ohio State Department of Education requires a semester course or its equivalent be taught at the high school level (9-12).	A. 1. Time allotted/week *Grade* K _____ 1 _____ 2 _____ 3 _____ 4 _____ 5 _____ 6 _____ 2. Health is taught as a separate course at the junior high level? (Circle grade[s]: 7, 8, 9) Yes ☐ No ☐ 3. Health is taught as a separate course at the high school level? (Circle grade[s]: 10, 11, 12) Yes ☐ No ☐ 4. How often do the classes meet? Junior high _____ Senior high _____ 5. How much time is allotted per class period?

Standards and recommended practices	What we are doing
B. The number of pupils assigned to health classes should be no greater than those assigned to other classes.	B. 1. Average number of students per health class is _____. 2. Average number of students per all other classes is _____.
C. Most authorities recommend that health be taught in a natural setting and that the sexes should only be separated if they are separated for other courses.	C. 1. Which of the following is typical in your school? Separate classes, boys and girls Yes ☐ No ☐ Coed classes Yes ☐ No ☐ Usually coed but separated for some classes Yes ☐ No ☐ If yes, which topics: Human sexuality Yes ☐ No ☐ Feminine hygiene Yes ☐ No ☐ Other (list):
D. Scheduling for health instruction should be like all other disciplines.	D. Health receives the same status on scheduling as other disciplines? Yes ☐ No ☐
E. A staff member, specialized in health education (major in health education) should be designated health chairman or coordinator and assigned the responsibility for coordinating the entire health program.	E. A health chairman is designated? Yes ☐ No ☐ 1. If yes, is the health chairman a specialist in health education by professional preparation? Yes ☐ No ☐ 2. If chairman is not a specialist in health education, check any of the following that apply: a. Has taken some health education courses and had experience in teaching health? Yes ☐ No ☐ b. Has attended a school health workshop at a college or university? Yes ☐ No ☐
F. An interdisciplinary committee of persons should be appointed to plan and evaluate the health program cooperatively. The health coordinator should chair this group.	F. A health committee is appointed? Yes ☐ No ☐ 1. How often does the committee meet? 2. The health coordinator chairs this committee? Yes ☐ No ☐ 3. The local health committee is represented by the following (check appropriate ones): Teachers ☐ Parents ☐ Administrators ☐ Physicians ☐ Nurses ☐ Guidance counselor ☐ Psychologist ☐ Students ☐ Others (list): ☐

Standards and recommended practices	What we are doing

School nutrition program — cont'd

G. The school administration should provide a setting conducive to health instruction, including an equipped classroom, movable furniture, supplies and materials and tables for demonstrations.

G. Our school utilizes:
Regular-sized classroom ☐
Movable furniture ☐
Materials and supplies ☐
Tables for experiments and ☐
demonstrations

H. The school should provide in-service education programs for teachers to assist them in conducting health instruction in an interesting and sequential manner.

H. How many in-service programs on health education were offered during the past year?
_____
   1. How many faculty attended each program?
_____
   2. List the grades represented by teachers attending: _____
   3. Were the in-service programs evaluated? Yes ☐ No ☐
   4. Topics covered (check appropriate ones):
      General health knowledge ☐
      New materials reviewed ☐
      Teaching ideas shared ☐
      Organization and curriculum development planning of program by grade level ☐
      Demonstration of use of audio-visual and other equipment ☐
      Other topics (please indicate):
   5. Were resource persons from universities, state, or local health agencies utilized? Yes ☐ No ☐
   6. If yes, name participating agencies.

I. The school administration should provide textbooks, charts, filmstrips, resource books, models, pamphlets, transparencies, and other aids which are authoritative, up to date, interesting and appropriate for the grade level in which they are used.

I. List source of textbooks?
   1. When were the health textbooks printed?
   2. Have resources been reviewed by health committee? Yes ☐ No ☐
   3. Which of the following are readily available?
      Textbooks ☐
      Charts ☐
      Filmstrips ☐
      Resource books ☐
      Models ☐
      Pamphlets ☐
      Transparencies ☐
      Others (list):

Standards and recommended practices	What we are doing

Curriculum planning

A. The health instruction program should be based on the problem-solving conceptual approach to studying and meeting the health needs, interests and problems of the students.

A. 1. Check ways students were surveyed to find their needs and interests:
  Questionnaires ☐
  Tests ☐
  Checklists ☐
  Personal essays ☐
  2. List ways the community has been utilized to find local needs and interests:
  _____
  3. Are morbidity and mortality statistics for the community studied and utilized?
  Yes ☐ No ☐

B. Curriculum planning should be carried out by the interdisciplinary committee responsible for the school health program.

B. Is the interdisciplinary committee assigned the task of writing the health education curriculum?
  Yes ☐ No ☐
  1. If not, who is responsible for the curriculum?

C. The health instruction program should utilize the conceptual approach such as: School Health Education Study, "A conceptual Approach to Curriculum Design," the ASHA Curriculum, the Ohio Department of Education Comprehensive Drug Education Curriculum.

C. Is the conceptual approach utilized?
  Yes ☐ No ☐
  1. Of the following, check those which have been reviewed by the health committee:
  School Health Education Study, ☐
    "A Conceptual Approach to Curriculum Design"
  American School Health Association's ☐
    Curriculum
  Ohio Department of Education ☐
    Comprehensive Drug Education
    Curriculum, K-12
  2. If none of the above are utilized, name others that have been used as references:
  _____
  3. Check the grade levels in which the conceptual approach is used:
  1-3 ☐
  4-6 ☐
  7-9 ☐
  10-12 ☐

D. The school system provides for use in the school a teaching guide, which contains:
  1. A statement of philosophy upon which the school health education program is based.

D. A health instruction guide is available and used in the school? Yes ☐ No ☐
  1. Is a statement of philosophy included in the guide? Yes ☐ No ☐

Standards and recommended practices	What we are doing

2. Health education instructional content, which includes a developmental scope and sequence approach to curriculum design, including the following:
   a. Concept emphasis
   b. Content
   c. Suggested teacher methods and techniques
   d. Student learning activities
   e. Evaluation
   f. Student/teacher resources and materials

E. A long-range plan should be developed for implementing the health instruction program outlined in the teaching guide. A definite time plan should be included.

2. Of the areas recommended in column 1, for inclusion in the guide, check those which are presently available:

	K-3	4-5-6	7-8-9	10-11-12
a.				
b.				
c.				
d.				
e.				
f.				

E. Is a plan available?   Yes ☐ No ☐
   Three years _____
   Five years _____

Curriculum content

A. In general, the health instruction program for the school includes the following large areas with careful consideration being given to proper grade placement and sequence.
   1. Nutrition
   2. Dental health
   3. Physical activity, sleep, rest and relaxation, recreation
   4. Personal cleanliness and appearance
   5. Body structure and operation
   6. Prevention and control of disease
   7. Safety and first aid
   8. Drugs, alcohol and tobacco
   9. Community health
   10. Consumer health
   11. Health careers
   12. Mental, emotional and social health, including aggressive behavior
   13. Sex and family life education
   14. Environmental health

A. Indicate in which grades each subject is taught by placing a check in the appropriate square. Please write in the grade level.

	K-3	4-5-6	7-8-9	10-11-12
1.				
2.				
3.				
4.				
5.				
6.				
7.				
8.				
9.				
10.				
11.				
12.				
13.				
14.				

(Note: The above data should be analyzed and plans made for removing duplication and adding omitted topics to the curriculum.)

Standards and recommended practices	What we are doing

Methods and instructional aids

A. The students whenever possible should be actively involved in planning the health education program.

A. Of the following student related activities, check those which are used:

Role-playing ☐
Group discussions ☐
Dyad (interaction between 2 students) ☐
Debates ☐
Panels ☐
Case study ☐
Independent studies and reports ☐

B. The health instruction program should include a variety of teaching techniques. Instruction should be geared toward skill development in seeking information, analyzing it carefully, drawing conclusions, and making behavioral decisions.

B. Of the following methods, check those which are used:

Lecture ☐
Field trips ☐
Resource speakers ☐
Demonstrations and experiments ☐
Surveys ☐
Problem-solving discussion ☐

C. The school library should contain current periodicals and other reading matter as resource material for health classes.

C. Of the following, check the ones available to the students and staff:

"School Safety" ☐
"Today's Health" ☐
"Journal of School Health" ☐
Public affairs pamphlets ☐
Science Research Associates booklets ☐
Materials from American Medical Association ☐
Ohio Department of Education Media Centers ☐
"Ohio's Health" ☐
Materials from Drug/Health Education Curriculum Center ☐
Materials from AAHPER ☐
Materials from the Ohio Department of Health ☐
Materials from voluntary health agencies (heart, lung, cancer, etc.) ☐
Supplementary texts ☐
Others (list):

D. Projection equipment, tape recorders, and record players should be available for use in the classroom.

D. The following are available within the school for use in the classroom:

16 m projectors ☐
Record players ☐
Tape recorders ☐
Slide projectors ☐
Filmstrip projectors ☐
Transparencies ☐

Standards and recommended practices	What we are doing
Methods and instructional aids — cont'd E. Educational media is utilized in the teaching of health education	E. Which of the following instructional television and/or film series are available: "Inside Out" NIT-AIT ☐ "Self-Incorporated" NIT-AIT ☐ "Knowing About Growing" BGSU ☐ "Feeling Good" NIT-AIT PBS ☐
Evaluation A. The school makes periodic evaluation of the health instruction program to determine if behavioral objectives for pupils are being met. This includes an appraisal of knowledge gained, interests and values modified and behavior changed.	A. The health instruction program has been evaluated within the last three years? Yes ☐ No ☐
B. Evaluation of the school physical and emotional climate is also included.	B. An effort has been made to appraise the school atmosphere? Yes ☐ No ☐
C. The evaluation includes the interdisciplinary committee or program for health, the combined efforts of classroom teachers, health educators, administrators and, where appropriate, pupils.	C. The team approach has been used in the program evaluation? Yes ☐ No ☐ 1. A North Central or similar team has evaluated the health program in the last five years? Yes ☐ No ☐
D. The results of the evaluation are used as a basis for curriculum revision and program improvement.	D. The results of evaluations are being used? Yes ☐ No ☐

Index